SHIRRANS' SOLUTION
The Gastric *mind* Band®

by

Martin & Marion Shirran

with

Fiona Graham

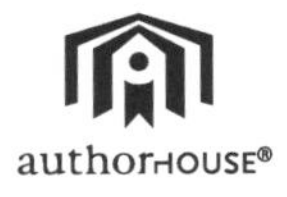

AuthorHouse™ UK Ltd.
500 Avebury Boulevard
Central Milton Keynes, MK9 2BE
www.authorhouse.co.uk
Phone: 08001974150

First published by AuthorHouse 8/16/2010.

ISBN: 978-1-4520-5251-9 (sc)

EATING DISORDERS

We are passionate in our belief that if you are totally committed, you will achieve the weight loss you desire with the Gastric *mind* Band therapy; but of course it needs your commitment as well.

Anyone undertaking any weight loss programme should first discuss their proposed actions with their GP.

As with people seeking gastric band surgery, at the Elite Clinic we ask all clients a series of questions before commencing therapy to ensure they are not suffering from any eating disorders such as anorexia or bulimia.

THERAPIES USED

You will see reference to several therapies, including **CBT** and **NLP**, throughout the book. **CBT** (Cognitive Behaviour Therapy) asks the individual to challenge the way their thoughts can be inaccurate – *thoughts* as opposed to *logical rational facts*. Once they recognise these 'sabotaging' thoughts they can begin to overcome them.

NLP (Neuro Linguistic Programming) encourages positive attitudes by using visualisation, the idea of 'seeing yourself' in another, different, better, mindset, with all the changes that might bring – becoming fitter, healthier, and so on. Once you can see the improvements, your negativity is easier to overcome.

Guided Imagery is a similar technique in which the client is encouraged to see into the future by taking them through alternative scenarios in their mind's eye.

Hypnotherapy works because any suggestions made while the subconscious mind is receptive during deep relaxation are far more likely to be 'accepted'; the subconscious is more influential in our behaviour than the conscious mind so in day to day life the suggestions can begin to take effect without any conscious effort.

Life Architecture is simply the name given by the principals to the therapy they have developed which is a combination of various therapies with each being used to underpin the other.

Pause Button Therapy is the name (EU Trade Mark Registration applied for) given by the principals to their method of allowing people to freeze time and fast-forward to see the consequences of their actions.

Throughout the book you'll see reference to Elite Clinics. This is the clinic in Spain owned and operated by the founders of the G*m*B therapy, Martin & Marion Shirran, and where they offer G*m*B alongside other therapies.

Height Conversion Chart- feet to metres

Feet	Metres	Feet	Metres	Feet	Metres
4ft 6in	1.37m	5ft 1in	1.55m	5ft 8in	1.73m
4ft 7in	1.39m	5ft 2in	1.57m	5ft 9in	1.75m
4ft 8in	1.42m	5ft 3in	1.60m	5ft 10in	1.78m
4ft 9in	1.45m	5ft 4in	1.63m	5ft 11in	1.80m
4ft 10in	1.47m	5ft 5in	1.65m	6ft 0in	1.83m
4ft 11in	1.50m	5ft 6in	1.68m	6ft 1in	1.85m
5ft 0in	1.52m	5ft 7in	1.70m	6ft 2in	1.88m

Stones & lbs	lbs	Kg	Stones & lbs	lbs	Kg	Stones & lbs	lbs	Kg
9 0	126	57.2	11 10	164	74.4	14 6	202	91.6
9 1	127	57.6	11 11	165	74.8	14 7	203	92.1
9 2	128	58.1	11 12	166	75.3	14 8	204	92.5
9 3	129	58.5	11 13	167	75.7	14 9	205	93.0
9 4	130	59.0	12 0	168	76.2	14 10	206	93.4
9 5	131	59.4	12 1	169	76.7	14 11	207	93.9
9 9	132	59.9	12 2	170	77.1	14 12	208	94.3
9 7	133	60.3	12 3	171	77.6	14 13	209	94.8
9 8	134	60.8	12 4	172	78.0	15 0	210	95.3
9 9	135	61.2	12 5	173	78.5	15 1	211	95.7
9 10	136	61.7	12 6	174	78.9	15 2	212	96.2
9 11	137	62.1	12 7	175	79.4	15 3	213	96.6
9 12	138	62.6	12 8	176	79.8	15 4	214	97.1
9 13	139	63.0	12 9	177	80.3	15 5	215	97.5
10 0	140	63.5	12 10	178	80.7	15 6	216	98.0
10 1	141	64.0	12 11	179	81.2	15 7	217	98.4
10 2	142	64.4	12 12	180	81.6	15 8	218	98.9
10 3	143	64.9	12 13	181	82.1	15 9	219	99.3
10 4	144	65.3	13 0	182	82.6	15 10	220	99.8
10 5	145	65.8	13 1	183	83.0	15 11	221	100.2
10 6	146	66.2	13 2	184	83.5	15 12	222	100.7
10 7	147	66.7	13 3	185	83.9	15 13	223	101.2
10 8	148	67.1	13 4	186	84.4	16 0	224	101.6
10 9	149	67.6	13 5	187	84.8	16 1	225	102.1
10 10	150	68.0	13 6	188	85.3	16 2	226	102.5
10 11	151	68.5	13 7	189	85.7	16 3	227	103.0
10 12	152	68.9	13 8	190	86.2	16 4	228	103.4
10 13	153	69.4	13 9	191	86.6	16 5	229	103.9
11 0	154	69.9	13 10	192	87.1	16 6	230	104.3
11 1	155	70.3	13 11	193	87.5	16 7	231	104.8
11 2	156	70.8	13 12	194	88.0	16 8	232	105.2
11 3	157	71.2	13 13	195	88.4	16 9	233	105.7
11 4	158	71.7	14 0	196	88.9	16 10	234	106.1
11 5	159	72.1	14 1	197	89.4	16 11	235	106.6
11 6	160	72.6	14 2	198	89.8	16 12	236	107.0
11 7	161	73.0	14 3	199	90.3	16 13	237	107.5
11 8	162	73.5	14 4	200	90.7	17 0	238	108.0
11 9	163	73.9	14 5	201	91.2	17 1	239	108.4

Stones & lbs	lbs	Kg	Stones & lbs	lbs	Kg	Stones & lbs	lbs	Kg
17 2	240	108.9	19 12	278	126.1	22 8	316	143.3
17 3	241	109.3	19 13	279	126.6	22 9	317	143.8
17 4	242	109.8	20 0	280	127.0	22 10	318	144.2
17 5	243	110.2	20 1	281	127.5	22 11	319	144.7
17 6	244	110.7	20 2	282	127.9	22 12	320	145.2
17 7	245	111.1	20. 3	283	128.4	22 13	321	145.6
17 8	246	111.6	20 4	284	128.8	23 0	322	146.1
17 9	247	112.0	20 5	285	129.3	23 1	323	146.5
17 10	248	112.5	20 6	286	129.7	23 2	324	147.0
17 11	249	112.9	20 7	287	130.2	23 3	325	147.4
17 12	250	113.4	20 8	288	130.6	23 4	326	147.9
17 13	251	113.9	20 9	289	131.1	23 5	327	148.3
18 0	252	114.3	20 10	290	131.5	23 6	328	148.8
18 1	253	114.8	20 11	291	132.0	23 7	329	149.2
18 2	254	115.2	20 12	292	132.5	23 8	330	149.7
18 3	255	115.7	20 13	293	132.9	23 9	331	150.1
18 4	256	116.1	21 00	294	133.4	23 10	332	150.6
18 5	257	116.6	21 1	295	133.8	23 11	333	151.0
18 6	258	117.0	21 2	296	134.3	23 12	334	151.5
18 7	259	117.5	21 3	297	134.7	23 13	335	152.0
18 8	260	117.9	21 4	298	135.2	24 0	336	152.4
18 9	261	118.4	21 5	299	135.6	24 1	337	152.9
18 10	262	118.8	21 6	300	136.1	24 2	338	153.3
18 11	263	119.3	21 7	301	136.5	24 3	339	153.8
18 12	264	119.7	21 8	302	137.0	24 4	340	154.2
18 13	265	120.2	21 9	303	137.4	24 5	341	154.7
19 0	266	120.7	21 10	304	137.9	24 6	342	155.1
19 1	267	121.1	21 11	305	138.3	24 7	343	155.6
19 2	268	121.6	21 12	306	138.8	24 8	344	156.0
19 3	269	122.0	21 13	307	139.3	24 9	345	156.5
19 4	270	122.5	22 00	308	139.7	24 10	346	156.9
19 5	271	122.9	22 1	309	140.2	24 11	346	157.4
19 6	272	123.4	22 2	310	140.6	24 12	348	157.9
19 7	273	123.8	22 3	311	141.1	24 13	349	158.3
19 8	274	124.3	22 4	312	141.5	25 0	350	158.8
19 9	275	124.7	22 5	313	142.0	25 1	351	159.2
19 10	276	125.2	22 6	314	142.4	25 2	352	159.7
19 11	277	125.6	22 7	315	142.9	25 3	353	160.1

BODY MASS INDEX (BMI)

Body Mass Index (BMI) was developed by 19th century Belgian statistician Adolphe Quelet, and is usually calculated by dividing your weight in kilograms by the square of your height in metres. The Imperial calculation is as follows:

$$\text{BMI} = \frac{(\text{weight in pounds} \times 703)}{\text{height in inches}^2}$$

If you weigh 13st 5lb (187lb) and your height is 5ft 5in, your BMI is calculated as follows:-

$$\frac{187 \times 703}{4225} = \frac{131461}{4225} = 31.11$$

The BMI figure of 31.11 is found by multiplying your weight in pounds (187) by 703 then dividing by your height in inches squared (ie 65x65, which is 4225).

Weight and height conversion charts are on the previous pages.

Or you can find a BMI calculator on the internet by visiting the following website:-

http://www.nhlbisupport.com/bmi/

BMI Definitions	BMI
Underweight	< 18
Healthy	18 – 25
Overweight	25 – 30
Obese	30 – 35
Severely obese	35 – 40
Morbidly obese	40 and over

A report in The Guardian newspaper in Spring 2009 said that researchers had combined information from 57 different studies of nearly 900,000 people, and found that the lowest death rate was in the normal BMI range, and the risk of death increases directly in relation to the increase in BMI.

We have spoken to some of Elite Clinics' clients for case study material and have changed some names and details to preserve anonymity where appropriate.

The Gastric *mind* Band ® therapy was developed over a two year period, and is the subject of ongoing research and development. The therapy, which incorporates many different techniques, should of course not be confused with any of the stand-alone hypnotherapy approaches to weight loss. One of the many components of the G*m*B treatment involves the use of a unique therapy registered to Elite Clinics, Pause Button Therapy, discussed later in the book.

While we have striven to make this book as comprehensive as possible, it can never replace the considerable benefits obtained by sitting on a one to one basis with a therapist.

At the time of writing we are in the advanced planning stages regarding the opening of additional clinics in the USA and the UK. For details of the clinics, locations and availability of sessions, please visit www.gmband.com

READER OFFER

Our work as therapists has led us to write this book but our passion is in helping people.

As a 'thank you' for your interest in reading about GmB, should you be interested in visiting one of our clinics for the GmB therapy, we'd like to offer you a preferential rate.

When booking, please quote the following code: 5251-92010
We look forward to seeing you!

Contents

1

THE LIGHTBULB MOMENT

The Gastric *mind*Band therapy was developed out of a chance remark, and has become a phenomenon in a relatively short time. A client of Elite Clinics' therapists Martin and Marion Shirran was putting on weight after they'd successfully hypnotised her to give up smoking. In an instant they regard as one of the defining moments of their lives, the couple say she jokingly asked if they could hypnotise her again, this time to believe she'd had a gastric band fitted, and they all laughed. That was in March 2007. Within a few hours, though, it had turned from a quip to a lightbulb moment – why had no-one thought of this **before**?

That weekend the couple put together a selection of ideas and therapeutic structures, and two years and many tests and trials down the line, Martin is 56lb lighter and they have honed the idea from a spur of the moment, throwaway comment, to a well developed therapy that has caught the imagination of members of the medical profession and overweight and obese people worldwide.

In this book you'll be taken on a journey of self-discovery, learning about your psychological relationship with food. As if you were a client sitting in their clinic, Marion and Martin will help you see the way you make the wrong food choices, the times when you eat for the wrong reasons, the many different triggers you and every overweight person has which has led them down the road towards obesity. Moreover the couple will give you the tools to make major lifestyle changes. They'll introduce you to diet terrorists and anarchists, and the associated chaos they cause those trying to take control of their weight.

You will also be introduced to the unique 'sting' that takes place when dieters eat in restaurants or at social events, and the highly detrimental effect it usually has on every dieter's life. These tools, along with many others, will help you start to change your flawed psychological relationship with food to a more positive, controlled, healthier one. After all, you can't live without food so now is a good time to learn to live with it.

As you go through the book, you'll be introduced to some of the couple's growing catalogue of success stories; people who'd been overweight for years, struggled with yo-yo dieting, virtually given up, thought they'd never successfully lose weight and certainly never dreamed they could keep it off. Read in their own words how unhappy they were and yet how now their lives have changed since visiting us at an Elite clinic. You're guaranteed to recognise most of the things they say. They describe the feelings that made them believe they'd never get to grips with eating normally and never succeed where they'd always previously failed – putting all the weight they had lost straight back on again. Their experiences with the G*m*B therapy will show you it is possible to get the weight off, keep it off and achieve your long-term goals.... with Martin and Marion's insight into the problem and passion for solving it through a vital learning process.

You'll also read about a client who came to the clinic for help having experienced a catastrophic surgical gastric band failure resulting in her almost losing her life and fearing she would always remain overweight. Not the miracle cure she'd anticipated!

This book provides the reader with the nearest thing possible to a course of G*m*B therapy in the clinic - covering every component including hypnotherapy. You'll hear in the couple's straight talking style how to identify your often-irrational food and eating issues, your bad choices and why it's not necessary to leap back on the yo-yo diet roundabout. In fact why you shouldn't diet at all!

Marion and Martin don't solely talk bluntly about your eating habits, they illustrate how no overweight person should carry on the way they are without being brought face to face with the appalling health risks attached to being overweight.

They'll ask you if your reason for wanting to shed excess weight is to fit into a bikini next summer, or to avoid losing a limb to Type 2 diabetes. Why you can't see the irony of driving around in a car with seatbelts and six airbags to protect yourself in case of an accident, while at the same time eating a bar of chocolate guaranteeing you carry excess weight which is statistically far more likely to kill you – from a stroke, or heart attack. How bizarre is that.

You'll be asked questions about your food choices, about your relationships not only with meals and eating now but also when you were younger. About all the triggers overweight people have which lead them to overeat. About the effect of you being overweight not only on you but also on your family and friends. About how you'd see yourself through someone else's eyes. How you might feel a year from now if you were slim. Soon you'll realise you're at a fork in the road in your life. A place where the choice of direction is entirely up to you. Then, finally, with their help, you'll see just how few changes you need to make to set off along a totally different pathway to the old, fat, bloated, unhappy one you're on now.

Most importantly of all, they'll make you realise this is possible. You can be that slimmer, fitter, healthier person next year – if you have the motivation. The Shirrans are passionate about their therapy. They are straight talkers, and they'll make it quite clear that it's your decision, your journey and you won't achieve a thing unless and until you're totally ready, totally committed. You have to believe you can do this, and the evidence from past clients says you can.

As has been said before, you can't live without food so now is maybe a good time to learn to live with it.

2

OBESE? ME?....

Obese. Obesity. I hate the words, with a passion. I always have and always will. I can remember lying in a hospital bed in Great Yarmouth, Norfolk; following stomach pains I'd been admitted to have my appendix removed.

The surgeon came to the ward to see me before the op along with four young trainee doctors. He was talking to them about me, my condition and the surgery which was to take place. But he talked about me as if I wasn't there. I was described simply as an 'obese male'. More than 25 years later I remember those words vividly. I remember thinking that at the time I thought I was a little overweight, but no – in that moment I was labelled as being clinically obese. Not pleasant at all.

However that's not unusual nowadays. No-one is chubby any more; people don't have a 'spare tyre', kids no longer have puppy fat – more often than not they're labelled. Classified as obese, a truly horrible word.

The problem of global obesity is of course no less real just because I don't like the word. I read recently that obesity is thought to be a bigger threat to the planet than global warming and terrorism combined. However as a word, as the effect it has on people, obesity is like that other dreaded word, the one that is even more frightening, the one guaranteed to bring you out in a cold sweat with simultaneous nausea. I'm talking about cancer.

No-one has a 'lump' any more, nor do they have a growth or tumour, just cancer. Just mentioning the word sends people into shock. I'm not a doctor but I imagine the word must send any possible sufferer's immune system into near total shutdown at the sound of the word – just at the time I would think they need their defences to be working at maximum efficiency.

I can remember a partner of mine having a lump in her breast; the doctor thought it was a cyst, which statistically they usually are; and over a few weeks, as expected, it disappeared. The same partner a year or so later had a lump come up under her arm. Thinking back it was never discussed as cancer in the lymph nodes, just as a cyst. Like I said, I'm not a doctor, but I wonder if the word cancer is not bandied about a little too freely. It would be interesting to know the negative effect on the immune system of the person just being told it could be cancerous. Would it not be beneficial to keep them positive? At least until they receive a full diagnosis... like I say, I'm not a doctor....

I mention all of this because in a similar vein, when clients come to the clinic we always strive to ensure that they are never overwhelmed by the problem of being overweight. We want them to be, and remain, 100% positive. The absolute belief and positivity in a person's ability to succeed is paramount in all change scenarios in life, not least in the field of weight loss. We are adamant that it's essential for our clients to continue believing that this situation, this problem they have with excess weight, can always be reversed. Sure we use the words obese and obesity, but reluctantly and only when and where it is appropriate.

So rather than saying 'well you're overweight, maybe even obese, you need to lose five stones and you'll take at least eight months, we position it differently. We'd say 'sure you have a weight problem, but you know you needn't worry, we often see clients with far more weight to lose than you. You can, with a little help and certainly no pain, fix it – not temporarily but permanently. We're here to help and show you how – right here, right now. That is, if you're ready, of course......

Just the same applies to you as you begin reading this book. As you start putting our therapy into action, positivity is vital. You can shift that excess weight. You can be healthier, fitter, look and feel better. The Gastric *mind* Band is here to help you, and you will be able to do it. Starting now.

Should you feel after reading the book that you'd like to attend one of our clinics, you'll find details on our website at www.gmband.com.

The G*m*B therapy we've developed will take you to the eye of the dieting storm, offering you an exciting new approach, introducing you to issues you'd never before considered to be connected to your overeating problems. Putting a spotlight on your complex emotional relationship with food and showing you how to rethink the whole issue of being overweight. In the therapy we deliver at the clinics, and in the pages of this book, we know you will, maybe for the first time in your life, have the tools and knowledge to finally take control.

3

YOUR PERSONAL REASONS TO SHIFT THAT EXCESS WEIGHT ARE...?

OK let's be frank. The majority of people who will read this book are probably overweight to some degree or another, and each will have their personal reasons for wanting to reverse the situation, whether it be health or vanity related.

Your reasons for wanting to lose weight may not be the same reasons as your neighbour, or his father, or his teenage niece.....everyone's reasons are different. It's often appearance, or wanting to wear nicer/different clothes, or to look better for your partner.

Surprisingly most overweight people rarely consider the amount of damage they are doing to their body by keeping it so unhealthily fat. Hopefully you will soon be starting to understand that in the same way as in all other aspects of your life, with weight too you need to accept the very important consequences of your actions.

You may not be super morbidly obese; maybe you just know you need to lose weight before it affects your health any further. You know it, we know it, and most of all you want rid of the very idea of it. But do you know what you're doing to yourself? Let's hope you do – or maybe let's hope you don't or you'd have changed your eating habits a long time ago.

Before you start on the road to a new you, it's important to lay bare the gravity of the problem. You may be familiar with some of it, but it may help you focus your thoughts and establish the right mindset prior to starting out on this very important journey.

It's not clever to dig your grave with your own knife and fork
(English Proverb)

Do you have a fear of death? It's such a powerful question. Are you scared of dying? Stop for a moment and ask the question again. Many people carry on blindly living their lives unaware of the gravity of what being overweight could be doing to the quality of their life ahead. In fact what it could be doing to their life expectancy. Think again about how the thought of a shorter life, or chronic illness, or death, makes you feel.

Of course many people live unhealthy lives and live to a ripe old age, but the trend is going the other way. Thousands of deaths in the UK are caused directly as a result of obesity; adult obesity rates have almost quadrupled over the last 25 years, and two-thirds of UK adults -that could be 30 million people - are now considered overweight or obese. The UK government says hospital admissions in 2007-2008 caused directly by obesity were up 30%, at over 5,000, including strokes and heart problems. According to the NHS Information Centre, the number of drugs prescribed to treat obesity rose by 16% to 1.23 million by 2007, at a cost of £38 million – so the scale of the problem is becoming recognised. But of course pills only treat the symptom, they'll never fix the cause.

The global obesity epidemic has been key in joint work by the World Health Organisation (WHO) and the International Obesity Task Force, who are now working to convince world leaders that the problem can, and should, be addressed – quickly. With an estimated 300 million people overweight/obese worldwide, they reckon that cutting obesity with healthier diet and more exercise will prevent up to 4 million cases of cancer every year.

Until 50 years ago it wasn't even considered important enough to keep records of obesity – it was that uncommon.

There are many many health downsides to being overweight. We can't possibly cover them all but here's a reminder of just four of them. It does not make comfortable reading – but it's something every overweight person whatever his or her age should take a close look at, however much you may not want to. It may be a good idea to create your own imaginary order of what you fear most?.........

Type 2 Diabetes: reckoned to be among the top five killers in most developed countries, over three quarters of people with Type 2 diabetes are overweight. High blood glucose levels associated with diabetes increase the risk of heart disease, stroke, high blood pressure, kidney failure and poor circulation which can lead to limb amputation. Damage to the retina is a common problem associated with diabetes, and can lead to blindness.

Stroke: according to the NHS, is the third largest killer in the UK. Usually a blockage or rupture of a blood vessel in the brain, strokes can leave a person paralysed down one side and affect speech and vision – among other things. Obesity is a high indicator of likelihood of suffering a stroke.

Cancers: Some 13,000 people in the UK every year could avoid getting cancer if they were a healthy weight. The WHO says obesity/overweight are the most important known avoidable causes of cancer after tobacco. Among types known to be linked to weight are colon, breast, prostate and thyroid.

Heart Attack: A fifth of heart disease in the UK can be attributed to obesity, and heart disease can cause heart attacks and angina. A heart attack is usually caused by a blockage or rupture of one of the main blood vessels around the heart. Usually extremely painful – however although a heart attack is by no means always fatal, after effects can include depression and catastrophic lifestyle changes.

This is a snapshot of the better known health risks of obesity. If you need any further convincing, there's a more extensive – though still not exhaustive - summary in Chapter 21 on page 283. Maybe you should read and digest the information. It may alter your level of motivation for change.

When it comes to eating right and exercising, there is no "I'll start tomorrow." Tomorrow is disease.

V.L. Allineare

Having read the brief highlights concerning diabetes, stroke, cancer and heart attacks, it's possible you may now have a different focus to your reasons for wanting to become slimmer. Whatever your personal goals or motives, we believe G*m*B to be an exciting new tool, not only in your battle with your excess weight, but also in the global battle against obesity. The fact that there has been extraordinary press coverage for our therapy has been great for us personally and professionally (not to mention very good news for those clients who came to us as a result and finally conquered their weight issues) but the stories in the media predictably focussed on the 'hook', the seemingly magical effect of the *mind* Band hypnotherapy session. Little if any mention was made of the rest of the therapy; you could be forgiven for thinking the whole approach was very 'lightweight' in more ways than one.

However there's much, much more to the Gastric *mind* Band therapy than just the one 'banding' session. There are many thought-provoking questions, answers, research, challenges, suggestions, techniques and lessons. We are totally serious and committed to the constant development of the therapy, and really hope the opportunity will arise to bring G*m*B to a wider audience through health organisations and professionals, both in the UK and internationally.

Obesity, being overweight, is a symptom of overeating; of having an unhealthy relationship with food. The G*m*B therapy aims to treat the cause of the problem. It's surely always better to focus on the cause of a problem rather than the symptom. That's how you get permanent results.

Summary:

- **Stroke**
- **Heart attack**
- **Diabetes**
- **Cancers**
- **The list goes on**
- **Think about it**
- **Turn the page and start doing something about it**

4

THE BIGGER PICTURE

There are many reasons why people become overweight. Being overweight is primarily the result of people overeating. Often, the reasons they began overeating are anchored in their past; maybe some emotional event caused them to begin eating for security, comfort or protection. The memory of the event remains sealed in the subconscious mind, even if they have consciously forgotten it.

The reason for the weight problem can be as simple as the fact that as a child the person was required by their parents to eat up everything that was put on their plate, maybe accompanied by the oft-quoted phrase 'Think of all the starving children in Africa'. Such sayings follow us into adulthood, even though the logic behind it is rather strange – how can the fact that we are overeating possibly compensate for the poor undernourished children in Africa?

When we grow into adults many of these ideas stay with us. Add in the mix of the stress and strains of daily life and the fact that we move – literally move our bodies around - less than ever before, and the result is us creating an obesity problem that is spiralling out of control.

While we yearn for the body beautiful – or at least the body socially acceptable – companies compete for our hard earned money, promising quick fixes, miracle solutions, shakes, pills and all manner of new fangled machines all promising something we hope we can achieve by short cuts – a healthy lifestyle and a body to be proud of.

It's not rocket science. We know that we need to lose weight and improve our health; we need to change the reasons and way we eat and move, and hopefully get away from the idea of ever 'dieting' again.

Dieting alone rarely produces permanent results, because diets do not address the important complex and sometimes highly emotional relationship that exists between overweight people and food.

Most "diets" cannot be sustained for more than a short-term period, because they are often very restrictive and difficult to keep to, so the diet becomes a form of self-torture that you go through temporarily, going against all your usual eating habits, whilst being deprived of many of your favourite foods. Deprivation simply creates stronger desire, so if you are following a diet that creates certain "forbidden" foods, you end up craving all the foods you are not allowed to have.

When you finish 'dieting' you revert to your "normal" eating habits, which in fact means overeating, and eating for the wrong reasons. You also tend to reward yourself with all the things that you have been craving so much during the diet, and as a result all the weight, if not even more, goes back on again.

Because dieting doesn't address the underlying, psychological craving for excess food, an overweight person ends up on a seemingly permanent roller coaster ride of yo-yo dieting, losing their self-confidence along the way and feeling more and more despondent about their continuous battle with their weight.

In this book we're going to help **you** put an end to this all too familiar pattern once and for all.

G*m*B Therapy as experienced at Elite Clinics

We feel that when reading the book, people might be interested to understand what the experience is like for those clients who visit our clinics in person.

This should give you some idea:

When a client elects to undertake the G*m*B therapy at an Elite Clinic, the treatment is normally undertaken over four sessions, usually over four consecutive days. Total therapy time 10 hours.

At the beginning of the **first session**, which can last up to four hours, the client is taken through a complete and detailed overview of the entire G*m*B therapy. They are told exactly what to expect, each component of the treatment is fully explained, and of course any questions that arise are answered.

This is followed by what we call 'Information Harvesting'. Over a two-hour period a vast amount of in-depth background information is obtained from the client. The detailed data is obtained and captured using Elite Clinics' own psychological weight loss profiling questionnaire. We have re-created the questionnaire for you to complete as you work through this book.

The first session, which is the longest, ends with a 20-minute hypnotherapy session.

—

Clients are requested to 'fast' for a minimum of four hours prior to attending the clinic for the **second session**.

During this session, the client is accurately weighed and their body analysed using a Tanita body analysis device. The equipment analyses information including body mass, visceral fat, muscle mass and BMI. This is followed by the client undertaking a test to establish their RMR (Resting Metabolic Rate, described in more detail in Chapter 12), this is achieved using a device developed in the USA known as Korr Metacheck. This session ends with a second hypnotherapy treatment.

—

The **third session** focuses on CBT, incorporating a full analysis of all the information previously obtained during sessions one and two. The client is provided with a range of explanations and demonstrations regarding why they eat and behave in certain ways. They are shown how easily change can be introduced. Many small but unique techniques are shared with the client which if they wish they can use for the rest of their life.

Session four involves many components, including a demonstration using an actual surgical Adjustable Gastric Band, plus film and animation. The session concludes with the actual 'Band Fitting', undertaken using deep hypnotherapy, and visualisation techniques. Professional studio lighting, sound effects and computer driven vortex aroma devices bring together a 'virtual reality type' experience.

At the end of the treatment the client is provided with a comprehensive manual, which covers in depth the four sessions. Additionally they are supplied with a set of four CDs one of which is a personalised recording of the client's own sessions. They are also given some visual aids to help them adapt to their new lifestyle.

www.gmband.com

Summary

- **Forget dieting…it doesn't help!**
- **Our face to face in-clinic therapy? It's a winning formula**
- **(and you've got most of it in your hands right now!)**

5

GIRAFFES, SPARROWS AND OBESITY

How is it possible for an overweight person to be in control of their alcohol consumption, but always give in when offered a bar of chocolate? How can a person resist trying cocaine all their lives, but regularly succumb to a Big Mac, and how does an ex smoker turn down the offer of a cigarette, but at the same time throw in the towel at the thought of a chicken korma and rice? They show restraint in other parts of their lives. If they just took that same element of control and put it into their eating habits, Eureka! Job done. All before breakfast! Now read on, and we'll show you how.....

Your reasons for wanting to shed excess weight could include a desire to impress your partner, physical appearance, low energy levels, fashion trends; or it could be a very real fear of coronary heart disease, Type 2 diabetes, colon cancer or any of the many other obesity-related health issues. For the moment, though, the simple question is this:

Why do people eat? Do we have dinner because we are hungry or do we have dinner because our watch says it's 7 o'clock? Do we stop eating because we're full or because the plate's empty? It's almost certainly the latter, so there's no actual physical connection with our body .... so has it become a family custom? Has it always been a tradition? Or is it a social event? Say you're alone - then why do you have dinner? Just because it's 7 o'clock?

It doesn't just apply to what you see when you look at your watch.... if you travel through a time zone and arrive when you 'should be' asleep, but the rest of the population's about to have lunch, what do you do? If you eat, ask yourself why.

Sad people eat when they are not really hungry; happy people watch a good film, listen to some music, write a letter or an email, take a walk or enjoy a long hot soak in a bubble bath, waking in the morning feeling refreshed, not fat and sad

To tackle your inherent problem with poor choices involving food and eating, you need to start at the beginning. You need to understand hunger. Ask yourself if you even know what it is to be hungry. Maybe we're all just too busy stuffing food in our mouths, and doing it so fast our brain never gets a chance to yell out 'hey wait, I'm not hungry' .... Let alone 'stop, I'm full! '......

Does anyone in the Western World recognise a true hunger pang any more? Has anyone even experienced one in the past 10 years?

A pound of fat = 3,500 calories. So you only need to be eating 135 calories a day more than your body needs and you'll be putting on 14lb a year. 135 calories...that's not a mega meal, it's less than a standard Snickers bar, a small glass of wine, less than a quarter of a Big Mac; it's only really one large apple a day more than your body needs and you'll be piling on a stone a year. If you've put on weight faster than that, you've been eating much more than your body needs – and it's showing in the most obvious (and visible) way – on the scales.

But the good news is that 135 calories is quite easy to skip. Just don't eat that bar of chocolate, have a glass of water instead of that wine. Just small steps each day add up to massive results when you're reducing your intake in just the same way as they added up to rolls of fat when you were choosing to eat when you weren't hungry.

Along with why you eat, it's about understanding the thought processes that led you to eat (and overeat). Understanding that just thinking – and eating – in the here and now won't achieve your goal.

We'll look at this in detail later in the book. That piece of chocolate cake may look good, but the taste will last maybe only two minutes. Just two minutes. Was it really worth it for just two minutes? But it's also about realising that eating the piece of chocolate cake isn't the end of the world. Just get back on the bike and learn that it's just a lapse. Make sure it never happens again, but more importantly take knowledge from it. Learn why and how the event occurred. Why you picked up the chocolate cake. Where were you? Who were you with? Then understand and realise that any lapse, any mistake, is not such a bad thing but a great way of learning how not to do it again.

—

**A piece of chocolate cake is a lapse and nothing else.
It's a single event. A one-off.
A relapse is reverting to filling your face with chocolate day in, day out, and not bothering to get back on the bike again**

—

Creating a new relationship with food is absolutely vital to the process of shedding your excess weight because try as you might have done in the past, you can't avoid it. You need to eat to live. You have to face food choices several times a day. Food is after all a major stimulus in our lives. It's vital to retrain yourself to understand how and why you made the wrong choices before and what you need to do to learn new, healthier habits for the future. Throughout this book we will be teaching you how to recognise your triggers, how to stop and identify the first thought that leads to your bad food choices.

> Once you've experienced that first thought, and you're within moments of reaching for food when you really do not need to eat – that is the perfect time to use our mental Pause Button. We'll explain more later in the book, but whenever you find yourself in these seemingly hopeless situations, all you need to do is imagine that you have a remote control for your life (similar to the one for your TV/DVD etc) so you can pause/fast forward/rewind as and when necessary. Using this you can see ahead to the consequences of your actions and avoid making the wrong food choices.

When people are shedding unwanted weight by changing their eating habits, they really ought to make sure they enjoy that whole journey. You didn't put the weight on all at once; don't expect to lose it all overnight. Of course have a target, a goal, but enjoy all the smaller steps along the way.

—

Tell yourself that you are going to lose one pound this week, NOT that you need to lose four stone before that wedding next Easter

—

Imagine an 18 stone person wanting to get down to 10 stone. It's going to be a long journey and will need a certain amount of determination and resilience. Think of it as if it were a long cruise, say from Southampton to Sydney. Arriving at Sydney may resemble in your mind getting down to 10 stone, but from the second they untie the ropes of the cruise liner at Southampton, the journey begins. There'll be many parties, many things to celebrate, many wonderful ports of call along the way. Enjoy them all, enjoy shedding every single pound.

If you've lost 4lb yet you still have 4st 12lb to lose, celebrate the fact you're now 4lb less than you were a fortnight ago. Then the next 4lb, or even the next half a pound; be positive rather than thinking how much more you want to lose and feeling negative. We'll be teaching you, reassuring you, that being positive has a knock-on effect on how you make your choices.

—

To travel should be as good as to arrive

—

To achieve a real change, you have to start to recognise things about yourself and your decision-making processes that you may never have given a thought to before. That way you have the best chance to identify what you need to do to make that change. It's important to learn your own personal triggers; everyone has them but everyone's is different. It could be the smell from a baker's shop, the fact you've had an argument with your best mate, or the fact you're lazing around watching your usual soap; all sorts of things. But recognising these triggers means you can avoid reacting in the wrong way and reaching for the doughnuts, or bar of chocolate, or whatever.

If you doubt you'll ever be able to get a handle on how thoughts lead to actions, and not only get an understanding of the process but be able to use it to change, read on!

What is a want? What is a need? What is a desire? What is a craving? Learn the difference and that's a big step. Recognise when you make Seemingly Irrelevant Decisions – for example agreeing to go to a party you're not that bothered about – but you know there'll be a good buffet to tuck into. Going home via a scenic route, which just happens to take you to a bar you and a mate like to visit for a pint and a curry.

Then there's something so many people will recognise: it's called Here and Now Thinking. You only see the next few seconds in front of you, to the pork pie, or the ice cream; you know that's really going to be yummy, that it's what you need right there and then....but you're not looking at the medium or long term consequences of what you're doing. You can get on top of it, but you need the tools and as you work through the book you will get them. Here and Now Thinking can be overcome, and we'll show you how.

We'll also introduce you to the actions of terrorists and anarchists, and how they create chaos in the minds of dieters the world over.

THE RESTAURANT STING & THE LAST SUPPER

For some reason, that is hard to explain, the majority of overweight people seem to have a problem when eating in restaurants. Many manage to faithfully follow a diet for weeks when eating at home, but for some unexplained reason they 'crash & burn' as soon as they walk in the restaurant door.

There are many reasons, along with a never-ending list of excuses for the collapse of their diet, of course the restaurant will often play the 'Sting', which often catches people out, but quite often it can be put down to what we call at the clinic 'The Last Supper' syndrome.

Dieters and often non-dieters alike, for some reason seem to treat the occasion as if it were their last ever visit or meal in a restaurant, they have to have it all, and have it tonight.

They feel compelled to have their favourite starter along with their chosen main course and not forgetting the house special dessert. It is as if they feel that maybe, this is their last chance, they cannot say no to the dessert, not tonight I am on a diet, but maybe next time, they treat it as 'The Last Supper'. Start watching them, you will see it for yourself.

We'll also introduce you to LFT – Low Frustration Tolerance – learning about that will help you tolerate hunger and stop you being frightened of it.

Getting an understanding of all these flawed ways of thinking, and more, amounts to you being given a great big yellow toolbox and a hard hat – a toolkit to understand all the ways you can change your attitudes to food. It's a hard hat to protect you against your own flawed thinking and against those dangerous terrorists and anarchists out to foil your best intentions.

There are so many elements to the psychology of eating; we'll be teaching you to pick out those bits that apply to you, how to stop yourself and freeze time before every meal to see if you really need to eat what you've chosen - because you've probably never done that before. We'll show you how your mind ambushes you and how to control it.

With the Gastric *mind* Band, it's this mix of approaches that makes it different. The underpinning of one therapy by another, in unique ways. Merging proven 'science based' therapies like CBT with NLP and Guided Imagery.....we call our combination therapy Life Architecture, which we think sums it up nicely. All these methods appear throughout the book – sometimes several times, just in different ways.

It's about you, no-one else, designing a plan for living – and enjoying – your life tailored to your own individual needs, fears, dreams and aspirations. No forbidden foods, nothing banned, no themes, daily calorie counting, fat points, none of it. Just a normal relationship with something you have to face daily just to stay alive.

So what of the giraffes? Simple – giraffes, sparrows, squirrels – virtually any wild animals you care to name – eat when they're hungry, until they're satisfied, then stop eating. Have you ever seen a fat sparrow? Do they sit there eating the seed on the ground until it's all gone and they can't fly? No, they eat what they need and fly off. Would a giraffe stand there and munch so many leaves it couldn't walk? Not a chance! Squirrels, for example, have got it sussed. They'll go out and collect loads of nuts, then sit eating. But do they eat them all until they're fat? No – they eat what they need then bury the rest for when they're hungry again. Obesity is almost exclusively a disease affecting the human species. The squirrel says 'enough: bury' ... Squirrels have got it sussed!

Not to mention illness...... we can all probably name a friend or family member who's died of cancer, or a heart attack, or liver disease. How many animals die each year from an obesity related condition? How many would be domesticated and how many wild? Think about what that might mean.

And what do we do? We sit there and eat, one, maybe two, courses then order pudding. No-one orders pudding because they're **hungry**, do they? How can they be? They've just had two courses, probably a glass of wine and a bread roll. Their stomach could stretch to the point at which it's painful – think about it, you know it can happen. Why would anyone do that?

So we've had three or more courses, then we go on to eat between these meals as well. We eat and eat even though we're not actually hungry. So if we're not hungry, why eat? How stupid are we?

'The only overweight animals you will ever see are the ones who depend on humans for their food supply, such as domestic cats and dogs'
Allen Carr

—

If you've been on diets before and they've failed, it'll be because the diet doesn't address what's going on inside your head - the whole concept of emotional eating, eating when you're bored or stressed or whatever. A diet never addresses that problem. In fact it's our belief diets can't work long term because you always 'go back' to your old ways unless you've changed your thinking. This book is all about giving you the tools, the defence mechanisms. You've got to be able to enjoy yourself and live in the real world.

There are plenty of people who've lost a considerable amount of weight with different slimming groups, or diet systems, then in the next year they put it all back on because none of them ever gets to the subconscious part of the decision making process. They don't address the real problem. In a way they address the symptom, not the cause. We'll teach you how to recognise and change those underlying habits, how to get on top of what's going on in your head and address your personal eating problems.

Where weight loss is concerned, motivation is as important as what you eat.

Motivation and the psychology of weight loss is as important as restricting calories, yet gets talked about nowhere near enough. Whether it's Weight Watchers, Cambridge, Hay, Scarsdale, whatever you like, surely motivation is the thing. We'll teach you to understand your motivation.....but at the end of the day it's down to you whether it is important enough to you to make the changes.

If you were told by the doctor 'you've got Type 2 diabetes, your toes are already looking a little bit grey, you're probably looking at amputation before Christmas unless you do something about your weight,' would that be enough, would your motivation be so high you wouldn't need us? If you had 100% recovery after a mild stroke and the doctor said you'd been lucky the next one could leave you paralysed, would you be able to lose weight?

If someone said they'd pay you £500,000 to lose all your excess weight, would you sign up for it and succeed? That's motivation. So why haven't you been motivated to lose weight before? Maybe there's a discrepancy between what you think you want to do and what you're actually doing.

—

You seldom get what you want in life;
You do, however, normally get what you expect

—

Our minds have great influence over our behaviour, and the human mind works best when it concentrates on a positive goal. We tend to talk about ***"losing"*** weight, but our <u>mind</u> thinks that if we lose something we can't rest until we find it again. A much more positive concept for your mind to accept is for you to see yourself not <u>losing</u> weight, <u>but getting rid of excess, unwanted fat</u> and moving closer to your target weight as a result. We will actively strive to get rid of rubbish and things we don't want in our lives any more.

Though 99% of diets should succeed, nowhere near that many are successful long term. It's been claimed that women spend TEN YEARS of their life on various diets, and that throughout their adult life, the average woman tries over 100 different weight loss methods – yet many do all this and lose NOTHING long term.

As long as whatever you want to accomplish is realistic, achievable and important enough to you, then there is no reason why you can't make it happen – the only thing stopping you is yourself!

Virtually all weight loss programmes can be successful if you stick to them..... Why don't people stick to them? They're not sufficiently motivated. They don't understand what's really going on. So you have to ask yourself the question 'Why am I doing this?' 'Why do I want to lose weight?'; answer truthfully, then you'll start to get close to discovering the solution. The problem with eating is very seldom down to the food or the stomach. It's psychological. You're eating for some other reason than hunger. You're bored, because it's 7 o'clock, because you're lonely, because you just found some leftovers in the fridge. The word hunger seldom slips in. When the person is offered the chocolate cake, in that split second she said yes the one question she never asked herself was 'Am I hungry'?

—

Hunger, Craving, Desire....
You have to understand the difference between the three. It's fundamental.

—

So why ARE you having dinner? Is it because you're hungry? If you're hungry, where do you feel the hunger? In your brain? In your throat? In your stomach? What does it feel like, this hunger thing? Let's try and re-experience hunger, let's go back and find out what the base symptom is. Medical research says hunger has nothing to do with the stomach. There has been research on people who've had their stomach removed, so they've only got a tube between their throat and their intestine. No stomach. But they still get hungry. So it's got nothing to do with the stomach. We're told the brain is detecting that the blood falls short in certain nutrients – amino acids, carbs, proteins, and sends the message that you're hungry and you are ready to eat. And when you're hungry you'll eat anything that's not poisonous. If you say 'I'm absolutely starving I've got to have a fillet steak', don't kid yourself. Those two things can't go together. If you're really hungry, an apple or a piece of toast or some simple grilled fish will do. If you really want a fillet steak, that's a craving.

—

The next time you reach for something to eat, stop BEFORE you put it in your mouth and ask yourself 'Am I hungry?' If not, what emotion or feeling are you experiencing that's prompting you to eat?

—

When you get the signal that you're hungry, your body is asking for certain things – fats, proteins, carbs, whatever. If you go and get a bag of crisps, it won't satisfy your body's needs: so an hour later your brain will say 'I'm still hungry, give me more'... and that cycle of eating junk but never fulfilling what your body needs nutritionally is the cycle of obesity, because people are just eating, thinking that stuffing junk food in their mouth, anything that's available, anything they fancy at the time, is going to take the hunger away and it doesn't.

Something you may not know is that the first sign of dehydration is hunger not thirst. So what do you do? You sit here, dying of thirst, say 'I'm hungry', and eat a cheese roll. Five minutes later, though, you'd be 'hungry' again because it wasn't food you needed it was water... so you'd eat another cheese roll. And be hungry again in five minutes. Getting fatter and fatter instead of just having a drink of water.

If you think you're hungry, try having a glass of water. If you're still hungry 10 minutes later then eat. If you're not hungry, it was simply that you were thirsty!

A newborn baby knows it wants milk. After 8 minutes or so it stops drinking. But it doesn't know its BMI or height to weight ratio, it just knows it's not hungry any more and it stops. And that's how simple it's got to be. If people ate only when they were really hungry we wouldn't have a problem. There's a saying 'sleep when you're tired, eat when you're hungry', and that's all you've got to do. You don't go to sleep in the middle of the afternoon because you're bored. You don't go to sleep mid morning because you've had a row with someone, so why would you eat?

When you do a day's gardening or something strenuous and you really put your back into it and finish the day with a long hot bath and go to bed: that sleep after muscular exhaustion, when you're really tired, is a deep wonderful relaxing sleep. That's exactly the same as sitting down and eating a meal when you're hungry rather than when the clock says a particular time. If you sit down and eat a succulent steak or lobster when you're really hungry, it'll be amazing. When you eat it for no other reason than because it's 7 o'clock it'll have a completely different appeal – try it sometime.

This of course is why we've got all these overweight children running about. Eating whether they're hungry or not. If we could get them to eat only when they're hungry, the changes would be immediate. There should be no place in society for behaviour like that; in fact there is currently some public debate about whether parents who feed their children a diet mainly consisting of junk food, ready meals and processed foods, resulting in the youngsters becoming obese, should be made to take nutrition education classes.

If you're not hungry why are you eating? Are you so sad that all you can do in your life is stuff food in your mouth? Can't you go for a walk? Go to the theatre? Paint a picture? Read a book? Watch a film? Watch the sunset? Listen to some music? Why do you have to sit down and continually eat all the time?

People are eating when they're not hungry. Eating for all the wrong reasons. Many are eating themselves to death.

So - you've been overeating for 10 years: maybe all your adult life. Now things are going to change. You know that arriving home looking and feeling good comes with a price, the price is a bit of effort: the slim person knows that. But how can eating what your body needs be a punishment? How can you say you feel like you're being punished because you're eating healthily?

You're giving your body exactly what it needs to run the best, the most efficiently, it possibly can; it may require a bit of an effort, but it's not punishment! Many slim people, interestingly, might say that having to see an overweight person would be a punishment. For you being that way and for them having to see it. Everyone that's fat wants to be slim. Anyone that says different? Well we say they're not telling the truth…..

We've spoken to a handful of past G*m*B clients, asked them all the same questions then done face to face interviews to tell their personal weight loss stories in their own words for this book. You'll recognise many of the feelings they admit to when they were overweight. It will be obvious they know full well how the weight loss – gain cycle leads to a feeling of hopelessness. What they'll tell you very clearly though is that the G*m*B therapy has turned their lives around and completely altered their relationship with food.

In the four G*m*B sessions, we will help you to see the ways **you** make the wrong food choices, the times when **you** eat for the wrong reason, the many different triggers every overweight person has, but specifically **you** have, which have led you down the road to obesity. Better still, we'll show you there's a fork in that road, and you're standing there right now about to make the choice that leads to a totally different, manageable, and yes, enjoyable, relationship with food.

Overweight people wear their problems for all to see in the shape of their body. Those with other issues – a drug addict, alcoholic, or someone with severe depression, for example, their problem usually isn't visible when they walk down the street. With an overweight person it's there for all to see.
It's very rare to find an overweight person who's happy with their life.
Obese people who say they're fine being overweight? I just don't believe them.

Martin Shirran

Summary:

In this book, we'll be looking at

- **the psychology of overeating**
- **recognising your own triggers**
- **questioning why you eat**
- **identifying your motivation for shifting excess weight**
- **understanding hunger**
- **the difference between need, desire and craving**
- **how you can show restraint in other areas of your life but not with food**
- **how thirst can be mistaken for hunger**
- **remaining positive over a long-term weight loss**

6

NITTY GRITTY – ANYONE FOR GASTRIC BAND SURGERY?

So maybe you've wondered about having gastric band surgery? You wouldn't be alone. Thousands are not only wondering but actually doing so every year. Statistics vary but there's no doubt the number of obese individuals has risen hugely in the past 20 years and the development of bariatric surgery has given an alternative solution to the problem which is being used more and more. However even people who've had a gastric band fitted acknowledge it's far from the miracle "cure" many expected it to be.

Surgical gastric bands were first developed by a Ukrainian, Dr Lubomyr Kuzmak, in the early 1980s. By 1986 he had implanted an adjustable silicone gastric band to address severe obesity. Professor Franco Favretti's team used Kuzmak's system and between 1991 and 1994 over 2000 gastric bands were implanted, though it was not suitable for laparoscopic (so-called 'keyhole surgery') procedures. Trials and tests for an adjustable laparoscopic band were completed by 1993 and the first two were implanted in Belgium and Italy in the first week of September. US trials started in 1995, but it didn't receive US approval until 2001.

Gastric bands are usually only offered to patients with a BMI of over 40, or a BMI of 35-40 if they have other health problems such as heart disease, high blood pressure or diabetes. A typical gastric band operation involves placing an adjustable silicone band around the upper part of the stomach to create a pouch. The band's tightness is adjusted by injections of a saline solution into a port located just below the patient's skin. As you eat, the pouch fills much more quickly than your stomach would, because it's a fraction of the size – about the size of a golf ball rather than the one litre capacity of a normal unstretched stomach. As a result you can generally eat far smaller quantities than without the band. This is designed to reduce the amount of calories consumed, leading to weight loss. From the pouch, the food passes slowly into the lower part of the stomach, through a narrow adjustable opening (picture two thumbs held together) created by the band, then normally through the rest of the digestive system.

The operation involves four or five incisions in the upper abdomen, and the band is fitted via keyhole surgery lasting between half an hour and an hour. Gas is pumped into the abdominal cavity to make space for the surgeon's equipment during the procedure. The band is held in place within the patient's body with stitches. The initial incisions from surgery are closed with two or three stitches. A fine tube runs from the band to an access point or 'port' secured under the skin around the chest/ribs, or sometimes the abdomen area. A few weeks after surgery, the band is adjusted by injecting precise quantities of saline through the skin into the port, and via the tube, to 'inflate' the band. There are often two or three adjustments – each requiring repeat hospital or clinic visits - in the first few months after the operation.

However this is a very basic description of the process. The full story of what happens before and after the operation is currently not fully understood by the general public – 'you are obese, you get a gastric band fitted, you can't eat very much, you lose weight, right?' And you lose it faster/better/more easily than any other reversible method, don't you?

The reality is rather different. It all starts not with the operation, but several weeks before. Patients are instructed to start following a strict diet to ensure the liver – which sits above and partly in front of the stomach – is not too fatty. Having an enlarged liver is a problem commonly associated not only with drinking alcohol, but also with over-eating.

For gastric band surgery, your liver has to be moved to one side for the operation to take place, and if it's enlarged, it can literally get in the way as well as increasing the risk of causing serious damage to it during the process. In fact it has been known for part of the liver to break off during surgery, leading to massive internal haemorrhaging.

The pre-op diet can, depending on the surgeon, mean a restricted diet low in sugar, fat and carbohydrates. With each ounce of glycogen (a form of sugar stored in the liver, and in muscles for energy) the body also stores 3-4 ounces of water, so if you are on this strict diet, low in starch and sugar, the body loses glycogen and water, thus shrinking the liver.

—

So having followed that regime, before you even reach the operating theatre you often lose up to a stone or more by reducing the amount of food you eat.

—

Once the band's in place, the soups and blended foods you are advised to eat after surgery give the swollen stomach area a bit of a rest. How long that lasts for varies, but it can be for about six weeks, so the weight continues to drop because you've gone from eating massive quantities (despite what people often say, it is EXTREMELY rare to become overweight without eating far more than your body needs) to following a restrictive diet for three weeks, then living on soup for another six weeks.

Work it out. Before the band comes into play you'd have lost anything up to 20lb. No surgery, just sensible eating!

At six weeks the person has their first 'fill' of the band. Saline solution is injected via the port, inflating the band to reduce the outlet and restrict the flow of food. It may take quite a lot of adjustment – everybody's different so the medical team gets the person to try to eat and drink while they're doing it to check if it's right. If it's too restricted, they may not even be able to drink water and they could vomit it all up. The surgical team has got to get it exactly right so the patient can eat little bits and feel the restriction but not to the point where they can't get anything down.

When a 'bandster' or 'bandit' (as gastric band patients dub themselves) has the right amount of fluid in their band so their weight is coming down steadily, they refer to this as finding their 'sweet spot'.

After the first fill the patients are slowly reintroduced to normal solid foods, and the size of a meal they can eat is about six tablespoons of food. Return visits to the clinic or hospital are required as often as necessary to have the fill adjusted to ensure continued weight loss. Obviously the weight loss is quite fast to start with, but once it's settled down, the figure overall, according to the WHO, averages out at between 1-2lb per week - no different from any sensible weight loss programme.

That simply replicates what our Gastric *mind* Band aims for and expects. You shouldn't lose any more than that over an extended period of time anyway. Not least because rapid weight loss can lead to the development of gallstones.

So the surgical gastric band only offers the same long-term weight loss as any surgery-free healthy eating plan. However it's not foolproof. The success rate is only 70%, in all likelihood the main reason for it not being 100% being because you can cheat on the band by how you eat. Obviously solid foods will stay in the pouch for a long time, making it harder to overeat because of the discomfort once the pouch is full - but softer things – e.g. ice cream, chocolate, will pass through quite quickly. So if you were a comfort eater in the past and prefer foods that don't take a lot of chewing before they disintegrate, you can still go through life drip-feeding yourself continually on mashed up junk food, or softened chocolate, ice cream etc., and the band won't actively restrict it at all. The same applies to alcohol, which as you'll learn when we discuss portion control and calories, is like drinking calories that are no use to your body whatsoever. These are known as empty calories. If you like to drink water during a meal, that's not advised after the fitting of the gastric band because it frees up the food matter to pass out of the pouch more easily. So you don't feel full for as long as without the water.

THOUGHTS FROM THE FORUMS

You might be surprised at patients' comments found on Gastric Band forums….

'To be totally honest, I have been eating what I like. I started out eating well and did change a few bad habits, but at the end of the day nobody gave me a brain transplant. I still think like a fat girl and always choose the cake over the fruit ….even to this day'

'….our worst nightmare – opened up for the op and it wasn't done cos her liver was too fatty'

'I had pain from trapped wind, from the air that is pumped into your tum to make it swell'

'I was under the impression the band would restrict everything I ate but this is definitely not the case. Cakes, biscuits, peanuts, yoghurts, crisps, pudding, mince, mashed potato, sweets, all easily eaten even with the band in.'

'....six months later and I've put all the weight back on and some extra....'

'some people thought weight gain was a thing of the past – oh no. The band is simply a tool, not a magic cure.'

'....she found various ways to cheat her band....'

'I know that if I only ate when I was hungry I would not put on weight...a lot of our behaviour becomes habit; it's retraining our brains and making the right food choices. Man have we a lot of work to do!!!'

So – you want to know what you'd be putting your body through and the potential risks and downsides of gastric band surgery?

There are many risks involved in any surgery when the patient is under general anaesthesia, ranging from infection, unexpected reaction to the anaesthetic, to developing a blood clot, allergic reaction to substances leading to cardiovascular problems, jaundice, slow recovery due to poor heart, liver or kidney function, and of course being obese makes undergoing any surgery intrinsically more risky. According to the American Heart Association, severely obese patients are at increased risk for pulmonary embolism, wound infection and other conditions.

—

Approximately 1 in 2000 gastric band patients die during or after the procedure

—

Obesity makes it hard for surgeons and medical teams to establish whether a person has underlying health problems because some symptoms are indistinguishable from aches and pains which might be simply due to their weight or a more serious problem. – e.g. chest tightness may be due to an underlying cardiac problem, or simply due to their obesity.

- You have to fast for about six hours before having general anaesthetic, sign a consent form confirming you understand the risks and alternatives as well as the benefits of the procedure, and you may have to wear compression stockings to help prevent blood clots in the veins in your legs. You may need an injection of anti-clotting medicine.

- Once the operation is complete, you rest until the effects of the anaesthesia have passed, then you may need some or all of the following: pain relief, catheter from your bladder (if you've had one you'll know the discomfort of this procedure), tubes running from your wound(s), fluids via a drip, post-op x-ray on position of the band, and compression pads on your legs.

- You'd be allowed home after about a day and have to drink clear fluids for the first 24 hours, then you would start on other liquids leading into pureed foods (like baby food) for a few weeks.

- You would have a follow-up appointment to check the healing wounds, followed by several repeat visits for band adjustments. The stitches? That depends on whether they're soluble – they disappear on their own in 7-10 days – or not, which means another hospital/clinic visit for them to be removed.

- You shouldn't drive for about a fortnight; full recovery can take three weeks.

Possible side-effects of a gastric band operation are as follows:

Post-anaesthesia sickness, bruising, pain, swelling of the skin around the wounds, feeling or actually being sick after eating, and requiring multi-vitamin supplements because of your restricted diet. If you are unlucky enough to get an infection which doesn't respond to antibiotics the band may have to be removed; there could be damage to other organs in your abdomen, or slippage - months or even years after the operation, there is always the risk that the stomach will move up through the band and the upper pouch will become enlarged. (The band can be re–fixed in the correct position.)

Leakage - This may be due to damage of the reservoir or tubing if fills are not carried out with extreme care or if two of the band components come apart. Again, this would necessitate replacement of the damaged component.

Erosion - Very slowly, and particularly if the adjustment balloon is tightly inflated, the band can work its way into or through the wall of the stomach and cease to be effective. In this case the band would be removed and replaced if possible. The band itself is made of silicone and there are no known side effects to this material inside the body. However it is possible that at some time in the future the band may need to be replaced simply because it has worn out or newer, better bands have been developed to replace current ones (hip replacement prostheses are replaced for these reasons).

Gallstones sometimes develop if you lose weight quickly and can require surgery to remove them – in fact some surgeons advise removing the whole gallbladder at the same time as having gastric band surgery.

Occasionally a surgeon converts from keyhole procedures to open surgery, requiring a bigger cut on the abdomen.

And finally, of course, an average of around 10 per cent of people with a gastric band may need another gastric band operation in the future and/or, having regained the weight lost, be recommended to have the far more serious, and irreversible, gastric bypass surgery.

In a review of gastric band patients at a Florida centre of excellence, 17½% of those sampled needed follow-up revisional surgery, ranging from repositioning to removal.

Acid reflux – many 'bandsters' seem to regard this side-effect as the norm, but in bad cases, people can experience burning sensations in their throat as a result of the simple act of lying down in bed at night.

From the mouths of those who've had the surgery, here's a quick reminder of how you might be feeling after a surgical Gastric Band operation:

'I thought I would just eat like before but feel full up quicker, but there is a lot more pain and discomfort involved in learning to eat differently and feeling full happens in the chest and not the stomach - a very strange experience'

'Let's not forget this is not a miracle cure.'

'There is a range of foods I cannot now tolerate - unfortunately none of these are chocolate, ice cream, cheese or alcohol, so there is still a lot of self discipline involved !'

'I've had incidents when I didn't chew enough and my food made a dramatic re-emergence'

'the best way to describe the mush stage is as though you were weaning a toddler'

There are three other key points. Firstly, provision of the Adjustable Gastric Band is generally limited to people between 18-55 with a considerable amount of weight to lose and resulting high BMI (body mass index) – usually above 40 (above 35 if there are additional health issues).

Secondly, as we said earlier, because people can 'cheat' the band and unless they've gone through psychological steps to change their relationship with food, it is not always the miracle cure so often believed.

Thirdly: in practice, many gastric band providers look at figures of between 50%-60% of excess weight lost over two years, but did you realise that with the Adjustable Gastric Band, success is not always defined as reaching your 'desirable', 'goal', 'proper' weight, but as losing more than 25% of your excess weight. So you could be 5ft 6in, 16 stone, BMI 38, be aiming at 11 stone to achieve a healthy 24.5 BMI. You could have a band fitted, lose 1½-2½ stone and be considered a success story – whereas in fact you'd be someone still 5ft 6in, still weighing 12½-14½ stone, still with a raised BMI (between 28-32) - defined as between overweight and obese, depending on whose scale you use - and still wishing you were a good 20lb lighter.

—

After the initial drastic loss of the first nine weeks or so, the average weight loss for somebody who's had gastric band surgery is between 5-10 lb per month

—

So… you've got the band fitted. What now? According to BOSPA (the British Obesity Surgery Patients' Association), there are six golden eating plan rules to follow if you are dedicated to obtaining the greatest benefit from your gastric band:

- **Eat three meals per day**
- **Eat healthy, solid food**
- **Eat slowly and stop as soon as you feel full**
- **Do not eat between meals**
- **Do not drink at meal times**
- **All drinks should be zero calories**

They suggest eating a healthy balanced diet including foods from each of the five main food groups, and there is quite a list of foods which aren't tolerated well or can cause blockages and/or vomiting. These include oranges, meat (needs to be chopped to the size of an end-of-pencil rubber before considerable chewing), broccoli, dried fruits, coconut, crisps, nuts, popcorn, soft white bread, pineapple, asparagus, and more.

—

To some extent the surgical gastric band tends to restrict healthier food.

—

So you could say the eating plan with a surgical Gastric Band is: Eat nutritious food slowly and don't graze or snack between meals. Think about it........If you did that anyway, you wouldn't need the band in the first place!

We've given some detail about gastric band surgery earlier. During the sessions in the clinic, Marion tells her clients more details.... some of what she explains is as follows.

The medical team may suggest removing the gallbladder while operating, because of your increased risk of developing gallstones. You can live without it, but it's quite common for people without a gallbladder to suffer from digestive problems such as bloating, gas, indigestion, constipation or diarrhoea, especially if their diet is particularly low in fibre, high in fat and refined carbohydrates or highly processed foods. It is also possible to develop stones in the liver even after the gallbladder is removed, which causes congestion and makes the liver sluggish.

Marion's got some interesting observations about other elements of gastric band surgery.....

Everything in the abdomen is closely packed together, and during the operation, the surgeon might inadvertently perforate the bowel or any other part of the body near the area of surgery.

Afterwards, if the band is over-filled, patients can end up choking when they try to eat. Or the band can actually start eroding into the wall of the stomach – which could lead to removal and gastric bypass surgery as an alternative. This involves stapling across the top of the stomach and diverting the intestines...however the first part of the small intestine is where nutrition is absorbed and even when eating a healthy diet, they need supplements to make up for the effect of the surgery, which basically alters the way the whole digestive system works.

If someone with a gastric bypass eats rich food, it travels through the body faster since there isn't so much intestinal tract left, so you can end up with uncontrollable diarrhoea – known as 'Dumping Syndrome'!

As for what happens after gastric band surgery is over? Marion's equally forthright.

The band may need to be tightened several times. The adjustments can be made using x-rays and barium meals so the doctors can chart the progress of the fill and see how much of a restriction there is.

After the first fill the patient can start eating solid food again – so after 6 weeks on soup the great temptation would be to have a big mouthful of food, chew it briefly and swallow it down but of course it would simply come straight back up again. They have to really focus all their attention on eating small amounts and chewing each tiny mouthful really thoroughly – a drastic change.

A lot of people underestimate how complex it can be getting the adjustment right. Each fill involves having maybe just an extra 1ml of saline injected into the port until the optimum level of fluid (the 'sweet spot') is reached. No further adjustment is needed then, until the person reaches their target weight, and at that stage some fluid is removed, so from then on the person can eat enough food to maintain rather than reduce their weight.

If a person is being sick rather a lot, the whole process of retching can cause the band to come loose from its stitches and slip out of place, so it needs to be re-positioned.

So you go from overeating to only being able to eat a portion of food of literally no more than about six tablespoons on a plate. It'll take a long time to eat even that small amount because you can only take mouthfuls no bigger than your little fingernail, or the rubber on the end of a pencil. Imagine eating a meal in which that's the maximum size of every mouthful you can take. You have to chew each mouthful at least 10 times before swallowing, otherwise the larger particles of under-chewed food can get stuck in the pouch and end up blocking the access to the stomach. End result? The body rejects the offending item and you'll be sick; better known as productive burping.

When you eat with a gastric band, the feeling of fullness happens high up in the chest, which ends up feeling like indigestion. People often end up rushing to hospital, thinking they're having a heart attack because of bad chest pain though in fact they only have indigestion. When you get stomach pains in the top part of your stomach, it's literally right next to your heart. Only the diaphragm separates them!

Suffering from acid reflux is a major problem for people who have had the gastric band fitted. It's yet another downside to having the actual surgery. There's a sphincter muscle at the top of your stomach to stop the acid coming back through which sometimes doesn't work properly. If there's a build-up of acid in your stomach it can then come back up into the oesophagus, causing a nasty burning sensation. This happens because there's only ever a small amount of food in that lower part of the stomach: the bulk of the food is in the pouch at the top, slowly drip-feeding through.

If the band is over-tightened, it's possible to have a situation in which the person can't even swallow a mouthful of water without it coming straight back up again.

The surgical gastric band has only been around for a few years so as yet no-one really knows the long-term implications.

In conclusion, if you've got your head sorted out, you shouldn't actually need to have this foreign body inside you for the rest of your life, if at all! You are relying on the band to do the whole job rather than relying on your mind. You've got to get your mindset right.

Having the operation doesn't help you build up a better relationship with food; it's just like a diet when you end up even more obsessed with food. You'll be forever thinking, "Oh, is that mouthful too big? Have I chewed that mouthful ten times before I swallowed it? Oh no, I haven't left a long enough gap between eating and drinking!

Imagine how difficult and uncomfortable it would be going to a restaurant with friends. To try to sit down and eat a meal in front of them, with all these things you've got to consider. You're always going to be on edge.

PRODUCTIVE BURPING.....
WHAT'S *THAT* ALL ABOUT?

The band is portrayed as being nice and easy and it's been really glamourised recently with lots of celebrities having it done. Everybody sees the end result and how great they look - but no-one knows anything about the whole process that's gone on in-between and how difficult it might have been, what that person's gone through, etc. No-one knows the background to it all. Because the medical profession wants the whole gastric band operation to seem very simple and straightforward, they don't even like to say to people "Look, you will be sick if you try to eat too much food or if you take a mouthful that's too big". They've actually created an expression for it to make it seem not quite so drastic. They call it suffering from "productive burping". They don't want to call it being "sick", "vomiting" etc. They're nasty words! The more you find out about the more it makes you realise that it's not as simple as you think and that it's not a quick fix at all. Far from it. In the end it doesn't really help people to build up a nice, relaxed relationship with food.

For many people, however, there's no doubt that the gastric band procedure has been life-changing. It is relatively safe and is now being carried out in most countries in the world. To some, maybe many, it has been a life saver.

As a post script, it is worth noting that there are no intrinsic dangers or side-effects from the triple therapy of the Gastric *mind* Band treatment. And of course there is no invasive surgery.

Summary

- **A gastric band is a successful way for some people to lose excess weight**
- **It is relatively easy to 'cheat' the gastric band**
- **The weight loss expected may not be any greater than that achieved using a healthy eating plan**

—

"Undergoing surgery to assist with weight loss is a serious procedure, not a quick fix"

Professor Peter Littlejohns,
NICE weight loss surgery appraisal leader*
*(*National Institute for Health & Clinical Excellence)*

—

7

SARAH WAS.............BUT NOT ANY LONGER.........

If ever there was a cautionary tale about gastric bands, it's that of a recent G*m*B client, who for reasons of confidentiality we'll call Sarah. She went through two life-threatening band failures and excruciating abdominal pain over a period of nearly two years because she remained convinced the band – which by that stage was going severely wrong - was the answer to her problems.

At 31, the 5ft 4in mum of three wasn't sure what she weighed – it was around 21 stone. But wearing size 26 & 28 clothes, she knew one thing. Her target was a size 10/12 and she believed the only way she'd achieve it was through surgery.

"I was huge", she says. "I'd just had my son and I knew I couldn't go through another year of getting bigger and bigger. My weight had always gone up and down, since childhood. I felt I had to do something drastic.

"With what I now know, I wouldn't recommend it to anybody. At times I had pain like I've never had in my life."

The story starts as a straightforward decision to go for a gastric band rather than bypass – which Sarah initially wanted because it's a permanent solution – to avoid potential side effects and more drastic surgery.

"I went to seminars, did the best research I possibly could" she says. "In the end my mum and I agreed that no way should I have a bypass, there were too many issues that could go wrong, and it had a higher death rate.

"So I borrowed the money and went for the band. At the time I believed it was the best thing since sliced bread, and rarely goes wrong. Once you get to where you want to be you can either have it taken out or just loosened. I was told it was virtually pain free, that I'd ache a bit after surgery but that I could expect to be up on my feet in a couple of days.

"To me that sounded perfect. I had a baby and two other children – I was constantly doing the school runs."

The cost started out as just under £8,700 and rose to £10,500 with repeat visits for fills. But as you'll hear, despite problems almost from the outset, Sarah was more than happy once the weight started dropping.

"Once I'd booked in, I was informed I had to slash my food intake for two weeks to shrink my liver, so I was on three low calorie diet drinks a day and shifted a stone, but felt really ill because I was used to such a high calorie intake. But there was light at the end of the tunnel – a reason for doing it.

"By the time I went in for the operation I'd lost about two and a half stone on my own."

When she came around from the operation, she was in considerable pain but despite being booked in for three nights, was sent home the following day, being told that it was to get her moving to avoid developing blood clots.

"Looking back, now I think I had the band fitted too soon after having my baby (three months before surgery), but the hospital said I could have had the op even sooner if they'd had a slot. Although at the time I felt really chuffed, I don't think my stomach was really ready. I should have waited a year. At the time I was so desperate it didn't matter what anyone would have said.... except they didn't, because Mum made a point of asking!"

Once at home her recovery never really went well. "I felt absolutely awful – couldn't pick anything up. It was excruciating. I started getting on my feet the second week, but not pain-free."

Then followed what she describes as the trial and error of discovering just what you can and can't eat. "That was hard, because you're still very tender and while you're trying things out you try not to be sick because you could hurt yourself. For me, everything used to bounce back up again. I had to eat very slowly, very small pieces, very small quantities. A coaster sized plate as a meal; mashed carrots and swede for example. Toddler food really. It was very hard work"

"When I look back I can see that I wasn't well, but I didn't care because I was losing weight. I just wanted to be able to go into a shop and pick something off the shelf – that was my ultimate dream, it was what I'd got in my head, what I was focussed on."

"I was being really good because I'd paid all that money. Through the support group I heard about people who ate chips, who melted down Mars bars.... I thought 'why? Why have you got to the point of undergoing surgery yet you still want to eat this stuff and then sit there saying you haven't lost a lot of weight'"

For quite some time, Sarah kept putting to the back of her mind how unwell she'd been feeling, but it became obvious things weren't as they should be one bank holiday weekend. "I felt really really ill; I'd drink and feel sick, I just couldn't eat," she says. "I started to get to the point where I'd have a sip of water and it would come up, then even putting water on my tongue I was gagging. I tried to get hold of the hospital but everyone was away. I couldn't even hold myself up, had to just lie on the bed. My husband had to carry me to the toilet. I could barely speak.

Luckily for Sarah, someone from a support group realised she was genuine and suggested a barium test.

"I rang the hospital and got an emergency appointment, and was told I was very lucky, my organs were shutting down because the band had somehow tightened. Apparently I even had the characteristic sweet smell you get just before your organs do that. If I had gone to sleep that night, I was told the chances were high I would have gone into a coma, probably died.

"As soon as they loosened it off, it was fine. At the time I was told this was the first case they'd ever had, but despite trying to consult my specialist about why this happened, no further action was taken."

So Sarah had the band adjusted, and despite misgivings about what might happen if it tightened again when she was not able to get to hospital, she got on with her life and her continued weight loss.

"Several months later the same thing happened again" she says. "They didn't have a clue why it was happening. Nothing had triggered it, but there seemed no research. At that point the hospital hadn't had a band that had gone wrong.

"Obviously these occasions made me very poorly; I couldn't do anything apart from lie in bed. It was hard for us as my husband is self employed, and had to come home to look after me, and take the children to and from school. He couldn't work so we were losing even more money."

"My children used to get very worried", says Sarah, "because even when the band was working 'as it should', I was constantly sick – I even had to pull over on the side of the road once when I was taking my son to school."

The sickness used to come over her very suddenly – and on top of that she suffered heartburn bad enough to take prescription tablets. At times she was also sick in her sleep. "That is absolutely terrifying," she says. "Your natural instinct is to swallow, but you can't for fear of choking!"

Sarah carried on with the discomfort, and takes her story up again two years after having the band fitted and some considerable time after it self-tightened. "I was still feeling unwell, but left it and left it. In 2007 I felt really ill. I'd got to the stage where every time I drank or ate I got horrendous pains in my upper back – it was excruciating. If I ate too much of something it felt like I was swallowing it 'down my back', I didn't know how or why.

"I got a cough, my chest hurt, everything hurt. I went to the doctor, had tests, I was convinced it wasn't the band.....it was a completely different feeling.

"I had tests, antibiotics – nothing touched it. It got really bad, and in the end I paid to go back to the consultant, which I begrudged. He said it couldn't be the band."

Sarah was given medication for people who have heart attacks, which she had to spray in her mouth before she ate, but experienced what she describes as 'instant migraine' and was unable to continue with it.

She eventually saw the consultant again (this time on the NHS) and was told she would have an endoscopy, a type of camera on a cable inserted into her stomach. "I was thinking 'hang on a minute, I've paid all this money, I'm in excruciating pain, I've just about had enough. We've been through everything it could possibly be and now it's looking as if it's got to be the band'" and she was told not to worry, it would be sorted.

After the endoscopy under general anaesthetic, Sarah received the bombshell news that her band had tightened and gone through her stomach wall into her top bowel, explaining the excruciating pain.

"I thought how could this possibly happen.....then all of a sudden everything else didn't matter and I was thinking 'you've failed me big-time, I'm going to be fat again'. I'd only just finished paying and it was going wrong. It was really selfish, I wasn't even thinking about what was going on inside me. I was about 10 stone then, wearing size 10 jeans (which I've still got!). I was absolutely devastated."

She was told the band had to come out as soon as possible and that it would be possible to insert a 'slip' – like a small-scale bypass – but in the end was told the risks were too great.

Sarah got to see the pictures taken of her insides, and was disgusted and appalled to see black and orange showing up. "I was pretty sure if something is black it's dead; and orange suggests serious infection's going on," she says.

Her story didn't end there, though, because having finally got booked for the removal operation in 2008 after several hiccups in the planning, she not only had to go through pre-op reduction dieting again but things didn't go smoothly after that procedure either.

"When I came round from the surgery, I experienced pain like I've never felt in my entire life," she continued. "I was all wired up, tubes in my mouth and nose and everything, I lay there and honestly thought I'd died. I was on morphine the pain was so bad"

And there's more... "My chest drains were left in too long and fused to my ribs" she says matter of factly. "I had to have five days in hospital.

"When I was at home recovering, I got a serious infection, I'd been feverish and hallucinating – one day I got upstairs but I was in agony, bent over to do something in the bathroom and heard a 'pop' and a load of yellow pus and blood poured out of wounds on my chest."

Having lived through the whole experience, Sarah did go down the road of investigating her chances of compensation, or at least seeing if she could persuade anyone to highlight her problems.

"I did all the complaining I could", she says, "and I spoke with staff at after-care, but although I was pointed towards counselling, I felt I just hit a brick wall. A solicitor advised me that taking the case to court would cost a great deal and it would have been the first one of its kind she had dealt with."

Since it all happened, she's traced other cases in the USA – though they've generally happened three or four years down the line rather than so soon after fitting. Most have then gone on to have another band or a gastric bypass.

"But I was told there was too much damage to ever have another band fitted" she says with a rueful smile. "At present I'm waiting to go into hospital to have another endoscopy to see what is going on; to be honest it really frightens me."

Not only is there the pain, but she is still restricted as to what she can eat. "I can eat most things, but still struggle from time to time with rice – it feels as if it is getting stuck in my throat. I also find it hard at times to drink and eat together: that brings on the same feeling of suffocation."

Still experiencing occasional breathlessness, pain in the area where the port was if she bends, and some back pains, she obviously regrets having the surgery in spite of her successful weight loss at the time.

"At the time it was the best thing since sliced bread," Sarah says. "But friends and family see it as bad news. For the first time I had the feeling food didn't rule me, but I paid a big price as well – three near-death experiences. No, I wouldn't recommend it to anybody.

Sarah came to Martin and Marion after her mum saw an article on the Gastric *mind* Band therapy in the national press. "I'd really given up", she says. I felt I'd been failed by the system, and I was really on a low. I'd regained much of the weight I'd lost and just wasn't interested. I just wanted someone to wave a magic wand. Once I arrived at the clinic and met Marion and Martin, I was feeling really upbeat from the start. – It gave me a really good boost."

"There's a part of me that will never regret having the band put in – to see I could really be slim again wasn't a fantasy. Feeling slim to me is my everything, it makes me tick. "But although I've had good and bad experiences of the band, it is a high price to pay, both financially and with your health. I'm lucky I'm here to tell my story. I wouldn't recommend the band to anyone."

"I feel really motivated, excited for the coming months and the new me taking shape! I've lost a stone so far, but I've recently had to change my medication, so I could gain pounds rather than lose them."

Her weaknesses, she says, were picking, a sweet tooth, burgers and fast food breakfasts.... not forgetting the odd curry!..... quite a typical catalogue of problem foods. She's not alone in having tried all sorts of weight loss programmes – but says bluntly what so many dieters experience, "you lose the weight then plonk it all back on and more."

"Amazingly, although I gave into a few temptations at Christmas, with what I learned at Elite I got back on track quickly and couldn't wait to get to the gym, so something has changed!"

"I am hopeful that this is going to 'cure' me of my bad relationship with food... I want to not have the nagging voice in the back of my mind day in, day out, arguing with myself as to whether I should eat all that pizza or just half etc. To have a better understanding of how this all works.

"I believe this can really work, really makes sense. With G*m*B I know I'll be feeling on top of the world again."

Sarah is finding comfort in all the CBT elements of the G*m*B, and of course she's far happier knowing nothing more can go wrong medically as a result. "It's safe with nothing at all to go wrong", she explains. "I also believe that hearing the views of someone who's been overweight and can share the same experiences as you is priceless.

"People who've suffered with being overweight bury their heads in the sand, don't want to hear about going to slimming groups because they've already tried it a million times and lost a bit of weight only to find later on they're gaining again.

"It's different getting encouragement which tells you about someone who's suffered not getting through turnstiles and funfairs, not been able to get the tray down on your lap on a plane, the fake happy-go-lucky brave face you put on to everybody else who says 'you wouldn't be you if you were slim'!"

When we spoke, Sarah was approaching the end of her sessions with Marion and Martin and had already started to recognise a change in herself and her eating habits.

"I've already changed," she said. "My lifestyle now consists of exercise, every day, and it's not a chore. It makes me feel good. The best thing is not being on a diet. This is a lifestyle. There are no forbidden foods. Have anything but in moderation, don't beat yourself up about it, pick yourself up and carry on. If you've decided something on your own – say to have a salad instead of a sandwich, you feel so good. I can't believe it's actually me saying this, but it's really how I feel. I'm in control...... at last!"

—

Nothing tastes as good as being thin feels
- Author unknown -

—

Summary:

- **Even when you do your research there are no guarantees**
- **Gastric Bands can and do go wrong**
- **G*m*B can offer new hope**

8

DEVELOPING THE GASTRIC *mind* BAND (MARTIN THE GUINEA PIG)

As we've said in the introduction, the idea for the Gastric *mind* Band came up purely by chance. A client who we'd successfully helped give up smoking using hypnotherapy, had begun to gain weight. She had a friend who'd just had a gastric band fitted at a cost of £11,000 and since she didn't want to spend thousands, and it was an operation she herself didn't want, asked couldn't we just hypnotise her again, this time into **believing** she'd had the operation?

At the time it just seemed a joke – we all laughed and thought no more about it but that evening we had to fly back to the UK, and at the airport, over a glass of wine, we started talking about it. Marion's reaction to the idea was clear. 'Why not?' By the time we'd arrived at Stansted we had exhausted the laptop battery and filled several A4 sheets of paper with the outline proposal for a treatment package which would conclude with the fitting of an imaginary gastric band. Effectively, by then we felt there was a good chance we could do exactly what our ex-client had suggested. As time went on we sculpted, added to and refined our thoughts and ideas, and developed the G*m*B therapy. This remains the subject of ongoing development even now.

Our lead guinea pig was Martin, the obvious candidate as he was overweight himself, though as things progressed we had an ever growing list of clients and friends all prepared – in fact some very keen – to help with the trials.

At first we just tried with hypnotherapy, but we found it too light, and of limited success. We then tried just using CBT, but that on its own didn't cut it. Next we tried hypnotherapy together with NLP but that didn't work the way we were looking for either. Gradually over the course of the following 18 months, all three approaches were used to underpin each other. Putting the three therapies together and underpinning each one with the other ticked all the boxes and did the job. This was a different ball game completely. We'd come up with the Gastric *mind* Band treatment that was achieved using the therapy we'd developed, the triple therapy that we call Life Architecture.

To get the most from the hypnotherapy sessions, we knew we had to play with clients' senses so we developed techniques and devices that would enable us to introduce the sounds and smells of the garden and beach during the relaxation into a hypnotic state. We added ways to include the taste of sea salt on clients' lips, the smell of ozone; we helped them to experience the sights sounds and smells of the hospital and ultimately the gastric band operating theatre.

If experienced in real life, those sensations are really memorable... during therapy the client gets the most from it if the virtual reality is as accurate as possible.

This book can never replace one-to-one hypnotherapy or treatment as experienced in the clinic. However, if you are sufficiently motivated then you will be focussed and receptive to the suggestions we'll be making to you in the same way as if you were sitting in front of us.

There was really only one way to be sure The Gastric *mind* Band worked – Martin tried it himself..........

MARTIN'S STORY

Martin, who is 57 and 5ft 8½in tall, weighed in at the start of trials for the therapy at 18st 12lb. He is continuing the process even now, but seven months later was 13st 11lb, with a 34in waist. A loss of 57lb.

(A number of before and after pictures of Martin appear on our website – www.gmband.com)

We asked Martin, as we have all our 'case studies', to tell us his weight history. "When I was about 11 years old I had to see the school doctor every couple of months. I remember I was 7 stone 7lb - it never changed. I was thin and stayed that way for a long time."

As time has gone on and more and more G*m*B clients have gone through the clinic, it has become clear from casework that being underweight during adolescence and then going on to develop an unhealthy relationship with food, leading to obesity, was not unique to Martin.

"By the time I was 16 I was what I suppose you would call overweight, and whilst I dieted on and off over the years nothing really changed except the usual I suppose: I would lose a couple of stone and then put on three. My brother and sister were never what you would call thin but neither did they seem to suffer with their weight, my dad was a normal weight and so was my mum until later in life.

"I suppose at my heaviest I must have been getting close to 19 stone. My weight has been a problem for nearly as long as I can remember. Like many, I suppose my weight has been an issue, a part of my life that I've reluctantly carried with me for ever. Looking back now, I'm sure that at certain phases of my life it was more important than others."

Asked to express how he felt about his weight, he explained: "I was never really depressed about it, sure it mattered and I went through phases of trying to do something about it; however I think maybe whilst certainly being overweight is an issue to blokes it has a different priority level to the way women feel about it."

"Everyone who goes through the treatment seems to benefit in different ways from the various sections and approaches, for me the CBT, the understanding, the psychological reasons why I ate and how I thought about food, is the part that has stayed with me the longest. Of course, as time has gone on I've developed new approaches not just for myself but that I share with the many clients we now see each week."

He is clear in his mind that the Gastric *mind* Band treatment has worked totally. "Yes it really has, I suppose I am in a different position to most other candidates, I have lived with the trials and discussions, sometimes 24/7. What worked the most? The whole thing. But in particular I am now more in tune with my body than maybe I have ever been in my adult life. I can now recognise hunger, real hunger. I live by the rule 'sleep when you are tired, and eat only when you are hungry'. It works for me."

He feels there's no doubt the gastric band element was important: "It definitely played a part. I know that clients' views differ on the overall importance of the op element in the therapy, but it does underpin everything we do."

"Asked to define how the process has changed his eating habits, he said he eats and drinks differently and for different reasons. "I look at everything and everybody differently now," he says. "I was saying to Marion only recently that I'd been trying to work out why, in certain circumstances, we, or more likely I, end up drinking more alcohol than I should. I was questioning why it always happens in the same company. Then it came to me. I think that group of people bores me, their conversation is not stimulating, and I was therefore self-prescribing, self-medicating, with what I believe to be an anti-depressant, namely alcohol.

"The answer to which parts of the therapy I feel helped me the most was easy and hardly needed thinking about. Without doubt the tools that have helped me and those that I still use today (and not just for dieting) include:

"Knowing how to identify the Diet Terrorists and Anarchists, those people who manage, often without any effort, to create total chaos in the lives of people trying to practice healthy weight control. I sometimes call it the Restaurant Sting.

"Let me give you some examples of what I'm talking about. On our way home from the clinic Marion and I occasionally visit a local Chinese restaurant, usually with the pre-arranged plan of having just one course between us. All is fine, unless that is, the owner's daughter serves us. 'Hello Mr Martin Hello Mrs Martin' is always her welcome, bless her; then before the menus arrive at the table, that we don't really need anyway, she sends over a complimentary, extra large portion of prawn crackers. We never ordered them, not sure we actually want them, but there they are right under our noses. If I have just one I know I am at risk of blowing my eating plan for the night. It's hard to have one prawn cracker, wouldn't you agree?

Of course this young Chinese girl is highly trained in the art of chaos; it's like she sees us getting out of the car and plans the whole thing, no-one else is getting jumbo portions of crackers put under their noses for free, just us. If I manage to get past the prawn crackers or not matters very little – this girl's good; very good. When the bill comes at the end of the meal it is always presented at the table along with two complimentary drinks from the bar, always the same thing, Bailey's on ice. 'Gotcha' I always think she must say as we walk out the door. The calories of the prawn crackers before you even looked at the menu, then those two Baileys - let's say 900 calories....

"Only recently we joined some friends for an Indian meal; it had not been a good week for me as far as food was concerned, I was determined to drink only water, putting myself up as the driver, and to only order a plain Chicken Tikka starter served as a main course, no rice or Indian bread. We sat down at the table and before I had even pulled my chair in the waiter brought a tray with poppadums over and put them in the middle of the table; there must have been two dozen, piled up like Mount Everest. 'Who ordered them' I asked. 'They're free' I was told. Great; the waiter returned two minutes later with a tray of chutneys to go with them. There were six of us, he could have put the tray anywhere on the table. He chose, of course, to put it right in front of me.....terrorist or what!

“I went back to the UK recently to visit my mum. I had only been there two minutes when she said, ‘make us both a cup of tea and sit down and tell me all your news’. A few minutes later when sitting with her she said ‘I bought us some of your favourite biscuits, go and put a few on a plate’. I haven’t eaten biscuits for ten years but what could I say to my 90 year old mother. When I opened her kitchen cupboard it was full of Jaffa cake biscuits, boxes of them. When I asked her why she had enough biscuits to feed an army she told me they were on a two for one offer at the supermarket so she had bought a dozen extra packets for me to take back to Spain with me for Marion and me to enjoy. ‘I remember years ago you used to love them, so I thought I would treat you.’ Another terrorist, and she’s my mum!

I was recently invited by a friend to join him at his mother’s for Sunday lunch; it seemed like a good idea so I accepted. He had not seen much of his family for a while and they all had a lot of catching up to do – which meant I spent most of the time in the kitchen talking to his mum while she cooked the Sunday roast and he was off chatting to his brother and sister. It proved to be an education.

She told me we were having beef with all the trimmings. I then watched her open the oven. When I asked her if the beef was cooked already she said ‘No, I just want to baste it along with the roast potatoes’. It was at that point I realised that maybe accepting this invitation was not such a good idea.

The meat was being cooked in an oven tin standing on a baking rack type of gizmo to allow the fat to drain off; I watched as she ladled all the fat that had just been drained from the beef back over it again. When she finished she started pouring the remainder of the fat over the potatoes. Over the next hour or so I watched in amazement as she re-opened the oven three more times and re-poured the fat repeatedly over the meat and the potatoes. I realised then that the reason people like roast potatoes so much is because of all the fat used to crisp up the outsides.

When the meat was cooked she removed it from the oven and finished cooking the vegetables, which she told me three times had been grown in their own allotment, and that they were fresh and completely organic.

While her husband carved the meat I watched as she took the oven tin from the oven, the fat, juices if you like, still in the bottom; she placed it on the stove, sprinkled some granules in and made the fat-based gravy to pour over everyone's fresh, organically grown vegetables....

"In the book you'll find details of Marion's now increasingly famous Pause Button technique, which you can use to freeze time, to give you precious moments to ensure you make the right choice, decision. I use it on a daily basis, along with the fork in the road therapy described later. Both have been invaluable to me, and like I said above, I use them in many other situations other than relating to food. So can you.

--

Changing a situation, or the dynamics of a situation, always has the effect of changing the result; if something is not working for you, change it. Today....

--

"I can now look back and see that my eating patterns had not been good - too much of the wrong foods, eating late at night and usually skipping breakfast. I now eat a healthy breakfast every day, one day fresh fruit, one day porridge made with half skimmed milk, half water, and I try to have my last meal as early as is possible. I don't, though, allow this healthy new approach to interfere with my social life.

"I started losing weight straight away - it was quite fast to begin with, then as I expected it gradually slowed down. I had a few plateaux along the way, I know how hard they can be to dieters, but I carried on, sometimes changing my diet, sometimes the time of day that I ate my main meal, and sometimes generally increasing my exercise level.

"I remember a period of three weeks when I thought it had all gone wrong; I was close to throwing my toys out of the pram. I had at that stage been regularly losing between 1lb and 1½lb a week. Then one Monday, at my regular weekly weigh-in, I was informed I'd lost nothing. My food intake had been on track and consistent, as had my exercise level. I insisted Marion changed the batteries in the scales. She did so – reluctantly! Same recording, same result..... Somehow she convinced me to carry on.

"She reminded me of all the hard work I'd already put in, the fantastic results we'd achieved week on week, and how good I felt about myself. So I carried on, and the next week when I was weighed I'd put on 1lb. I doubt anyone other than someone familiar with long-term weight loss will ever know just how depressed I was at that stage.

"I agreed I'd give it one last final week. At the regular weigh-in the following Monday, the scales indicated I'd lost 4lb, equalling 1lb per week. So I was back on track."

With regard to the notion of being able to 'override' the Gastric *mind* Band, Martin says: "I was able to over Christmas, I adopted the 'some meals matter and some don't' approach, I pre-planned it and relaxed the tension over the holiday period.

So did he believe the Gastric *mind* Band part of the treatment? "Absolutely. A hundred and ten per cent."

"The G*m*B treatment is about introducing change, sometimes major change, into someone's life. It is certainly not always easy, and sometimes it's seemed like a thankless task but the results are lifelong and so, so, worth it."

"I was asked about the most memorable recent changes/experiences I have had since losing the weight. There are two that will always stay with me and both occurred on the same day:

"We were at the airport waiting for a flight; it was busy and we were sharing a table with a couple and their two children, one of whom was sitting next to me. The lad was drinking what turned out to be a chocolate milk shake with an ice cream float in it. To cut a long story short, it was spilled. I had virtually all of it in my lap, milky chocolate and a load of melting ice cream. It wasn't the child's fault but nevertheless I was not a happy bunny – I had a two and a half hour flight and a two hour drive ahead of me when we landed – I knew I would not look or smell very pleasant. Marion said 'there's a Levi/Wrangler shop over there, why not just go over and buy a new pair of jeans'. I ran over to the shop, picked up a pair of 33in waist jeans and put them on and gave the cashier mine to throw away; I wasn't going to carry them with me, not the way they smelled.

"I cannot remember the last time I could do such a thing, just go into a shop, pick a pair of jeans off the rail and put them on. Anyone who is overweight and reading this will know exactly the significance of that event.

"An hour or so later, on the flight, we bought a couple of drinks and the stewardess leaned over and undid my tray catch and put mine on it. I smiled to Marion and explained how amazing it was not only to have the tray down with drinks on it, but also to have a space between my stomach and the tray; it was amazing. Only a small thing, but you did ask!

Summary:

- **So why *had* no-one thought of this before?!**
- **It's the mix – Life Architecture - that's made the difference**
- **If you are motivated, anything is achievable**
- **Although the results will never be identical, you can get a very similar experience to our Gastric *mind* Band clinical therapy by reading this book and reinforcing the key elements through self hypnosis**
- **A plateau is a plateau, nothing more. Work through it.**

9

THE SESSIONS – A LIFE-CHANGING SEQUENCE

The Gastric *mind* Band therapy is actually a process – a unique process of learning about yourself and your eating patterns, unlocking the underlying reasons why and how these have developed. It involves learning new eating habits, understanding how to make better food choices and live the rest of your life with a healthier relationship with food.

At the clinic, the treatment is carried out over four sessions, made up of 10 hours of therapy time - obviously ending with the unique Gastric *mind* Band element. All our clients find different parts of all four affect them in different ways. You'll find you pick up on specific anecdotes, rules, thoughts or observations which 'get to you' most successfully. There are so many of these, sometimes you'll think they're repeated. They are. Sometimes they're repeated with slight adjustments. It's no bad thing to be reminded in as many ways as possible of just how you've been tricking yourself, cheating yourself, allowing your mind to give the go-ahead for all sorts of behaviours that have ended up with you overweight, unhappy and looking for help to get out of the mess you're in.

Everyone reads a book the way they choose, but with this one, if you can keep to reading it in the right order, re-tracing your steps as and when necessary, you'll make best progress. The sessions, in particular, run in a sequence – identify your problems with food, identify how much you should be eating, spot the errors you've been making and ultimately cap the process off with the Gastric *mind* Band session. The progress is obvious and you'll make the most of your experience if you can work through logically.

Session One:

Session One is all about building up the picture – harvesting personal information, poking you with deliberately awkward questions, creating a personalised history, an overview. Why do you eat? Why are you overweight? It must be tiring carrying all those extra calories and pounds of fat around. We ensure you start to question everything you eat, everything you put in your mouth. Take 'before' photos – there can be nothing stronger than having a photo of Big Fat You on the fridge as a permanent reminder. It'll also help you see progress as your eating habits change.

Visualisation - imagining a fork in the road; either another year overweight, not liking yourself, feeling sad. Probably getting fatter. Or the other route, visualising a positive, slimmer future. Close your eyes and go forward to next year, see yourself at your chosen target weight and size, or as a perfect size 10: what do you smell like, what do you feel like, what do you wear at work? Which shops do you buy clothes in? Do you still avoid mirrors? How much energy do you have, how much confidence have you got, what sort of things are people saying to you, how has your life changed, where are you going, what are you going to drink, what are you going to eat, how has it affected your relationship with your partner.....

Session Two

Session Two involves ensuring you understand metabolic rates, calories, portion control, what your body needs and what it doesn't. The role of exercise. Looking at 1lb of fat. Comparing the density of fat and muscle.

Visualisation: picture yourself sitting down to eat a healthy, balanced meal. Thinking through the process of producing smaller meals. Serving on smaller plates. Focus your attention on your food. Eat slowly, mindfully. Smaller mouthfuls, swallowing before you take another mouthful. Placing your fork on your plate occasionally. Checking if you're really hungry before anything goes in your mouth. Then picture yourself at target weight, focussing your attention on the positive feelings that go with being slim. If you find yourself reaching for food when you're not hungry, your subconscious mind will distract you to do something else - ....

Session Three

The hunger question. Defining fullness. Questioning everything you put in your mouth. How did you get to be this size? How do you maintain your current weight? Work out how many calories you would need to eat to maintain your current overweight size – you're obviously eating that much and you may have a shock! What is your motivation for losing weight? Does this include health issues as well as other more emotional aims? Wants, needs, desires, cravings. The difference between lapse and relapse. Lose weight by 'chunking'. Everything you do starts as a thought. Creating new habits.

Session Four

Revising all previous sessions - what you have learned and achieved so far. How much you can and should eat, and why.

Looking at what happens now.

How the restriction of the band will help you reach target and maintain a smaller food intake.

The Gastric *mind* Band – Taking a closer look at the surgical gastric band illustration and learning about the operation and its side effects.

Visualisation: Picturing a band being wrapped around the top of your stomach. Clenching the golf ball in your hand at the same time as you picture the band being put in place. Squeezing the ball tighter as you imagine the band being clicked in its final position. Feeling the golf ball as it signifies your new smaller stomach capacity; recognising the restriction on your stomach and being unable to eat as much as before. Being satisfied eating much smaller portions. Eating only in response to hunger rather than for any other reason. Making healthier eating choices. Eating more slowly and mindfully. Recognising that this is a whole new way of life.

And when you next eat, you notice the difference...........

10

SESSION 1
WHY DO YOU EAT?
WHY ARE YOU OVERWEIGHT?
BUILDING UP THE PICTURE

The Gastric *mind* Band therapy is not a diet, it's a toolbox for achieving a change in your relationship with food and how you have habitually used it for emotional reasons rather than what it should be for – fuel. G*m*B's a way to understand yourself better and recognise the choices you've been making, how they've shaped your food shopping, your eating and ultimately your body. And it's a way to be able to change those choices starting today. No, not only once you've finished the book, but today, at the end of this chapter! To achieve this, you need to be honest and help build the total picture of why you have a weight problem. Why you eat, when you eat, what you eat and just how often have you been kidding yourself?

—

If hunger isn't the problem in the first place,
then eating will never be the solution.

—

The questions that follow are taken from the questionnaire that was created for our one-to-one therapy at the clinic. Read through them first, maybe more than once, and then go back and answer them. They're designed to help you find out for yourself just what your eating habits and patterns are doing to you and why.

Be honest - you're not cheating anyone but yourself if you don't give truthful answers. Write them down. It's these replies that provide the road map for your personal Gastric *mind* Band journey. Knowing those answers, seeing them written down, will ensure that maybe for the first time you will know more about yourself and what choices, what behaviours, you most need to address.

Keep that information safe. You may think that once you're on the road to a healthier relationship with food you won't want them any more. But there are two very good reasons for filing them away. Firstly so you can go back weekly (daily if you need to) and see if you're making the right changes. Secondly, there'll come a time when you know – you just know – your life has changed. When that happens, in the same way as a 'before' picture is a brilliant incentive to lose weight, a catalogue of your old, bad, eating habits will be something to look at and be pleased you've put behind you. It'll remain as a constant mental 'nudge' never to return to those wrong ways.

You may feel like asking for help from a close friend or family member to ask you the questions; that's ultimately up to you but never forget this is your journey, no-one else's, you do not need to be judged, you need to make your own decisions for your own reasons. To be successful you have to build what may be a painfully honest picture of your weight history and then and only then can you think about addressing change.

Good luck!

This section is structured in such a way as to encourage you to ask some pretty heavy, maybe even awkward, questions about yourself, your past and your beliefs, to prod you and to get you thinking. Be alone, if you wish be quiet and allow yourself the quality time it warrants to explore yourself in detail, and to discover how the years behind you have moulded you into the person and the shape you are today.

It would be beneficial to record your answers in a notebook for you to refer back to as your journey progresses.

It is important to read and think about all the questions in order – they're in a particular order for a reason. You should be open and honest with yourself to gain the most out of this.

Before you start, however uncomfortable it is for you, you need to get on the scales and find out how much you weigh now, and make a note of this. You need to know the starting point of your journey. You should also have an idea of the weight you want to be and make a note of this too. It's also a good idea for you to make a note of your current clothes size and the size that you're aiming to be, but of course you should be realistic. The controversy about size zero celebrities and models is contentious for good reason. Don't hanker after the bad flipside of being overweight. Underweight is as unhealthy as fat.

The medical profession uses a formula called the Body Mass Index (BMI), based on the relationship between a person's height and weight, to work out whether they are of normal weight, overweight, or obese.

To work out your own BMI you need to know your height in metres and your weight in kg and then you can use the formula and conversion charts at the front of the book. (see page viii)

Current BMI
Desired BMI
(Recommended BMI to be of normal weight is 18.5 – 24.9)

So let's find out something about you………

Do you have a date in mind for you to reach your target weight / size? *(remember to make your expectations realistic – ideally you should aim to reduce your weight by between 1 and 2 pounds per week) Grab a calculator and calendar to ascertain a realistic goal date.*

Do you have a particular outfit in your wardrobe that you'd like to be able to wear again? *(The significance of this is that part of the visualisation therapy involves you projecting your mind forward in time to when you are your ideal weight and size. You would then picture yourself wearing these particular clothes, focussing on how good you're feeling about yourself – proud and confident, slim, attractive, fit, healthy and full of energy etc. In psychology it's called "going there first" – athletes regularly use this technique to picture themselves giving their best possible performance)* If you don't have any "slim" clothes, then just think about what sort of outfit you're going to enjoy buying and wearing. How you will look. And more importantly, how you will feel.

Ok it's only two questions but let's stop there, if you have a realistic date in mind, write it on a scrap of paper now. Hopefully have an outfit that you would like to be wearing, so let's say it's six months from now, maybe it's around Christmas, so let's go there right now, try and project yourself forward. When you have finished reading this paragraph, take yourself somewhere quiet, be alone, close your eyes and see yourself, really see yourself. It's 7pm on Christmas Eve, you are going out to dinner with your partner and a few friends, you are at your target weight, what will you look like, how much energy and confidence would you have, what fragrance will you be wearing? How would your partner and friends see you and behave towards you, would your voice be full of achievement and pride - take the time to go there, build the picture in your mind. If you could have that right now, all of it - spend as much time daydreaming about it as you wish – or, of course, you could have a bar of chocolate, or a bag of crisps, which would you choose? It's your choice.

Your Childhood & Background –

Although we may find it hard to believe and accept, many of our mannerisms, traits, habits, etc., were learned and developed during our childhood. Think carefully about your childhood – ask yourself if you had any reason to develop any issues related to food and eating as you were growing up. The questions below may help to bring to the surface any possible problem areas.

The more time you spend thinking about these issues the better. Some people have spent two or three days on this section of the questionnaire alone. Go on, take some advice. Re-read the paragraph which starts 'Ok'. Go on….read it again.

Who brought you up? (parents, grandparents, other…)

When you think back was your childhood happy?

How was your relationship with your family? Did you feel loved/ wanted etc?

Were there any problems at home with parents/ step-family/siblings? /divorce?/splits etc

Were there any rivalries in relationships within the home?

Any problems at school - bullying etc? Did you go to boarding school?

How were mealtimes at school?

Were you healthy as a child? Were you overweight as a child?

How were mealtimes at home? Was it a pleasant, relaxed, family time or were there rows, stress etc?

Were you brought up to clear your plate at every meal and was food ever used as a reward when you were a child? – *For example, did your parents ever say to you if you clear your plate you can leave the table, or if you finish your dinner you can have an ice cream?*

Do/did your parents have a weight problem, or any other members of your close family?

If you have children, are they overweight?

How is your current relationship with your close family?

Do you have any problematic relationships in your life at the moment? If so, how do you see it improving?

Do you have any problems currently with your partner or have you ever experienced any problems with previous partners? (e.g. abuse etc)

Do you or your partner have any children from a previous relationship? If so, are there any problems with step-children on either side?

When you think about the questions above, your upbringing, childhood and time at school, what do you remember? What were mealtimes like, were they fun, or stressful, how about school dinners, did Mum and Dad encourage you to clean your plate, "eat it all up then you can have some pudding?"

What about now, how are meal times? Are they happy family times or rushed and treated as unimportant events?

The answers to these questions may explain how you came to eat for emotion rather than hunger, but realistically now you have to step well away from that history and create your own healthier new history.

Weight History

Take time now to chart your weight ups and downs over the years, going back to the very first time you were aware of your weight being an issue for you. Include details of any diets that you've followed in the past, what worked best for you, what didn't and why. Think about when you were at your lightest and your heaviest and how long you stayed at each weight. Set your notes out along a time line (what it sounds like – draw a straight line on a sheet of paper, birth to current day, noting significant events good and bad, and your weight at the time) Then add in any information you can think of relating to what exactly was going on in your life at that particular time and how you were feeling – ie whether you were happy or unhappy, feeling content or lonely, carefree or stressed out, getting married or splitting up etc. This should help you realise how different events and emotions have influenced your eating habits over the years.

Maybe you should consider taking a break now, take some time, give yourself time for the information to sink in. You may wish to discuss certain aspects of what you've written, or to check that your recollection of your childhood was accurate according to other members of your family. You'd be surprised how often your recollections of events differ from those of others.

So now let's look at your current eating habits.

Do you enjoy eating? If yes, why? It may seem a funny question but it's worth asking yourself is it the taste, the sensation or the chewing, or the fullness feeling that follows?

So often people never really think about the question above, if you really do enjoy eating ask yourself why, think about it, if you're reading this book it's likely that you have an unhealthy relationship with food. Try to ascertain if you eat when you're bored, depressed or lonely, and why you have been led to believe that food can overcome these feelings.

Do you enjoy cooking? Planning the meal, shopping for the ingredients?

How often do you eat out?

Do you tend to eat more when eating out? (Are you aware that it's quite common even for slim people to eat up to 20% more, compared with eating at home?)

Who does the food shopping in your household? Who prepares and cooks the food?

Who is ultimately responsible for your being overweight?

That is a question that very few people ever really think through, consider the accurate answer....

Do you eat regularly?

Do you eat breakfast?

How many meals do you eat per day?

Which is usually your main meal of the day?

Do you tend to eat quickly?

There's an excellent book by Lee Janogly called 'Only fat people skip breakfast'. How true a statement, over 90% of clients that visit the clinic to lose weight don't eat breakfast. When you ask them why, most say it's because they are not hungry, and why would you not be hungry if you ate the correct amount of food the previous day and had just gone without food -in effect fasted - for up to 10 hours. It's a fact that people whose weight is of normal proportions always eat breakfast, they often wake up hungry, and would not consider leaving home without breakfast.

It's strange that the same people who say they really enjoy food and eating, want to shovel it down as fast as possible getting very little pleasure from it.

The majority of our clients confirm they are fast eaters, it seems that the last thing they want is to eat slowly, savouring every mouthful, wanting the experience to last as long as possible. You can slow down your eating by holding your knife and fork in the opposite hands.

Do you ever find when you're eating with a group of people you're the first to finish?

Overweight people tend to be fast eaters. You should be aware that when your stomach sends the signal to your brain that it is full, it can take up to 20 minutes for the brain to receive the signal, so if you eat too quickly you will have already finished your meal before your brain has had a chance to register that you are full, and so you end up feeling uncomfortable because you've eaten too much.

Are you constantly thinking about food/the next meal? Do you feel as if your whole life revolves around food?

Do you tend to finish everything on your plate? Do you finish off other people's food? (e.g. your children)

Do you eat large portions at mealtimes?

Do you ever feel really stuffed after a meal?

So, imagine you're sitting down to your favourite meal. Would you eat your favourite thing on the plate first or save it till last?

It may seem a strange question but it's a fact that people with a healthy relationship with food eat their meals in a different order to people who don't have that healthy relationship with food. The slim person thinks when they see the meal in front of them 'I may not get to the end of this meal and I know that the thing I eat first when I'm hungry I'll enjoy the most so I will eat my favourite thing first. If I'm full before I get to the end and have to leave something on my plate, it really doesn't matter.' The majority of people with an unhealthy relationship with food, of course, will tend to save the best till last. They use it as a magnet to draw themselves to the end of the meal to ensure they hoover up everything on the plate – whether they're uncomfortably full as they approach the end of the meal or not, they'll always carry on until they've eaten their favourite part.

What sort of things do you eat regularly?

Sweets/choc biscuits	Cakes	Crisps/Savoury Snacks
Pasta/Rice	Bread	Fried foods
Cheese	Fruit	Vegetables

When you really think about it is it possible that with just a little more thought you could make healthier choices when buying and cooking food, choices that would take you closer to your goal, to that place, that time that you pictured a little while ago when we asked the first couple of questions? That time when you'll feel fitter, healthier, slimmer, wearing those clothes you've so longed for?

Be honest with yourself: Do you think that you eat healthily overall?

What are your favourite foods?

What foods do you NOT like?

Make a list of what you would eat on a typical day .....*(remember to be completely honest with yourself and include absolutely everything, even the odd snack; include all drinks. Remember every time you finish your kids' tea. Each nibble you grabbed from the fridge as you walked past or prepared a meal for someone else.)*

Do you like to finish off a meal with a dessert? Why? It's an accepted fact than when people in a restaurant order a starter and a main course then the chances of them ordering a dessert because they're hungry are remote. They may give in to peer pressure, or be intimidated by the waiter, but they're seldom hungry.

What's your favourite fruit? *(it would be far more beneficial for you to start reaching for a refreshing, nutritious piece of fruit, rather than a calorie-dense dessert that is probably full of refined sugar)*

If you're going to snack on something, what would you reach for first? *(think about whether you are a sweet or savoury person)*

Do you feel there's any particular food group that's causing your weight problem? And are there any particular foods you would like to cut down on, or cut out altogether?

Have you ever given up anything before? (e.g. sugar/milk/alcohol etc)

Of course if you have given up something in the past then these small changes that you are starting to make will be easy, like a walk in the park.

Real hunger versus desire and craving

Do you know the difference between hunger, a desire and a craving to eat?

If you haven't eaten for a few hours and have an empty sensation in your stomach accompanied by rumbling then this is REAL HUNGER. If you've just finished a big meal and still want to eat more (seconds or a dessert etc) then this is simply a DESIRE to eat food just because it's available – you aren't actually hungry any more. A CRAVING is a strong urge to eat a specific food usually in response to a trigger such as smelling it or seeing someone else eating it etc. If you are reaching for food and it's only between 20 minutes to 3 hours since you last ate something, then this is likely to be just a desire to eat rather than real hunger.

Do you ever eat when you're not hungry?

Think carefully about what your particular triggers are that start you off reaching for food and make a list of all of them – For instance – do you graze in between your meals, constantly picking? Or while you're watching TV? Do you ever eat just to please someone else (e.g. when eating in a restaurant, or as a guest in someone's home maybe because you don't want to "offend" them)? Or do you eat to distract yourself from something else maybe? Are you a comfort eater – do you eat when you're feeling bored or stressed, happy or sad, celebrating or commiserating etc etc?

Are you a secret eater (when everyone else is out of the house)?

Do you prefer to eat on your own?

Do you eat more when you're on your own compared with when you're in the company of other people?

Do you ever get up during the night to eat?

How much of the following do you drink per day?

Tea	Coffee	Water
Coke/fizzy drinks	Sugar-free drinks	Fruit juice

Do you take sugar in your tea/coffee?

What sort of milk do you use?

Full cream   Semi Skimmed   Skimmed   Soya   Other

If you drink tea or coffee with milk or sugar (or even both) grab a calculator and multiply the number you drink each day by 365, then multiply that by the combined calories in your drinks. You will be amazed how they mount up and even more surprised how by just making one small change you can achieve a big result, example, a person who drinks five cups of tea or coffee a day with semi skimmed milk consumes 15 calories x 5 cups per day x 365 days in a year, a staggering total of 27,375 calories a year, of course if they took a spoonful of sugar as well the figure would rise to 54,750, a weight gain or loss of over 15lbs a year!

Next we need to build up a picture and understanding of your current lifestyle.

Do you enjoy your job?

Do you have a lot of stress in your job?

How much and what type of alcohol do you drink per week? (number of units)

Where and when do you drink? (e.g. in the evening with a meal/at the weekend etc)

Are you concerned about the amount of alcohol you consume? (calories/health etc)

How would you feel about reducing your alcohol intake? Would it affect your social life?

Do you take any exercise currently? What sort of exercise do you do?

Average number of hours per week?

Do you have any plans to increase the amount of exercise you do? (Remember that the more you move about the more calories you are burning)

Take another break and read the following story: it might help you with some of the questions coming up.

Regrets, Martin's friend James has a few....

It was on a Sunday morning that the phone rang. I was told that James, a friend of mine for quite a few years, had been taken to hospital in Manchester with a stroke. James was just 41 – it doesn't happen to people that age? Does it?

To be truthful James was overweight. He was 5ft 7in and probably weighed around 18 stone. Apparently he had got up in the night to go to the toilet and he found he'd lost the use of his right arm and leg and collapsed on the floor.

Before the stroke hit, other than being overweight, James was an all round good guy. He ran his own successful business, he had travelled the world and always enjoyed the high life. He liked the best of everything.

That stroke was 15 years ago; the use of his right arm and leg never returned to any degree where he could manage to look after himself at home – let alone return to business.

Mentally it left him with a few problems as well; his memory would just fade away, then return. After a few years struggling to live with his mother he was eventually allocated accommodation in a sheltered housing unit where he still lives, alone. His once executive car has been replaced with a wine red mobility scooter; ironic really – his tipple had been red wine.

Recently he told me he so wished someone, anyone, had warned him of the risks he had been facing. He said "If only I could turn back the clock, allowing me to change, put things right, lose weight, cut down the drinking, take some exercise, anything to get my life back. Of course it'll never happen......"

Recently we had someone in the clinic who'd had a heart attack; luckily they made a full recovery. They said the same thing as James – "if only someone had told me a year, month, week or day before, I would have done anything not to live with this fear of it happening again. If only."

He said that despite his consultant telling him that subject to him adopting a few lifestyle changes he could live a full and normal life, he still lived as if he was a disabled person. Every time he woke in the night having fallen asleep on his arm he woke his wife to phone for an ambulance as he thought the numb arm was a symptom of a stroke. Whenever he got indigestion or started sweating for no apparent reason he called an ambulance expecting the worst. He was only 46, and he and his wife had not been abroad on holiday since. In fact he said he preferred to stay close to home – it seemed safer. Of course any physical manoeuvres in the bedroom were now confined to the couple's memories.

Why tell these two sad but true stories – well virtually every day we see someone at the clinic because they're overweight but haven't had either a stroke or heart attack.. Neither have they got Type 2 diabetes or colon cancer. Up to that point they'd been lucky. Luckily until now, they'd got away scot free. When I listen to them and watch the sadness in their eyes as they tell their stories about the effect their excess weight has had on their lives, I often tell them James' story and the other client's tale too. I explain that if they take on board the therapy, work with us and shed the excess weight we can give them their very own 'Get Out of Jail Free' card or winning lottery ticket. The therapy will give him or her the ability to freeze time, make those changes and new choices in life. There is no reason nor any need for them to go crashing through the glass wall; no more than there is for you.

Ok, you've had a break, read the two cautionary tales.... On with the questions.

What are <u>your</u> main reasons for wanting to get slim? What concerns you most?

Really take your time to answer this question because you will be using these reasons as part of a powerful motivational technique:

Once you've written down the things that are so important to you, you should regard it as a sort of contract with yourself – this is what you want to achieve and why – it's much more effective when you put something in writing, rather than just thinking about it and then pushing it to the back of your mind again. You can then keep copies of this document somewhere handy, so you can whip it out and instantly refresh your memory about exactly where you are aiming to get to, whenever you're in a situation where you are feeling tempted to eat something that you don't need. Use your reasons to decipher what is more important to you – the short-term instant gratification of eating, or the long-term benefits of getting slim.

Feelings about being overweight

Has being overweight affected your self-confidence?

Do you feel that it has any effect on your relationship?

If yes – how?

Do you enjoy being overweight?

Can you think of any benefit in maintaining your current weight? (e.g. maybe your weight has been a protective shield from any unwanted attention)

At the clinic we find most people when relaxed are happy to talk in detail to us about the innermost feelings they have regarding their weight, the often-negative effect it has had on their confidence, and the part it plays in their relationship with their partner or other family members.

Making the Commitment

Whilst some of the questions below may seem strange, you should spend a considerable amount of time thinking them through and considering how the answer to one question affects your thoughts on the next.

Are you concerned about your health and the implications of your weight not only on yourself but your family and loved ones?

Are you happy with your life?

Do you consider you have a lot of stress in your life?

What makes you really happy and conversely what makes you sad?

If you could change one thing in your life, right here, right now, other than your weight, what would it be? This question is probably one of the most important of all. You cannot spend too much time thinking about and analysing the answer you're going to give.

How long do you want to live?

Why?

Are you afraid of dying?

Who is important to you?

Who are you important to?

Are you committed to losing weight?

What is stopping you?

It is well documented that the use of fear in therapy seldom helps achieve permanent change, however if you were at the clinic being asked these questions we would ensure that you were aware of the risks of diabetes, stroke and certain cancers that go hand in hand with obesity. Maybe James' story will serve as that particular wake-up call. (Go back and read it again if you're in doubt)

When you sit down and talk about the risks, the pain, the desperation many people go through regarding their weight, and you ask them 'is the burger or whatever really worth that?' Can they really think it's that good?' Losing weight is not rocket science, it is not in itself expensive, it comes in all honesty with very little real pain, its benefits can last a lifetime, and virtually everyone can achieve it.

Are you prepared to accept the consequences of your actions?

The final question maybe sums it all up, are you prepared to accept the consequences of your actions in life? If you are, and you are ready to make a few - some only temporary - changes, then really there is no reason why your journey should not start right here, right, now.

—

Learn to hold yourself accountable, for all your actions.

—

Face to face, in the clinic, we would expect it to take around four hours to catalogue someone's history, to harvest all the information we would need. Because you're reading the questions from the book it means you're not talking to someone, hearing their responses, getting their feedback, having the question reflected back in a different way, etc. However as you complete this on your own, it's important to be thorough and completely honest, thinking right back to your childhood where appropriate because, as we said earlier, many issues, bad habits and the seeds of distorted thinking often stem from that time in all our lives.

Once it's all thought about and you've written down your answers, take some time and reconsider. Change as many of your statements as you wish and as often as you wish. Make sure you've been straight. It's not only your own life that will be affected. How could the issues the questions ask you have affected your eating habits? Your behaviour around food?

Once you've decided your answers are accurate, you're in a position to move on. Now is the time to start to look ahead. There's no more looking over your shoulder at the past. Now's the time to draw the line in the sand.

Here and now, at this very moment, you're at a crossroads in your life. You've obviously had enough of being overweight, feeling frumpy, unhealthy, struggling to climb stairs, fed up with your limited choice of clothes. Feeling embarrassed in front of your husband/wife/children's friends. Feeling depressed at the very sight of a mirror.

You've got to the decision point. It's crunch time.

You don't need reminding you did this to yourself, but you're open to suggestions as to how to change. You've probably now admitted there's something wrong that dieting hasn't sorted out. You're almost certainly at the end of your tether, and are beginning to see that this delving down is the only way to bring many forgotten issues to the surface. That's why honesty was so important. If you've been saying you live on salads but are actually a burger and fries junkie, it won't help you one bit because you'll end up completely off track.

If you were looking at yourself through someone else's eyes – how much excess weight are you carrying? What would you advise? What would you do? What would you think of that person? What would you say if it were your brother, sister, or your best friend? If you're upset by these thoughts, that's not unusual. But you need to see yourself as others see you, get to that place – because in these four sessions what we're trying to do is get you to the right place for you (not us) to bring about change.

We don't want to be judgemental – you've probably spent enough time judging yourself and putting yourself down, you don't need any more of that. You need to decide you've got to the end of all the negativity, and begin feeling better about yourself and putting a positive twist on things.

—

'Right, that's it. I'm sick of it. I want something different now.
It's crunch time. I'm not playing the victim a day longer'.

—

So you're at the fork in the road of your life. It's up to you. Will you decide to keep heading down that same old road? It's the easiest thing in the world to do, you wouldn't need to make any effort at all. Because it's such a well-trodden route it's the path of least resistance.

Imagine this as your FORK IN THE ROAD

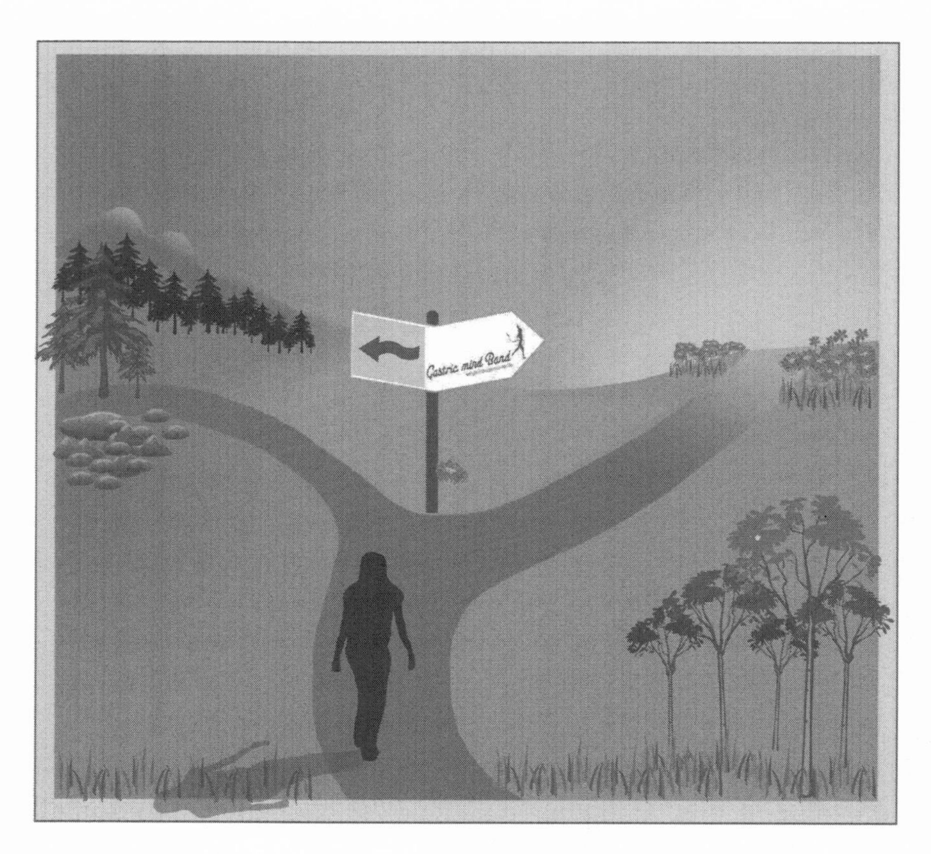

Stand at that fork in the road and just stop and think. Think what you'd feel like a year from now if nothing changes. You carry on doing exactly what you're doing. You'll have had another year of being overweight, feeling bad about yourself, comfort eating, looking older, feeling terrible, getting out of breath. If nothing changes in your life just how fat will you be next year? Don't be under the illusion you'll be the same as you are now because you won't. It'll be worse. It always is. Maybe much worse.

But to feel like that for another year is not why you're reading this. Take yourself back to the fork in the road and have a look at how it's going to feel different if you take the other road. Make a little bit of effort. Make a few changes. So a year ahead on this road, you can see all the positive things – you're lighter than you were a year ago, you're fitter, you look in the mirror and you look a lot younger, you have so much energy, your clothes fit you, you're feeling good about yourself, if you've got a partner they're looking at you admiringly, everything's great in your family, your relationship, everything's so much better and there are loads of positive things to focus on.

If you think calmly and deeply enough about the two options – another year the way you are at the moment, versus the positive, vibrant new year after making a few changes – you might find yourself getting quite upset at the thought of how things have been and how they could be.

Maybe you're doubting you can make the change? And what are the costs? Well financially they're probably close to zero. Physically it won't resemble having hot pins poked in your eye. You know it won't hurt. It may feel strange for a little while because you're changing those old habits. But eventually it will become the norm.

In fact, with regard to change, we all go through it in much the same way - there's actually an academic theory called the Stages of Change Model, which says that everyone makes changes in their life in essentially the same pattern, but taking vastly different times to do so. It's not unusual, in fact quite normal, to start doubting you even need to change!

The pattern of behaviour change is:

1. **Pre-Contemplation** - at this stage a person has not yet acknowledged that a problem exists or that there's a problem that needs addressing.

2. **Contemplation** – now the person recognises there's a problem but is often not yet clear as to whether they want to/know how to make a change;

3. **Preparation/Determination** – the person is preparing to make a change.

4. **Action/Willpower** – at this point change in behaviour is being introduced/practised

5. **Maintenance** – keeping up the new behaviours which are the focus of the change.

6. **Relapse** – in which you return to your old behaviours, bringing about a sense of failure, but which it is possible to use as a learning tool, just as we are trying to teach you to do - understanding why you went wrong and how not to 'fail' again as you continue your change.

—

Don't fear failure. Learn from it. See it as an education.
Martin Shirran

—

All of this will sound quite familiar to many overweight people who have shed excess weight in the past. Often you get through one or two parts of the sequence, only to slip and go back into an earlier stage, and get swept into a cycle. Everyone's cycle goes at a different rate, maybe going through different stages in varying amounts of times, and as we've just said, overweight people trying to lose weight will be only too familiar with what they see as a vicious circle rather than something they have to go through before they'll achieve what they want.

Some people consider there is a final part of the pattern, Transcendence, in which you are 'past' the change process and making that lifelong commitment to permanent change. We are confident that with the Gastric *mind* Band therapy this is exactly what you will achieve.

So. You're ready. You're prepared to make that little bit of effort, make those changes, because even a few months along the line you'll know it's so worth it. You'll feel fitter, healthier; you'll have a whole different mental attitude towards food which will make your life a lot easier. From this moment on you can now start to make positive and permanent changes.

And for some of you, the changes will be at least as much about your health as about your dress size. About avoiding diabetes, heart attack and stroke as much as about how you feel in your swimwear on the beach. Some of the health issues associated with obesity include colon, stomach, kidney and breast cancer, osteoarthritis, high blood pressure, gallstones, infertility and depression. Younger people tend not to prioritise these concerns, and think more about their appearance. Once you're a parent of teenagers, though, your thoughts run to 'can I keep up with them when they play football on the beach?' Will I live long enough to see them married/have my grandchildren?' 'Will I be healthy enough to enjoy my retirement (if I get there)?' and all the other associated health fears of mid-life.

The top ten reasons clients visit us at the clinic:

1. The unbelievable fear of discovering that the aircraft seat belt is not large enough to go around your stomach, and having to ask the stewardess for an extension, followed by the worst nightmare of all - her using the call button to attract the attention of a steward at the back of the plane and calling down the aircraft for an extension seat belt please for the lady in seat 6A.
2. The total utter embarrassment and shame of being pleaded to by your daughter or son not to walk them to school anymore because the other children in the playground, poke fun at them because of your size.
3. Chafing legs, being utterly fed up with having sore thighs caused by them rubbing together when you walk.
4. Having just returned from yet another horrid family holiday where you were uncomfortable on the beach having spent the whole time forced to wear a wrap around your waist to cover up the rolls of fat.
5. Wanting to go to a restaurant and not be aware that everyone else is watching what you order and what you eat.
6. Sick of being totally fed up not being able to bend over to cut your own toenails.
7. Noticing that on the plane the empty (or half empty) seat next to you was the only one not taken, this was after the stewardess had asked you when you boarded if you were pregnant, you were not of course, but it would have been an excuse.
8. Realising that your bathroom scales no longer go up to your weight.
9. To be able to have a bath – that is, to fit in it - and be able to get out afterwards without thinking you may have to ask for assistance.
10. To just once be in the wonderful position where you can go to a so-called 'normal persons' clothes shop, rather than have to buy your clothes from the XXL catalogue

When I think of people reading this book, I think of people I've seen sitting in front of me at the clinic, all in exactly the same place in their life. Yes they may be morbidly obese, yes they may have some illusion that being slim will make them feel more attractive and save their marriage.

But in reality what I actually see is someone who's just 29 years old but could be about to have a stroke, resulting in them not be able to go to the toilet on their own any more because they can't clean themselves.

I see the downsides. If you think about having Type 2 diabetes and maybe losing the sight in one eye, maybe both, or losing a limb....if you think about them long and hard, I want to ask the people: 'Do you really still want that pork pie?'

That's the fork in the road you're at right here right now. The pork pie and all the downsides of obesity, the heart disease, colon cancer – or to be slim and healthy next Christmas?

Check it out for yourself. Google it. I'm not creating an unrealistic scenario, they're very very real. The connection between Type 2 diabetes and obesity is off the scale. Similar to the connection between smoking and lung cancer – but the diabetes hasn't had quite the same level of publicity. If you carry on eating like you have been, getting fatter and fatter, you may find yourself getting closer to Type 2 diabetes, which many now say is developing into a disease of choice.

Martin Shirran

So you're ready to make the change. You've answered those questions, you've been honest about what issues you bring with you to where you are now. You should have a clearer idea how you got to be overweight in the first place.
The more times you revisit the questions, and your answers, the better.

People – we, you, just about everyone – have 'stuff' – emotional baggage. Sometimes it takes a while just to peel away the layers of the onion – stuff like 'I eat because my husband won't talk to me'.

With some people it really stands out that it's obviously an issue from childhood that their weight problem stems from – maybe they were always told to clear their plate whether they were hungry or not. Maybe food was scarce because of lack of money, was of poor quality and had to be eaten up. Maybe there are more deep seated psychological issues. With others it can be a build up of various things that have happened in their life but there's usually a trigger. It's rare for there to be nothing. With some people it's just a change of lifestyle. Going from working fulltime, running around after people; bringing up children, being active, fit and on the go and then suddenly retiring and doing nothing and not actually reducing the amount of food they're consuming. They're not fit and active any more, the children are grown up and left home, and there's a complete change of lifestyle. Could be they've moved and they're exposed to a different lifestyle or have more time on their hands.

Sometimes ladies have been fine all their life until the menopause then they start to have problems. You can actually build up insulin resistance so your body finds it difficult to process refined carbohydrates so because they don't get processed properly your body just absorbs all the calories from them and it just turns to fat. It's bordering on diabetes which means you have to be very careful about the intake of refined carbs.

Very often people who are overweight eat quickly. Not always but the majority do. Some 90% of overweight people who come through our clinic doors admit to eating too fast. When you eat quickly you can consume more food than if you eat slowly because by the time your brain gets the message that you're full it's too late because you've stuffed everything into your mouth already. So even something simple like slowing down and eating mindfully rather than just shovelling everything in mindlessly and not paying attention to what you're eating, which is a simple change, can have a big effect. A lot of this is about every small change developing into a large cumulative effect. You don't have to make huge changes in everything.

Do you eat too quickly? Try staying in the moment, smell the food, enjoy the taste, the texture, the smell, the appearance.

Another downside about eating too quickly is that to get the most from food you love it should stay in your mouth, where your taste receptors are, as long as possible. You won't get the most from it if it's already down your throat and on the way to your stomach.

To help people learn to eat slower we always recommend they start by swapping cutlery hands for a week. Just when you get the hang of it, switch to chopsticks – even if you're eating beans on toast! The following week revert to your old way – you'll find you are already eating more slowly. The fact you've had to keep sweeping up the mess from eating in an unfamiliar way will have taken up some 'non-eating' time too – plus will burn some extra calories!

Small changes often lead to big results. A male client who came to the clinic told us of his three cup a day coffee habit – complete with two teaspoons of sugar for every cup. We worked out that without doing anything else at all other than dropping sugar or using sweetener, he would create an annual calorie deficit of 37,000 calories. That means he would lose over 11 lb a year just by cutting out the sugar.

The same thing applies with using vinegar to dress your salad rather than lashings of olive oil – once again a small change adds up to many thousands of calories a year – and that's possibly many pounds in weight from a simple substitution. Another client wasn't overeating that much but liked to have a couple of vodka and cokes when she got home from work. We showed her how it contributed 148,000 extra calories to her intake every year, and that just by cutting them out that would give her a weight loss of over 40lb over 12 months with no other changes. Just cutting out those drinks. Guaranteed. Did she need us to tell her that? Small change, very big result.

—

Be honest: Do you eat mindfully or mindlessly?

—

Do you think about the colour or texture of your food? Or where it's come from or what processes it's gone through? Does this mean you're eating mindfully or mindlessly? Do you analyse the tastes and textures of the food in your mouth as you're chewing it? Do you think the way you eat, whether mindfully or mindlessly, might make a difference? Your taste buds are in your mouth, not your stomach so the longer the food stays in your mouth the more pleasure you obtain from it.

The enzymes in your saliva start to break food down before you've even swallowed it so chewing it as much as possible actually helps the whole digestive process. Not only will you be tasting the food better but you're helping your body do its work the most efficiently it can.

If people eat too quickly, they'll maybe take a mouthful of chicken, whatever, chew it twice, gulp it down – it's gone but often they'll end up with problems like indigestion/wind, because so much air is being gulped down at the same time. This means the body has to work that much harder to process and digest the food. Why make your body work harder than it needs to? If you really taste it and chew slowly, eating mindfully and concentrating on the flavour and texture of what you're eating, not only will you make things easier for your digestive system, you'll also find you appreciate your food more.

Gradually you'll realise that healthy food, if chewed thoroughly and totally tasted and enjoyed in the mouth, actually tastes a whole lot better than unhealthy foods. If you take a bite of a big sticky bun and eat it slowly, so it spends a lot of time in your mouth, you'll start noticing all the fat coating your tongue and sticking to the roof of your mouth, and the amount of refined sugar you can taste. You'll realise there's little if any texture. It may take a while, but your tastes will gradually change to switch away from the more tasteless 'junk', 'beige' foods.

On the theme of colour, it's quite widely believed that one of the easier ways to ensure you have a healthy diet is to eat as many different coloured foods in any meal as you possibly can (not counting multi-coloured cereals or sweets of course!) ... and writer Michael Pollan has highlighted the theory that it's not wise to eat any cereal that colours the milk – sensible advice if you stop and think about it.

A classic, mentioned earlier, is clearing your plate. Even if you're absolutely stuffed. As a child you were brainwashed 'think of all the starving children in Africa' and that actually stays with you until adulthood. Do you eat regular, proper meals, or just graze continually?

Big people seem almost frightened of feeling hunger. They'll just pick at bits and pieces all day long because hunger feels like a life or death situation. 'It's not good to feel hungry' so I'll just keep on eating..... so they never get empty, never get hunger pangs, so they get completely out of touch with their body's natural signals. If somebody is eating and it's not a response to hunger, that's an emotional issue, eating for head hunger rather than stomach hunger.

Feeling hungry is perfectly natural. It's simply your body's way of letting you know that it's time for you to eat something.

—

Don't fear hunger, try tolerating it!

—

Once you start to understand the notion of real hunger you'll also realise there are different 'grades'. If you fancy an apple, is that hunger or are you making excuses? Well yes it's hunger, but it's obviously not full-blown 'I need a meal' hunger. If you eat a piece of fruit, that should really be enough to tide you over for another couple of hours or whatever, until you need a meal.

Sometimes people like to have fruit - maybe several pieces - during the day. Is that fulfilling hunger for a little while or eating too often? We believe there's no harm at all in having a piece of fruit or a yoghurt or something, but ONLY if you're feeling hungry; be careful with fruit! It is delivered to your mouth complete with its own natural sugars.

Some people can go longer than others without eating. Don't just eat for the sake of it. Eat it if you're feeling a bit peckish. If people are cutting down massively on their portion sizes compared to what they're used to eating, they might find after two, three, four hours, they might need a little something but not everyone does. Some people will just have their meals and not need anything in between at all.

A little known fact: you CAN eat too much fruit! When you eat other sugars, insulin is released which means the brain knows when we've had enough to eat. High insulin levels quell appetite. Fruit contains fructose, though, which doesn't stimulate insulin or leptin – the hormone that makes you feel full; so theoretically you could eat excessive quantities of fruit without ever feeling satisfied.

If you allow yourself to get totally ravenous, then you're more likely to eat too fast and be tempted to overeat. It's better to have a piece of fruit or something small every so often because every time you eat your metabolism kicks in. You shouldn't go for more than about three or four hours without a little something. Your body starts shutting down, going into starvation mode – inhibiting calorie burn, slowing metabolic rate.

You need to work through the issues of when and why you eat. Is it when you're bored, stressed, sitting watching TV, picking at food between meals, it during the day, in the evenings, on your own, when you're sitting around aimlessly because nothing's going on? Is nothing going on because you haven't chosen to do something, make something happen?

What would you think if a friend of yours was drinking a bottle of cough mixture every day to overcome sore feet caused by wearing tight shoes? Strange? Weird even? Cough mixture for sore feet... wacky, eh?

If another friend who's overweight tells you they eat a family size bar of chocolate before bed every night to take away their loneliness – strange? Wackier still, maybe?

Another friend tells you they're taking laxatives on a daily basis to ease their toothache? Strange indeed.

Taking cough mixture for aching feet does of course seem an unusual and unbelievable remedy, but is it really any odder, or less believable, than a person who eats cheese sandwiches in the evening because they are lonely? Sadness, being lonely, feeling anxious are just emotions. Signals to change something in your life. They are never an instruction to eat two rounds of cheese sandwiches.

People with an unhealthy relationship with food seldom eat excessively because they are hungry; it is amazing how many eat because they are feeling depressed, lonely or tired – having a distorted view that such feelings, emotions can somehow, as if by magic, be overcome by food.

Say you've had a row with your best friend. What do you do... go and have a bar of chocolate, that'll make you feel better. How do you feel after you've had the chocolate? Still upset with your friend. Even more upset with yourself for eating the chocolate. You just need to work through those issues and say in that situation what would have been more helpful? Did the chocolate actually help you? No it didn't because you were feeling upset before you had the chocolate. You ate the chocolate. Then after the chocolate's finished you feel bad about yourself because you've had the chocolate that you didn't need, and you still need to cry your eyeballs out because you've just fallen out with your best friend.

All you needed to do in the first place was have a good cry, pick the phone up again and apologise to your friend and sort it out with her and forget the chocolate. Why did you need the chocolate? Where did that come in? How was that a logical thing to do? It's important to know that no food will ever overcome an emotion.

If you'd used our Pause Button (described in more detail in Chapter 11) when you felt like picking up the chocolate bar, you would have given yourself time to see how much more angry, upset and depressed you'd feel after eating it and given yourself the time to opt out of unwrapping it – way before you got close to biting into it.

—

Food doesn't solve anything other than satisfying your body when it's hungry:
Eating doesn't overcome emotions.

—

Hopefully by now you'll have been laughing at yourself, seeing all the places where you've been going wrong – the chocolate (or whatever you reached for) only comforts you temporarily, for the few minutes or seconds it takes you to eat it. You do get a feel good factor, but that doesn't balance out the whole guilt feeling afterward, the beating yourself up about it because you didn't need it anyway and now you've stuffed up your diet and you're going to put weight on and you're feeling bad about yourself so you're going to eat even more, so you're getting into that whole negative cycle....

Maybe your problem is dealing with 'bored' moments. There's always something you could do instead of eating. What do you enjoy doing? Reading? Working on the computer? You could pick up a book or walk around the block, or email some friends or something, find out about a new hobby, there are plenty of things to occupy your time rather than looking for food for that emotional crutch. Food doesn't solve anything other than satisfying your body when it's hungry.

If you enjoy a meal with friends, food is really only the catalyst for spending time with people you like; something to do while you chat, laugh, joke, and so on. Food isn't what makes the meal, despite what so many cookery writers and food programmes might have you believe. Sure sometimes food should be memorable – historic even, as Michael Winner would say. But it's the company that really makes the event special. In great company you could take an hour eating one plate of salad and have a better time than eating a heavy three-course meal with boring people and experiencing that guilt trip later.

There's a pattern which in CBT terms is called Low Frustration Tolerance. Whether it's drugs, alcohol, food, gambling, you say the person has LFT to that particular issue. They get a craving to have a cigarette, or go to the betting shop, or have a doughnut, and as soon as they have that thought they respond to it immediately because they see it as a command which has to be obeyed. They can't work their way through this craving, it's their LFT to that particular thing. They may have high tolerance to all other things in their life. For an overweight person it may be that they've never smoked, say they'd never touch cigarettes because they're dangerous and horrible. But food cravings are what they have LFT to. If you see a food advert, even if you've just had dinner, would you maybe get up and go and have something to eat?

It's really just that one person can handle a particular frustration better than another. Marion would not give in to a doner kebab at lunchtime where Martin would have ('not any more!')

As with all these psychological issues relating to food, there are techniques to help you overcome them. With LFT the first thing is to recognise what it is – for you it may be that you are eating salad but give in to having some bread which you didn't really need, you just automatically picked it up. It may be that you automatically took a toffee offered to you – you didn't think, you were just happy to have that toffee. Try to see all your decisions as treading a path – the less you use that path the more overgrown it will become. Equally the more you use the alternative path, the one of not 'giving in' to your LFT, the more that path will open up like a motorway until the old one is clogged with weeds and the new way develops into a superhighway.

Stress and boredom both come up often with a lot of people. A slim person when they're stressed can't eat whereas a stressed overweight person will eat constantly. And if a stressed overweight person eats, it's because for whatever psychological reason, they're thinking that the food is going to help them feel better. Once you develop a habit like this, it becomes so strongly ingrained in your mind that it comes naturally and you'll do it automatically without even thinking about it. Eating too much is a habit. But habits can be broken!

The easiest thing in the world is to keep on doing what you've been doing. That's like doing it on automatic pilot. To actually make the changes, create new habits, requires a bit of effort, which in turn requires motivation. But once you've done something, made new choices, thought different ways, a few times, it gets easier and easier.

If you are resistant you can make things hard to learn, but you can teach yourself if you want to. It's down to motivation again. If you've always driven on the left and you suddenly have to drive on the right, you can do it, even if you doubt yourself and your ability to unlearn your existing way – but.you have to concentrate for the first few times, maybe a long time. After a while it becomes second nature, and having to drive on the left again would be a struggle – but you could do that too, it just takes the concentration and motivation.

If you drink alcohol, it may play a far greater part than you realise with regard to your weight problem even if you don't drink very much, because it's easy to overlook the number of calories you're consuming. On top of that, the body can't store alcohol at all so has to process it, even before processing food. So if you're having food and alcohol it'll metabolise the alcohol first, get all the calories straight from that and if you're eating as well, and your body's reached its calorie requirement for the day, the food won't get processed properly and it will be stored as fat.

Alcohol increases your appetite, so once you start drinking you are also likely to eat more food. All of which isn't a problem if it is under control; also, if you're at your normal weight you can afford to consume more calories than someone who's overweight because if you're trying to lose weight you have to create a deficit. Someone at normal weight is just eating to maintain their weight as it is. There is one additional problem with alcohol and that is the belief that it reduces a person's metabolic rate for up to 24 hours after consumption – a frightening thought!

You need to identify your top five reasons for wanting to change your eating behaviour. Just review them.... the following list of suggestions may help but if they're not for you, come up with your own.

Reasons for changing my eating behaviour	
I'll look better	I'll be able to keep up with my kids
Other people will find me more attractive	I'll feel more comfortable and self-confident during sex

I'll do more things in public, such as swimming or dancing etc	I'll reduce my risk of developing Type 2 diabetes
I'll be able to shop in 'normal' clothes shops	I won't be so hard on myself
I'll be physically fitter	My self-esteem will be boosted
I'll enjoy trying on clothes	I won't be so introverted
I'll feel better in a swimming costume	I'll stand up for myself more
I'll have less hang-ups about my appearance	I won't feel so out of control
I'll be healthier	My life expectancy will go up
My energy levels will increase	I'll feel more comfortable eating in company
I'll no longer be embarrassed to take exercise – and when I do it won't be uncomfortable	I'll reduce my risk of developing coronary heart disease
I'll like myself more	I'll be able to wear a smaller size
My family won't comment about my weight or what I'm eating	Mirrors won't frighten me any more
I'll be able to buy some fancy new underwear	I'll reduce my risk of developing colon cancer
I'll be more willing to find a new job or make other life changes	I'll have more confidence

So what have you identified is most important to you? Your health? To wear a bikini next summer? To change your shape before the next 'big' birthday? Just to feel better about yourself? Everyone's reasons will be different, or in a different order, but what matters are yours and yours alone, and those reasons will be your motivation.

Write them down on an index card and keep them in your handbag or wallet. Then if you're tempted by a bar of chocolate, or you're about to sit down to a meal, whip the card out and remind yourself. Maybe even read the card at the start of each new day.

It'll remind you 'This is what's important to me right now. I want to be able to do this because......'

Writing them down makes an amazing difference. It's like making a commitment, almost a 'legally binding document with yourself'. People find it helpful. It really works. Sign it at the bottom if you like and just keep it handy to keep reinforcing all these positive things. So if you've got a cream cake in one hand and the reasons not to eat it in the other...use the Pause Button, as discussed in detail later in the book, and give yourself time to think of your reasons. ....What's more important, is it this quick sugar fix which will last five minutes max, then you'll feel bad about yourself for the rest of the day because you don't actually need this, or is it the long term benefits of shedding your excess weight – you can weigh it up in your mind.

Each time you are about to take a mouthful of food, the question is 'is this going to help me achieve what I want, or hinder me?' If you're hungry, it's going to help. Go ahead and eat. But if you're not, and it's going to hinder your progress, why on earth would you be doing it?

If you're reaching for something to eat, stop and think. Will this piece of cheese, this packet of crisps, this doughnut, help me slim down to 10 stone; will it help me move closer or further away from my goal? Which do I want more? If I want the food more, go ahead. But if the most important thing in my life, my decision, is to slim down, why am I making it harder for myself by still eating the wrong things that aren't going to help me achieve that?

Non-one is actually holding you down and forcing all that extra food in your mouth. Everything is your choice, ultimately your decision – you can either choose to keep on eating too much or you can choose to be slimmer and healthier. Realistically you can't have both, so make your choice.

—

Think of the process not as losing weight, but gaining a better life

—

Some diets actually promote the idea that feeling hungry is a negative thing, and even go as far as saying 'if you follow this diet you'll never feel hungry'. We don't like that idea. Hunger isn't something to be afraid of; you just need to understand it's a natural part of life. As we'll say again, the 80s character Gordon Gekko wasn't right. Greed's not good. We say it's definitely not good. Hunger's good! Learn to live with and accept hunger and you'll learn to live more comfortably with food.

—

You can't live without food, so it's vital you learn to live with it

—

What we're striving to do is help you create your own formula for changing your eating habits and your relationship with food. Diets tend to mentally mess you up and make you more obsessed about food than you were before. It's only if you deal with the underlying issues you've identified from the questions that you'll be able to make a permanent change.

You have to get out of the dieting mentality. If you're going out with friends it's essential that you have the tools to behave differently when you're making food and drink choices. You have to have a normal life, normal social engagements, without the 'I'm on a diet I can't do anything' way of thinking, without the rest of your life just put on hold.

'A diet isn't something you do for life, it's some kind of purgatory you go through for a certain number weeks and at the end you heave a big sigh of relief and think 'thank god for that' ....And then go back to the eating habits that got you there in the first place.'

Marion Shirran

From now on you should be asking yourself a question, stopping yourself every time you're about to eat: am I eating this because I'm actually hungry? Is it because I'm bored, sad, lonely, stressed because I've had a row with my boss at work? If not, put it down! Question – what's going on in my head, why am I eating this? Why? Question everything during the first few days and weeks until you get into the new pattern/routine. Again, these will be moments to use our 'Pause Button' idea.........

Living like a slim person lives, which is what you'll find yourself starting to do, is actually a much more relaxed lifestyle because the thing about food is you obviously can't say you're never going to eat again like you could with smoking. So you're faced with these choices every day, several times a day, for life. You've got to develop a good relationship with food. A lot of big people have this complete love hate relationship with food because every time they eat something they feel guilty because they know they shouldn't have and it was the wrong thing and the wrong time and they've got completely out of sync with the whole concept of enjoying eating.

There's nothing wrong with enjoying your food. It's quite a big part of our lives. You've got to face food and eat several times a day so why on earth would you make it a tortuous procedure when you could make it something that's really enjoyable? You could be enjoying eating things that make you feel fit and healthy rather than sluggish.

I eat to live, to serve, and also, if it so happens, to enjoy, but I do not eat for the sake of enjoyment
Mahatma Gandhi

—

This is the perfect opportunity for you to end your struggle with food and replace that "love/hate" relationship with a much more relaxed one. You will discover how eating really can be an enjoyable experience.

—

Of course, the quicker you eat, the less you'll actually taste your food and conversely, the longer the food stays in your mouth the more you'll appreciate the taste of it and maybe reduce your desire for it. That's actually how people's tastes can change. Those cakes and biscuits they used to eat, once they begin to notice the texture and flavour in their mouth there's a good chance they'll decide 'actually it doesn't taste that nice at all, I'd rather have an apple!' People do have these light bulb moments when they just change in an instant, because with typical comfort food they haven't been eating it for the flavour they've been eating it for the effect – soothing ice cream, chocolate, melt in your mouth.... It's nothing more than a quick sugar fix. It's no coincidence that comfort food is almost like baby food, stodgy mushy stuff... They think they're eating for the flavour, but it's more often than not just the sugar hit.

Having identified your problems with food, and identified your main reasons for wanting to change your eating habits and lose weight, pluck up the courage to find a 'before' photo – keep it in your wallet or purse. Maybe have one made as a fridge magnet. Attach a copy to the start of the questions, maybe. Then a few months, maybe not that many weeks, down the line, you can get another picture taken, make sure it's in the same clothes so you can see the difference as your weight changes - and see the benefits before your eyes, as they happen.

They're brilliant for motivation. If you can go one step further and stick it on the fridge, nothing is better. When you get to target weight the one thing that'll stop you piling the pounds back on is being able to say 'that was me on the beach, all those rolls of fat.'

It helps to get a picture of people's ups and downs, how long they've stayed at a particular weight, then put some on, lost it again .... Sometimes people avoid the scales because they know their weight is going up and they don't want the reality, they bury their heads in the sand. Then they find they've put on more than they think. When you're in control and you weigh yourself regularly (say monthly) you'd never allow that to happen.

When you start to shed the excess weight, don't make the mistake of expecting to expect <u>too</u> much <u>too</u> soon... you may well lose weight easily and quickly from the very start, many people do. But it will help if you don't set an unrealistic target and an unrealistic deadline. It might have taken you years to become this overweight; you can't expect to lose it in a couple of weeks.

If you've got a lot of weight to lose, your initial target may still be within the overweight range but what matters is that for you it'll be the lightest you've been for a long time (or ever). Once you're there you can re-assess if you want to keep going or you're happy at that weight. For somebody who's never been slim, it can be difficult to actually imagine being within the normal parameters of the BMI.

All these elements are compelling on their own, and when you put it together the mix could be seen as a proverbial 'kick up the backside'.....do you know your BMI? Is it outside the normal range? Well let's be clear. Telling you in no uncertain terms that you should reduce your BMI is not so much a kick up the bum as much as letting you know you're at high risk for Type 2 diabetes, coronary heart disease and also high risk for colon cancer to name but a few.

Please focus on whether you want a burger along with diabetes or you'd rather have a piece of grilled fish and be slim by Christmas. It's your choice, of course. The questionable pleasure of the burger will last 5 minutes or so, the associated diabetes could be with you for life, what's your decision.

One should eat to live, not live to eat.
Molière (maybe he was quoting Cicero ...)

* **Measurements** We always suggest you measure your problem spots, maybe hips waist bust, tops of arms and legs, every couple of weeks – it's up to you which bits you measure, probably best to be where you're looking forward to seeing the numbers go down! Because of the different density of muscle and fat, you may not see your weight dropping because you're building muscle if you've starting getting more exercise. Knowing your body is changing even if your weight's plateaued out is a valuable lesson, which can stop you getting disillusioned, keep you on track. Measurements can be as important as scales!

According to a 1951 survey, a woman's average waist size was 70cm (27.5in). By 2004 it was 86cm (34in)

Another of the ways to determine obesity is using the waist-hip ratio. Divide your waist measurement (inches) by your hip measurement (inches). The ideal, a figure of around 0.7 for women and 0.9 for men, is a strong indicator of general health.

Marion has been slim all her life. Because of her professional training and years spent in conversation with overweight people, hearing their thought processes, fears and doubts, she understands only too well how the whole process of weight loss can become obsessive.

'I weigh myself, yes.... You can tell by your clothes if you're altering at all. My weight never alters by more than five or six pounds at most, just that much up or down and that's about it. 'When you're trying to lose weight, I'd say weigh yourself no more than once a week. People who've been on diets become absolutely obsessed with the scales, weigh themselves every time they go to the loo, take all their clothes off .... It can get obsessive. For me to try and get inside their heads I've experimented and weighed myself several times a day and your weight does fluctuate by a huge amount. From morning to evening I can put on 3lb; it's water and food, etc. It's not that you've put weight on, it's what's inside you. But people get so worked up about that with the whole dieting mentality. They'll see their weight creeping up during the day and that makes them spiral out of control and think they're failing!

You should do it at the same time of day, the same situation each week then you get the right accurate picture. I'd say I weigh myself every few weeks – though a bit more often at the moment just to try to get inside people's heads to see what they're going through.'

Summary:

- **Learn to live comfortably with food; you have to face it more than once a day**
- **Hunger is not a dirty word**
- **Don't expect too much too soon**
- **Eat mindfully & slowly, & really taste your food**
- **Food solves nothing except hunger**
- **Don't fear failure, learn from it**
- **Take responsibility for all your actions**

SESSION ONE
SELF HYPNOSIS

In the Gastric *mind*Band sessions undertaken at the clinic, obviously hypnosis is a key part of reinforcing the suggestions and images mentioned during the therapy conversations with clients. The best results will be achieved at one of our clinics with a therapist, but as a reader - **if** you have the motivation for change - you can achieve similar results, experiencing that all-important boost to the subconscious through self-hypnosis.

This is done by relaxing yourself deeply and thinking yourself through an exercise in which you visualise and reinforce the positive elements of change you're trying to make. There are quite a few 'Positive Thoughts', specifically targeted and listed for each of the hypnosis sessions.

Please note that self-hypnosis should never be practiced when driving, operating machinery or carrying out any other activity that requires your full attention

Hypnotism is an altered state of consciousness characterised by a feeling of extraordinary relaxation and "letting go", with a heightened awareness and focus and increased suggestibility. As experienced from the inside, you are conscious, but detached as though you are observing what is happening to you rather than being in charge of it. It's as though you've temporarily got out of the driver's seat of your body and mind and are taking a turn as a passenger.

When in this state, your body and mind are very open to suggestions. The state of mind required for hypnosis is a perfectly normal, natural state of mind (the alpha state) that everyone is in every day of their lives. When we are engrossed in a novel, a television programme, or a daydream, to such an extent that our awareness is fixed on the specific subject of our attention, we are in this state of mind. This relaxed, highly focused state of mind generates the brainwave state known as alpha. When you fall asleep at night, alpha is the state of mind you are in right before you fall asleep. And once you fall asleep, your alpha state deepens before you drift down into the theta brainwave state—the state of mind where light sleep and dreams occur. Alpha is also the state of mind most associated with hypnosis.

You can learn to hypnotise yourself and provide suggestions to yourself. Your self-induced hypnotic state will not be as deep as is possible when you are hypnotised by someone else, but this is necessary because you need to remain in control enough so you can continue to make suggestions to yourself. Self-hypnosis methods can be used to reduce feelings of anxiety, and promote feelings of confidence and self-control. You are going to use it to reinforce a belief in your ability to change your eating patterns for life.

Read your Positive Thoughts and make sure you feel completely focussed on what you are trying to achieve before you set about relaxing, so you don't have to 'wake up' to refer to notes or remind yourself what you meant to concentrate on. It's the subconscious you want to target, and that is best addressed when deeply relaxed.

Choose up to 3 suggestions that are relevant and appropriate and read and revise them. You need to be able to repeat them silently to yourself at least 3 times when you're deeply relaxed. They are your messages to your subconscious to change your behaviour for life, starting now.

If there are more than 3 appropriate suggestions, then you can alternate and choose a different set each time you do this session.

You may decide you'd prefer to have all the key elements in your subconscious armoury, and allow yourself as many sessions as necessary to target all of them. Keep to the same pattern of choosing three suggestions, relaxing yourself then repeating them mentally at least three times each.

Set aside a time each day and a private, quiet, relaxing area to sit or lie down. Make sure you will not be disturbed, and that all phones are turned off. If you like incense, its scent can help create a specific atmosphere which will become recognisable to your subconscious each time you practise your self hypnosis. Soft music can be playing, use the same track each time. (The use of candles is not advised.)

Lying flat on a bed or couch with arms slightly away from your side is a good starting point. If you choose to place a pillow under your head, it's better to use a fairly flat pillow so your head and neck aren't strained at all. Make sure not to cross your feet. If you choose a comfy chair to sit in, place your hands flat on your lap or, if your chair has comfortable arms, place your arms on the arms of the chair. Keep your spine straight and, again, don't cross your legs or feet.

You now need to 'talk' yourself into a state of deep relaxation.

Pick a spot (real or imaginary) on the wall or ceiling in front of you so you have to raise your eyes slightly in order to fix your gaze on it. Keep staring at the spot and mentally repeat to yourself at least three times "As I count from 5 down to 1, my eyelids are feeling heavier and heavier and when I get to 1 my eyes will close and I will completely relax."

Then slowly, mentally count down from 5 to 1, taking a deep breath in between each number. As you reach the number 1, close your eyes and allow yourself to let go and relax.

Now starting either with the tips of your toes, or the top of your head, focus your attention on each part of your body in turn, and gradually release all the stress and tension and relax every muscle one by one, while mentally repeating to yourself, "Relax", "Let go", "Deeper and deeper relaxed".

Then imagine a beautiful staircase with 10 steps leading down to a special place where you will feel totally safe, comfortable and relaxed. (It can be anywhere you want it to be, whether it's a country garden, a tropical, deserted beach, or just your own bedroom).

Now count down from 10 to 1 and when you get to 1 picture yourself in your special, private, safe place. Spend a few moments allowing yourself to experience all the sensations, familiarising yourself with any sights, sounds, smells, feelings and tastes. The more senses you bring in to the visualisation, the stronger the experience will be.

Now see yourself standing at a fork in the road of your own life, deciding which path you're going to choose. The left fork is a slippery slope downhill – the low, easy road – the path of least resistance – which is the same old road you've been going down for many years. The right fork goes slightly uphill – this is the high road, which will take a little bit of effort to follow, because it means making some changes, but also brings many positive benefits.

During the next few minutes you're going to take yourself on a mental journey – firstly head down the left fork and project your mind forward a year........

(choose at least three suggestions per hypnosis session from each segment)

1. Remind yourself how bad you feel being out of control, overeating and being overweight
2. Visualise the rubbish littering the slippery slope, snack food and sweet wrappers..... and all the emotional pain that they are causing
3. Catch sight of your reflection in a mirror, looking much older and even bigger
4. Recognise that if you take this road you'll be unhappy, your loved ones will be disappointed, your health will be suffering
5. Feel the weight not only around your body but of the disappointment of letting yourself down, of feeling terrible, of feeling a failure
6. Now bring yourself back to the present day

Then

7 Take a look at the road on the right and realise it is the road to success, the path to freedom, self-confidence, good health and a longer life.

8 The road will lead you to a place where you´ll feel better than you have your whole life, in control, not governed by your food choices.

9 See yourself in a year's time after choosing to head up this road, feeling fantastic, fit, healthy, energetic, proud, confident and successful.

10 Spot yourself in a mirror and notice how you look so much younger, you're wearing new clothes, getting admiring glances from your partner / proud looks from your family.

11 Recognise that this is a permanent change – a new way of life

Then

12 Realise you're actually still at the fork in the road, but absolutely sure beyond any doubt whatever that you're ready to make the change.

13 The long-term rewards of being slim and healthy far outweigh the instant gratification you used to get from eating the wrong foods for the wrong reasons.

14 From now on you will always check to see if you are hungry before you put anything to eat in your mouth.

15 You will never again use boredom or stress as a reason to eat.

16 You will become free to be happier and healthier for the rest of your life.....

travelling the high road of success

Now..... Count yourself up from 1-5 suggesting that you have enjoyed a wonderful relaxation and on 5 you will open your eyes, feeling refreshed and energised.

If you decide to do your self-hypnosis before going to sleep, you can suggest that on 5 you will move into a normal and natural sleep... until it is time for you to wake.

11

NICKY's STORY

> *"This hasn't slotted into my life – it is my life. I'm thinking like a thin person"*

Nicky, a statuesque 6ft tall, is single, 43 years old and at her heaviest weighed 23 stone, needing size 26 clothes.

We asked her to describe her weight problems: "I've always struggled with my weight", she starts. "At junior school I remember being taken to the nurse and put on diet tablets to 'help me'. I lost a couple of stones when I was about 16 but did not maintain the loss, and probably remained around 17 or 18 stone for the remainder of my teens/early 20s.

"Each Christmas I would gain 10lbs and never lose it again. I was relatively successful with Weight Watchers in 1999/2000. I got down to 18 stone from probably around 20 stone at that time. I maintained that for about a year then regained it with another three stone on top.

She finds it harder to be precise about how her weight has affected her because it's been wide ranging. "It's very hard to hide when you're 6ft tall, and 20 - 23 stone," she explains. "It has affected my life in many ways, not letting people get close to me, not doing 'girlie holidays' as I never wanted to share a room with thin friends - but I can't say it totally stopped me doing what I wanted.

"So I wouldn't sit in on a Friday night just because I was fat, but equally I was glad to get home without having been insulted while I was out. I always used to go out and wonder if I would be able to sit in a chair and travelling on aeroplanes was my worst nightmare. I would often book two seats just so that no one sat next to me and I'd have more room.

"Relationship-wise, I have always picked the wrong man - now that can happen if you are eight stone and stunning, but generally I think I always just used to be grateful that anyone would go out with me. Now that's gone but when I was much younger it did play a part."

Over the years, she's tried many ways to lose weight. "Previously I had sent off for weight loss tablets via the internet, and my old GP later prescribed some for me, but even though I had them I wouldn't take them if I was eating fatty foods as I knew what would happen (not pleasant). So I bypassed these. I've also had depression, my weight being part of the problem, and have had medication for that. All these added up, that's why I started to look for some solutions to my problem. I've done Weight Watchers, Rosemary Conley, Slimming World, and other local clubs too."

Then she came upon Marion and Martin's Gastric *mind* Band. "I was Googling the cost of a gastric band operation, and found the Gastric *mind* Band site by chance," says Nicky. "Realistically I'd only half considered the surgical gastric band. The cost and the risks involved would probably have meant I would have continued considering it, but not seen it through to the operating table."

She sees the Gastric *mind* Band as her last resort. "Yes, it is," she confirms. "Because although it's much less than a surgical gastric band, it's still quite a lot of money to pay out.

As for whether it works? "So far yes" she says. "When I started I was about 23st 1lb, and today I'm 20st 7lb. The weight loss has been steady, I only put on weight one week and lost that and more the following week. In the past, gaining weight would have signalled the return of eating anything and everything. This time it has not."

She reserves judgement about the *mind* Band element.... "At the end of the day you believe what you want to believe," she says. "It may be that if I had just had four sessions of CBT and hypnotherapy that I would have achieved the same result as the time was right for me to do this. However, thinking about the band does make you reflect more and think twice.

Martin's straight talking worked for Nicky. "Yes, he was straight with me... for example, my food weakness was cheese - so he broke down in graphic detail how cheese was made and all the fat involved, and I think since that session I have had 3 lots of cheese in 4½months. Prior to that I was eating probably 500g of cheese a week or more."

"He came up with different ways of thinking.... for instance, I said that I enjoyed vodka and tonic and he said to try drinking vodka neat and you won't like it. I did and I don't. So why have the vodka - why not just have the tonic. That kind of thinking."

She feels the process has changed her. "It's started to make me more confident" she goes on. "People around me always assumed that I am happy and buzzy because that's what they expect a fat person to be, when really I am quite shy. So now the process has changed me because I don't pretend any more. If I am fed up for a day then that's it - no big deal, but I don't feel I have to be happy all of the time.

"Eating-wise? I drink 2 litres of water a day, I don't pick at chocolates or biscuits in between meals, rarely drink cola (something I also used to do)."

So how did the Gastric *mind* Band help you achieve your weight loss? "I started losing the first week," she says," and lost all over Christmas period also and have continued to lose. It's been pretty consistent. On the weeks where I have lost say 4 or 5 oz instead of 2lb, then I can normally think – 'oh yes friends were over' or 'I went for a meal' and I can generally replay where I had more than in other weeks.

"I enjoy my glass(es) of wine each day and if I stopped that then I think the weight would come off much more quickly, but at the moment I don't feel ready to do that and am happy with the progress I am making. I've just moved house too, and there's going to be a gym on site in the complex and I will be able to go down on the treadmill early in the morning so again I think this will speed up the loss."

She says she hasn't actually tried to override the *mind* Band. "If I go out to a restaurant I will have say a portion of chips or fried rice but I have them, don't eat all of them and the balance is maintained." It's also proving easier for her to maintain a balance and not 'panic' if she eats a bit more sometimes. "So far I haven't found myself falling off the rails really, but on the odd time when I have had more than normal, it just seems automatic now not to have as much for the following 2-3 days to get back into a routine.

"What I could find a struggle, if that is the right word, is if I am not planning my meals, or if I am caught out - say being out when I had planned to be in. I like to know generally what is around the corner without too many surprises."

Asked to describe how her eating habits have changed, she says her patterns before would have been relatively healthy but with large portion sizes. I'd get fed up at not losing any weight and thinking I was eating healthily and then head to the chip shop or Chinese take away. Then another 'healthy week' would follow and that was pretty much the cycle.

"I did work in an office where there were always cakes/biscuits etc around so that didn't help. Now I am home based so don't have those kind of temptations in front of me each day. I also eat breakfast now on a regular basis and before I never used to bother."

She admits to having been a snacker. "I always used to pick food at night - crackers, cheese, peanuts etc. Now I don't do that. If I fancy something then I will have a thin slice of Serrano ham and be happy with that. But most of the time I don't."

She's got clear memories of the 'operation' under hypnosis........I did feel as though I had gone down for an operation and the tightening effect when I woke up, but I can't say that I was feeling my body for any evidence, no!

"I felt the tightening of the operation, but I didn't wake up thinking 'where've they put it?'. But when you're in that relaxed state you do feel a clenching sensation almost as if someone's pulling at you. The smells, and the senses, made it feel as if I were going down for an operation for sure. However I didn't feel sore or anything. I did feel a restriction on eating, and still do."

"I think it's mostly in my mind. All the other sessions lead up to the fitting of the band, and the operation is just the icing on the cake to seal the ideas in."

The various ways we approach people's bad food habits obviously hit home in many ways with Nicky. She tells her story like this:

"A lot of people have been slim at some point in their life but that never happened with me. I was 7lb as a baby but after that I've never been slim. I've done all the clubs, all the systems, everything except faddy diets. I didn't go down that road, but pretty much everything else. I had tablets off the internet, tablets off the doctor, but I managed to get around that because I simply didn't use them when I knew I felt like eating bad things that were going to make me have diarrhoea if I'd had the tablets – I just didn't have the tablets. It was an easy way to bypass it. I guess none of these things worked because I wasn't in the right headspace...

"Maybe it's just that now the time was right. In a way this was the last resort, because although I looked into having a Gastric Band I don't think I would have actually had the operation; mostly for fear of the surgery when it's not strictly a lifesaving operation.

"It was the beginning of November when I went to Martin and Marion, and I was due to go to a few parties etc. – anyway I made the appointment thinking I might be wasting my money starting before Christmas. On the other hand at least if I started I wouldn't be doing myself any more damage – and that's what I decided. Which is what I did.

—

I lost weight all through Christmas and New Year, which is unheard of for me!

—

"So I went away for Christmas, went to my parties. Despite the festivities, in the house, food wasn't an issue at all. There wasn't the volume of crisps, nuts, sweets, etc., like in the past. We had a Christmas cake which I'd already bought before I went to the clinic, and it lasted right through till February. I just had a little bit when I felt like it. I didn't think 'oh there's the Christmas cake, I'll have a slab today'. Which is how I thought before.

"It's completely changed my thinking. Changed my portion sizes – totally. Before I would have just put rice in a saucepan, not measured it, and it would come out and fill the plate. Now I have a quarter of a cup – half a cup for me and my Mum and it's absolutely plenty. I think back to the volumes I was putting in – it's not just eating less it's cooking less in the first place.

"When I worked in an office I'd never have breakfast before I went out, thinking I'd grab something on the way, so it'd be a Starbucks and a muffin ….. it was just every day the same pattern, or a sandwich from the canteen, sweets and things on the trolley….

"Now I don't even think to buy the stuff. I get up at 8, have a coffee and some cereal and start some work, maybe get engrossed, look at my watch and think 'no I'll work on for a bit', then an hour and a half's passed and about 1.45 I'm really ready for some lunch so I make myself a sandwich. Before I'd have had two bread rolls, now I'd have one. With salad on the side, not the crisps I'd have before. The crisps I do buy are baked rather than regular ones. Things like that – slight changes - where I used to have a big bag of Kettle Chips all to myself, because I used to love them. Well I **still** love them - I just don't think about getting them. I go down the supermarket aisles and just don't go to pick them up at all.

"With cheese, which is my favourite food, what I tend to do is maybe if I'm out have a jacket potato with cheese on, or I'll have some chips because I don't ever have them at home. But I don't eat them all, that's another difference.

"I think what I've noticed now is that I'm not thinking about it. With other systems you're constantly thinking you've got to fall within points, or it's a red or green day and as soon as you've gone one morsel over you think 'Give Up' because you've blown it; you've already failed.

"This time I haven't wanted to binge, really I haven't. I enjoy my wine. If I gave that up the weight would drop off. I'm cutting down on it, but I didn't want to deny myself everything. But I haven't binged. Yes I've been out and had a three course meal and thought afterwards oh I wish I hadn't had that pudding because I didn't need it.... but the next time I've gone out I didn't have the pudding because it wasn't necessary, or maybe not have a starter because I fancied a particular pudding. So I think it just seems to be a natural thing and not forced at all.

"Before, as a habit at night I would eat crisps every evening, whether I was hungry or not. At 9 o'clock I would get a bag of crisps out of the cupboard. If I do that now it's because I think I really fancy that bag of crisps **tonight** whereas before it would be an automatic thing. I'm not stopping myself having things. I don't feel deprived. Now I eat more fruit, and drink **so** much more water.

Now I've come so far I don't want to go back. I can't say it restricts me because I've been out and had meals, had profiteroles., but I'm not bringing them home and eating them at home as well. I can't remember the last time I bought peanuts. Pistachio nuts are better, they're more difficult to eat. Sunflower seeds too!

And it's having wider effects than just on weight loss. "This has made such a difference to me," says Nicky. "My joints don't ache as much because there's less weight on them. I don't feel as tired each day, I do much much more than I did before – because I just can. I used to get indigestion a lot and now I don't at all.

"It's natural, it all flows, all gels together. Whereas before I wouldn't do something because I'd have been tired, or hot, or just couldn't, now I <u>can</u> be bothered and I <u>want</u> to be bothered.

Nicky explains her view of the difference with the Gastric *mind* Band: "Other methods – diets - are forced, you're having to follow to the letter or feel a failure. With this it's not a diet, it just becomes a natural part of your life.

"Whereas before it was a failure, you've broken the rules. You know you're not going to lose weight that week. You haven't followed their guidance. There's no point. But with this you haven't broken any rules because there aren't any rules to break.

—

It feels as though this is how slim people probably are

—

"When I stayed in a hotel I had the full English breakfast, I thought 'bring it on'! And it was absolutely delicious. But it's not something I would do every day. And certainly not something that I'd get home and continue to do. It was nice for a change because I fancied it two of the four mornings I was there. But the other two I had toast and cereal and that was fine too. So one breakfast doesn't make a failure – you enjoy it and take it for what it is. But having said that I didn't have a big lunch, I just had some fruit as we were walking around town.

"I was a bit fed up because my friends hadn't noticed I'd lost any weight – and I'd lost two stone! ….. before, that would have been a trigger to feel 'what's the point' – but it was just a day, and I came back and was fine. Got back to what is now normal. Before I would have come back laden with cheese, and sabotage what good I'd done… Yet now I don't want to stop, I don't think there's anything to stop. That's where it's different. I've just changed.

"I always thought because I cooked fresh food I was cooking healthily – I cooked fresh, and healthy (or so I believed). But I was cooking for an army, enough chicken for the whole street…. And you still eat it. But you cooked it healthily so that's fine!

"Being so tall I really struggle to get trousers – the shop I want to get trousers from only go up to a size 20 so my aim was that….. for me that would be a big thing. Maybe I'll stop then, maybe I'll think that's what I wanted to do, maybe I'll just carry on and see how it goes. I like my clothes, I'm not a huge follower of fashion but I'd like to be able to go into Next and pick up a size 18 or 20 and know it would fit me. Whereas now I can just about get into a 22. There's still work to be done but it's going in the right direction because my biggest was a 26 – I've dropped two dress sizes.

"Now I'm thinking soon I'll be able to go into that particular clothes shop and buy something whereas before it would have been I'll go to Tescos and get fresh cooked jam doughnuts which they're just sprinkling with sugar….. If I wanted a Tesco doughnut now yes I'd have one, but one not six. There's nothing I feel I'll never buy again. If I fancied anything I'd have it but it would just be a one day blip. The M & S Food Hall wouldn't present me with the same issues as it used to because…. It's almost like checking in with yourself. You've come this far, It's not worth it. You busy yourself with something else and the moment's gone.

"I can't say anything bad about G*m*B. I've been losing about 2lb a week, which is absolutely fine. One of my big targets was to be a size 18 for my birthday, so that within a year of starting I'll be a completely different size and shape. It's nice. It's exciting. It's a completely different way of thinking. I don't look back, if I've had that bag of crisps or meal out I've enjoyed it – it's not a disaster.

"With portion sizes, the change was quite instant too. I weighed things out for a couple of weeks then after that I judged it by eye, then once a month I'll weigh it back out again and see if I'm creeping back up - but I haven't been. Previously my portions had been so out of reality!

Nicky had so much to tell us about her Gastric *mind* Band experience that rounding up her tale seemed harder than losing the weight!

"Having a little jar of fat, looking at 100 calories*, that played a big part for me....it's just horrible. It's not a hard decision to make. I don't think there are any downsides. No surgery. No pain. It's changing my life and my lifestyle. I got overweight because I ate too much of the wrong things and didn't exercise enough. I've done all the diets and clubs and now I don't feel I'm following anybody's rules apart from mine. But along the way my rules have changed in the things I want to buy. By default the way I'm thinking about food is making me lose the weight which is making me more confident so it flows through. I'd sum it up as effortlessly good. (*See Chapter 15)

—

I don't feel I'm following anybody's rules apart from mine......
It's working and long may it continue!

—

Summary:

- **G*m*B can change your thinking**
- **The little jar of fat is horrible**
- **If you busy yourself with something else, the moment to choose food disappears**
- **There aren't any rules to break**
- **Enjoying food isn't a disaster**

12

SESSION 2: UNDERSTANDING WHAT YOUR BODY NEEDS

What your body needs, long term, is an energy balance. Energy **in** equals energy **out**. Simple. If you consume the same amount of calories that your body requires to keep you alive and carry out whatever activities you do, you'll maintain an even weight.

If you consume fewer calories than your body requires to keep you alive and sustain whatever physical activity you do, you will lose weight. If you consume more calories than your body needs, you will gain weight. With barely any exceptions, almost always involving some medical complication, that's the way it is. Eat more than your body needs, get fat. Eat less than your body needs, lose weight. Easy peasy.

You've been consuming more than you need, maybe a lot more, maybe for a long time. Now, to lose that weight and learn to maintain an even weight, you need to start by consuming fewer calories than you need. Get the long term energy balance right and your weight, and your sense of well-being, will change for the better.

Total energy usage is determined by four components.

Basal metabolic rate, BMR, or the more frequently used resting metabolic rate, **RMR** which represents the number of calories needed to sustain the basic functions of your body at rest. (ie keeping organs functioning and regulating your body temperature. Nothing else.)

Thermic effect of food (TEF) which represents the calories expended in processing the food that you eat.

Thermic effect of activity (TEA) which refers to any and all calories burned above and beyond BMR/RMR. Chores, just sitting up in a chair, and exercise all contribute to TEA.

Finally, there are all the variables, changes due to factors such as fever, increased or decreased food intake, greater muscle mass because maintaining muscle uses more energy than maintaining fat, hormonal changes, fidgeting, etc. However none of these individually or added together, makes any major difference to the overall picture.

In the clinic, we use two independent high-tech instruments to measure clients' resting metabolic rate. Our reasoning for this is that we struggle to understand how anybody can seriously expect to be able to control their weight if they don't know how many calories they're burning. If you feel you'd benefit from knowing yours, the tests are available relatively cheaply now. At the Elite Clinics in Spain, we charge €55 to do the tests. However it is possible to do a basic calculation to give you a rough idea what your RMR is.

Generally, RMR can be estimated by multiplying your body weight in pounds by 10.5. So someone weighing 150 lbs has a RMR of around 1575 calories/day.

It really does help to have this figure in mind, because if you're working on allowing yourself around 1710 calories a day but your body actually only needs 1575, that's 135 calories each and every day that over time you'll be storing as excess weight without ever understanding why. In fact you would put on a stone during the course of the year – and say you didn't know how!

A small miscalculation could add up to a massive – seriously huge – weight gain. Let's look at an example. You eat half a Snickers bar a day on top of what your body needs. Not the whole one, that would be greedy. So half a Snickers a day. Of course it could be a couple of apples, a small sandwich, but those 135 extra calories you put in your mouth. Every day. How much weight do you imagine you'd put on at the end of a year? A few pounds? No. A stone. Fourteen pounds. So start that when you're 20 and by the time you're 40 you could have piled on 20 stone just by having a snack.

Scientists are currently exploring any possible connection between genetics and metabolic rates; there is some research on mice to suggest there may be a link, but until it's located and proved in humans and anyone develops a way of altering the body's genetic coding to boost what is currently only hereditary low metabolism, we have to work on the knowledge currently available.

CALORIES

With the Gastric *mind* Band, no-one expects you to count calories day in, day out, for the rest of your life. There's better stuff to do! However it's useful to have calorie values firmly in the back of your mind as a reference point, so for example you know just how disastrous it might be to choose a profiterole over a fruit sorbet every time you have a dessert. How having a frequent double burger and fries could set you back when compared to grilled fish and salad.

So without getting hung up about it, let's start by looking at how many calories you must have been consuming to get to the weight you are now.

If somebody has a sweet tooth, and loves chocolate, they probably don't even realise, don't even give it a thought, that a little chocolate bar, not a family sized one, can be 255 calories. They'd think nothing of eating something like that, maybe more than once a day. It might only amount to a minute of mindless nibbling. Do that every other day and, just like the apples, if it's on top of what your body needs you'll be looking at an extra stone on the scales in a year's time.

You could have a nice piece of grilled fish and some vegetables or something for about the same amount of calories, and that's an actual meal – whereas a chocolate bar is just a snack. Nobody would think of calling that a meal. It's not rocket science.... Yet it's amazing, people don't seem to understand. They look at the calorie content of healthy foods, things you'd have as a meal. But not all the snacks, cakes, biscuits, etc., because 'that doesn't count, it's just a snack and doesn't matter'... so they've no idea how many calories are in say one digestive biscuit – and deceive themselves. Maybe eat a whole packet over the course of a day, maybe even as much as 1900 calories, but convince themselves that they haven't eaten much today. Yet they might have actually eaten a whole extra day's worth of calories!

People with an unhealthy attitude to food tend to believe completely illogical concepts. CBT calls these 'sabotaging thoughts'... Believing these sabotaging thoughts that are not helpful at all such as whatever you eat if you're standing up, eating on the hoof, maybe like when you're out shopping, doesn't count. Doesn't matter. Because it's not actually a meal. People actually believe these things, they've trained themselves to believe these illogical thoughts.

We had one of our clients return to the clinic for what we call an adjustment session; she told us she was not impressed with her rate of weight loss, she was averaging less than a pound a week, occasionally she would go a couple of weeks and lose no weight at all.

I asked her to take me through a typical day, and then to recall the previous evening, She said "OK let's take last night as an example, my husband and I went to a lovely fish restaurant, we had a really nice, low calorie healthy evening. I passed on the starters, and just had a main course. I ordered grilled fish served with salad, I knew that would be around 275 calories, I had it once before and worked it out. We ordered a bottle of white wine, I had about a glass and a half, my husband had the rest, the whole meal was well within my calorie limits, and that scenario is not unusual, but still I am not losing weight at any acceptable level"

She was of course correct, grilled fish with salad and a glass of white wine should be fine. A while later her husband arrived to pick her up, he asked me how things were going and I told him that I was at a loss as to why his wife was not losing weight based on what she had told me about last night's visit to the restaurant. He asked me to go over what his wife had told me she had eaten, and then he told me a different story about the previous evening. And even though her story was different I am sure his wife was not lying; it is just maybe selective recall!

He told me that firstly before going to the restaurant they had visited a bar around the corner for a pre dinner drink, "oh yes she said I forgot about that" he said that along with a large glass of wine she had quite a few dips into the bowl of peanuts. When they arrived at the restaurant they were offered complimentary tapas while they were looking at the menu. He said he noticed that she put both oil and vinegar on her salad, which she conveniently remembered at that point. Apparently when the bill came they were, as is the custom, served with complimentary liqueurs, they both had an Amaretto on ice.

When we calculated the calorie value of the little 'extras' they added up to be close to 900 calories, three times as much as the low calorie grilled fish meal……

It's only when somebody points these things out that people say 'oh I've been really stupid haven't I'… but it takes someone to point it out. They might go along merrily saying I haven't eaten anything all day. Well yes, actually I've had a bar of chocolate, a McDonalds, chips, a milkshake when I was out shopping…maybe munched some sweets I found in my pocket….. but they don't count it as a meal because they are walking around while they're eating it! It would take a long while to burn off all those calories, as we'll show in the charts that follow. You could make up a whole fruit salad for less than that bar of chocolate. It's such a simple thing, but you really have to question everything you're eating, and question your choices

A calorie isn't always just a calorie. Many people don't realise that a calorie varies according to what sort of food you're eating. Overweight people often don't seem to realise. Your body can't process everything and absorb all the calories from the healthy foods that contain plenty of nutrients, vitamins and minerals and fibre, because fibre passes straight through. Take a carrot, for example - say worth 13 calories – not all those 13 calories will be absorbed by the body because some of it, the fibre, will pass straight through taking with it the calories it contains; some research suggests it takes fat with it as well.

Whereas when we eat highly processed foods containing white flour, white sugar and so on, the more refined the food is, the fewer nutrients and less fibre it has, so your body just absorbs all the calories but gains very little nutritional benefit in the process. So just by shifting the balance towards healthier foods you'll not only be consuming fewer calories, but will also feel satisfied for much longer.

If you eat highly refined foods full of empty calories you will not feel satisfied for very long, and as a result you are more likely to overeat.

—

When you think about reaching your goal weight, about how much energy and confidence you will have, the clothes you will wear and the self-respect you will gain, just how important is it to you? Do you really want it enough? Face up to the fact that until now it has not been as appealing or important to you as the pork pie, so what's got to change? What's going to motivate you this time? You need to find out.

—

It is useful to have an idea of roughly how many calories you are consuming in different foods and drinks. Without this knowledge – and you don't need to be an expert, just have a good idea – you could end up continuing to delude yourself you're eating healthily!

Calories provide us with energy. We obtain a set number of calories from each gram of carbohydrate, protein, fat and alcohol we consume.

One Gram of:	**Number of calories:**
Carbohydrates	4
Protein	4
Fat	9
Alcohol	7

Never forget 3,500 calories = a pound of fat

To give you an idea of what the calorie values of some common foods are, we've compiled a list. It's a fairly random selection of fruits, vegetables and other foods – you can easily obtain full calorie counter lists if you choose to. But this will give you a general idea of what to avoid and what to eat more of! *(and don't forget to check the labels of shop-bought foods – sugars & fats are often very high on the list of ingredients)*

FOOD	CAL	PER
Cucumber, raw	10	4oz
Carrot, raw/steamed	13	1
Tomato, raw	18	4oz
Raw cabbage	25	1 cup
Asparagus, steamed	27	1 cup, 5oz
Beetroot, raw/boiled	36	4oz
Pineapple	48	4oz
Orange	59	1 average
Grapes	60	4oz
Apple, Granny Smith	62	1 average
Pear	65	1 average
Apricots, dried	100	6 fruit
Banana	112	1 average
Cheddar cheese	115	1oz
Hazelnuts	175	approx 1oz
Potato crisps, cheese & onion	184	40g
Brazil nuts	193	1oz
Walnuts	194	1oz
Mars Bar (Standard Size)	280	1
Coconut, fresh/raw	285	3oz
McDonalds quarter pounder with cheese	515	
Well done 8oz fillet steak & chips	550	

WHAT'S YOUR POISON?

Did you know that a large glass of wine (250ml) contains the same number of calories as four fried fish fingers?

Alcohol is a multi faceted problem for people who are in the process of reducing their weight.

1. Alcohol can't be stored in the body like carbs, protein and fat, so your body will metabolise any alcohol first, before it starts on whatever food you consume. As alcohol is high in calories, your body will quickly reach the number of calories it needs for energy from the alcohol and then whatever food you eat at the same time will amount to excess calories and so will be stored as fat.

2. Alcohol is believed to **increase** your appetite.

3. Alcohol lowers your resolve so you are more likely to reach for something to eat that you really don't need.

4. Drinking alcohol slows down your metabolism for up to 24 hours.

Take a look at what you might be quaffing this evening: (and bear in mind home measures tend to be significantly larger than standard ones)....

DRINK	CAL	PER QUANTITY
Vodka/gin/rum/whisky	55	25ml
Sherry	68	50ml
Champagne	76	100ml
Orange juice with bits	90	200ml
Dry white wine	230	250ml

Red wine	235	250ml
Coke, Coca-Cola	142	330ml can
Lager	230	1 pint

OK, so now you're getting an idea just how many calories you could be taking in – in all probability it's more, maybe a lot more, than your body needs. If you actually work it out, maintaining your present weight could mean you're eating 2,800 calories a day, or even more – quite a shock? But it doesn't stop there. Maybe in the past few months your weight has actually been increasing. So the calories you must have been consuming would be worryingly high.

Well of course you don't want to maintain this weight, you want to decrease it, so you need to be consuming far less – 500 calories a day less than you need for healthy maintenance in order to lose weight at 1lb a week. Remembering that a pound of fat equals 3,500 calories........

So what to do about it?

There are many ways to look at how to deal with the calories you eat, obviously starting with eating fewer than you have been! Two of the most interesting are to see how long it takes to burn off a certain amount of calories doing different activities, or to see how long it would take to 'pay for' a particular food you like! Here are some examples:

ACTIVITY	CAL USED PER HOUR (average)
Yoga	176
Golf	288
Swimming	297
Aquaerobics	373

Mowing the lawn	390
Hill walking	417
Cross trainer	441
Skating	448
Digging	476
Boxing	571
Cycling (@15mph)	616
Skipping	636

FOOD	CAL	ACTIVITY	MEN	WOMEN
Red wine (175ml)	119	Digging	15mins	18mins
Coke, Coca-Cola (330ml Can)	139	Rowing machine	30mins	35mins
Cheese & Onion Crisps, Walkers	184	Frisbee	30mins	35mins
Tomato Soup Heinz (400g Can)	228	Basketball	45mins	50mins
Pot Noodle, Chicken & Mushroom	384	Tennis	60mins	70mins
Chocolate Chip Muffin, Morrisons	476	Mountain Climbing	48mins	58mins
All Day Breakfast	715	Walking @ 4mph	120mins	145mins

PAYING IN ADVANCE

Of course, there's another way of helping yourself with this energy balance and food choices – increase your activity levels.

Say this Sunday afternoon you feel really good about yourself because you've just gone for a walk so you've had some exercise, you've got the whole feelgood factor in your brain, there are tons of endorphins released, so you think – great I've worked off 300 calories doing that two hour walk, so now here's the burger.... You've worked it off, you've earned it, you deserve it, you've 'paid for it' in advance, you can eat this burger and at the end of the day you'll still be within your calorie intake. You haven't done any damage. You'll be right on track, no problem... you won't have put any weight on, you won't have lost any either but you'll be just level and balanced. So. Do you really want to spoil it by going ahead and eating the burger, or would you rather say no actually I'd rather be in credit with my calorie burn and feel good about myself and give the burger a miss. I'll have a bottle of water instead. The idea being that you've worked so hard to burn it off that when you weigh it up it's not really worth spoiling it. It takes a fair amount of work to burn off 300 calories because our bodies are really very efficient with the number of calories that we use.

If you're looking for a little incentive to move more, you could always buy yourself a pedometer.... UK Government guidelines suggest everyone should be walking 10,000 steps a day to maintain good health – and that doesn't take into account any attempt to shift excess weight.

Vitamins, minerals and water add to the nutritional value of the energy sources listed, but don't contain any calories. Foods and drinks that contain little or no nutrients other than the nutrient that is providing the calories are considered to be a source of "empty calories" – i.e. they are high in energy (calories), but low in nutritional value as they lack health-promoting "micro-nutrients", such as vitamins, minerals / antioxidants and also fibre.

Food and drink containing 'empty calories' include: Deep fried foods such as chips; refined grains such as white bread and white rice; sweets and foods containing added refined sugar; sweetened drinks and fizzy, canned drinks; alcohol – all wine, beers, spirits etc.

There are quite a few foods described nowadays as 'Superfoods', which we are advised for various nutritional reasons to include in our diets: try to incorporate as many as possible of these and unprocessed unrefined foods, and you should gradually start to feel the health benefits, which can include improved energy levels, immune function, raised mood and reduced likelihood of heart disease.

Some examples of these so-called 'Superfoods', foods which between them contain high levels of antioxidants, fibres, vitamins and minerals, include acai berries, teff grain, figs, dark chocolate of 70% or more cocoa solids, olive oil, salmon, natural yoghurt, baked beans, apples, goji berries, broccoli, bananas, brazil nuts, lentils, quinoa, watercress, garlic, spinach, apricots, wheatgerm, ginger, onions, avocado and raisins. There are others, of course, but if you pick some from this list every day and find out more for yourself, you'll be on the right lines!

—

How many calories do you think you need? If you've sat at home all afternoon watching television, you certainly don't need a massive meal....you might need a good brisk walk to get your metabolism going...

—

ps.... You've been sitting down reading this book for what?
An hour or so?
Any idea how many calories you've used?
If you weigh 11st.....just 70 calories
or 12st 7lb .....80 calories
or maybe 15st......95 calories
Not a lot, really!

Summary:

- **Work out your metabolic rate to estimate what you should be eating.**
- **Eat more than your body needs, get fat. Eat less than your body needs, shift weight. Easy peasy.**
- **Think of alcohol as empty calories**
- **Get moving**

13

PORTION CONTROL

Time for another reality check. Just knowing how many calories are in pasta, for example, is only half the deal. It's really easy to underestimate exactly how much you're eating. It's often self denial and deluding yourself, no more no less. Sitting there and saying 'I don't eat that much' - get a grip! You don't put weight on by not eating much. You're obviously overeating and not realising or overeating but refusing to admit to yourself just how much you're overeating.

Marion and I decided to try out a little test on some friends in the early days of the G*m*B therapy research. We explained that we were doing research and all we asked is that they came to our home for dinner and filled in a little questionnaire the next day. We were trying to establish when people were satisfied with a meal. Each of the three couples was served an identical fresh pasta meal; the only difference was the portion size. we used three sets of plates, varying in size from what I would call small to recognisably large restaurant pasta dishes. The portion sizes were calculated to fill the plate/bowl of the night. On night number one we served a portion of the size we would normally have for dinner after work at home around 80 grams each. The plates were cleared, everyone enjoyed it. On night two Marion produced portions for the next couple which were weighed at 160 grams, once again the plates were cleared, the food enjoyed, on the final night Marion produced portions in pasta bowls loaned by our favourite Italian restaurant, we used their portion sizes which were an amazing 260 grams, guess what, yep you are right, the plates were cleared, the food enjoyed. …One of the questions we asked them was did you go home feeling sufficiently full? All three couples said yes even though the last one's portion was nearly three times the size of the first. Do we eat until we are full? Until we are tired? Or maybe until the plate is empty, regardless?

When you've been calculating what to eat, or what you have eaten, you might say, oh I'll have a spoonful of this, a little bit of that, but if you actually physically weighed and measured the portions you were eating, you'd probably find you were eating about two or three times more than you would actually admit to. Even things like a bowl of cereal: have you ever actually measured how much you usually eat? You might be thinking it's only 200 calories including the milk; we know from clients visiting the clinic that in reality you're probably having double the recommended serving so before you're even out of the door you've consumed twice as many calories as you think you have. If you're doing that every day, with every meal, all those guesstimates and miscalculations add up and they're showing on the scales right now.

He that eats until he is sick must
fast until he is well
English Proverb

People's opinions on breakfast vary, but if you wake up not feeling hungry, it's because you must have overeaten the previous day and still have that food in your stomach. Overnight is normally the longest you go without eating, on the basis of 8 hours in bed and maybe 3 or 4 hours after dinner and before bed. That's quite a long time to go without food. OK you're not doing much, you're just resting but if you wake up in the morning and you're not hungry, there's something not right and you're eating too much.

—

There are some who say:
Breakfast like a king, lunch like a prince, dine like a pauper…
And some nutritionists might agree, on the basis of how

and when energy and nutrients are needed and used during the 24 hour period!

Clinical trials have proven that a high-protein breakfast, such as eggs, keeps hunger pangs away for much longer than a carbohydrate-based breakfast such as toast or cereal. Porridge is officially the most satisfying cereal: It has a higher protein content than other grain and is also a good source of soluble fibre.

—

It's so easy to fall down when it comes to portions, and dressings, etc. You might say you just had a salad. Great – hardly any calories, very nutritious. What did you put on it? Only a bit of oil and vinegar.......but if you checked just how much oil you'd probably be quite surprised – if you are over-generous then there could be more calories in the dressing than in the whole of the salad in the first place. So you'd be deceiving yourself by thinking you're having a healthy salad. We're not saying don't put oil on your salad, it's about being aware. We need to eat some fat, and olive oil's good for you, it's just getting the balance right. Just because something is healthy doesn't mean that you can consume unlimited quantities of it.

Another classic is the amount of butter you put on your bread or toast. If you love butter fair enough, but make sure you have it for the flavour, not the quantity. A teaspoon of butter is 37cal, a tablespoon 111 – and it all adds up and shows on the scales.

Even healthy things like nuts and seeds are very high in calories so it's easy to get carried away - in a small 4oz bag there'd be around 600 calories. And you wouldn't count that as a meal, would you - you'd probably think of it as just a little snack! So again it's all about being aware of quantities. Just two tablespoons of nuts amounts to a standard portion of protein, according to government guidelines – that's roughly a small handful (around 1oz, or 150 calories). NOT a whole bagful!

Do you like ice cream? A normal scoop of ice cream would be about 150 cals but an ice cream lover may eat twice or three times that amount. Which in one fell swoop would be quite a chunk of your daily energy requirement; and eating it with a spoon straight out of the container from the freezer – don't say you haven't done it? - means you have no idea how much you're having. Take it out, measure it into a dish, put the rest back, and when that portion's gone it's gone! The temptation for someone struggling with their weight is made worse by not recognising when you're full so with that huge container of ice cream you run the risk of keeping going and going until it's all gone.

Doesn't dried pasta look small! So you put a bit more in - then when it's cooked the temptation is to eat it up rather than waste it. But a portion of pasta should be about the size of a woman's fist – much better not to cook too much in the first place! It's not uncommon to eat three times that amount, and that also happens in Italian restaurants. You have this massive great pile on your plate.....you just don't need that much. Then of course it's all covered in high calorie sauce (until you start to change your menu choices!), probably three times as much as you need of that too.

One piece of food while hungry equals
a big box of food while full
Vietnamese proverb

If you don't have measuring spoons and measuring cups and scales, you really don't need to go out and buy a whole new set of kitchen equipment to gauge what portions you should be eating. Be clear about it, many, maybe most, people – and certainly overweight ones - don't have a clue when it comes to serving out a teaspoon sized knob of butter, or a teaspoon of olive oil, or a handful of walnuts, or a half cup of ice cream.

If you want to avoid waste – and who doesn't in these harder times – buy less food in the first place: you won't have those leftovers facing you in the fridge! Excess food will be wasted anyway in the end, whether it passes through your body first and then to the toilet, or goes directly in the bin and goes for landfill. Don't treat your body like a bin. You deserve better.

The good thing – no, not just good – it knocks diets into a cocked hat - is that once you've got a grip of portion control, you can eat <u>whatever</u> you want to eat. For the rest of your life. You don't need to have forbidden foods. Do you understand? Read that again. In fact we'll say it again. **You don't need to have forbidden foods. Eat whatever foods you want to eat.** Point being, if you understand portion control you can eat whatever you choose. If you're aware of what's high in calories and you particularly want to eat it, as long as you have a small portion of it, in the end it's not going to do any damage. Then looking at the bigger picture, if you're eating sensibly 90% of the time, you can 'afford' to eat a bit more of the calorie-laden foods the other 10%. It's all about achieving a balance, a reasonable combination of healthy foods with a few, less healthy, ones when you <u>occasionally</u> feel you want them!

You know that if you're going to eat out and have two courses, wine and whatever, you're likely to eat about 20% more than the average meal you have at home so you can 'budget' for that over the course of a week. You know Sunday's going to be a blowout? What you do is go easy on Saturday and the Monday afterwards – a couple of days either side compensating balances it out. Eating out doesn't have to be a disaster, but it requires that you see the overall picture.

See every encounter with food as a game, a contest; there will always be a winner or a loser, so don't be the victim all your life.

In the end, we try and instil in people the understanding that there's absolutely nothing wrong with enjoying food and eating. You can love food and follow the G*m*B system. We do. Marion – yes, slim

Marion – loves food, loves cooking & the wonderful stimulus that eating and dining, for example with friends, give.

You don't need to deprive yourself of anything. If you want something you have it, BUT you know you're only eating because you're hungry, which makes it OK. It's when you're eating food when you're not hungry that the problems start. The main reason why people feel guilty about what they've eaten is because they know they weren't actually hungry in the first place. When you are eating for the right reason (ie when you are hungry) then there is no need to feel guilty about it. As long as you're eating an overall balanced healthy diet you can have all the extra things as well, in moderation. It's all about moderation and portion control.

If you live with a diabetic you may be familiar with their cry 'but I've got to eat more often....' - Yes, diabetics are often told to eat more often.... But not a double burger and double portion of fries and a supersize coke, though – a biscuit or something small.

LUCK OF LIFE PORTION CONTROL

So if you're going to get to grips with how much you put on your plate, or put in the pan in the first place, are you going to use scales? You can if you like – some people prefer to be painstakingly accurate to learn for themselves. Others find visual aids exactly that – a simple and helpful tool to allow you to imagine, for example, the size or shape of something.

So we've compiled a list of objects to help you picture what amount of, for example, meat, you should prepare for yourself. Or how much rice, how much butter on your toast, etc.

Can you picture the following? A domino, dice, pack of playing cards, cheque book, golf ball, tennis ball, walnut, hazelnut? All should be familiar objects. Sometimes it's easier to gauge an amount if you can visualise another object that is the equivalent size and dimensions, and these are the ones we use.

1 Teaspoon = a dice, a domino, the tip of your thumb, or a hazelnut in its shell

1 teaspoon of butter spread on your toast contains 37 calories, whereas a tablespoon has 111 calories.

A slice of bread with the teaspoon will have butter thinly spread all over, no gaps. The tablespoon will not be spread but rather pasted thickly on.

¼ cup = a golf ball

Nuts. ¼ cup of walnuts (¾ oz) contains 155 calories.

1 teaspoon of oil (a domino) has just 45 calories, whereas a tablespoon contains 135 calories, so being over generous with your oil and vinegar dressing can end up doubling the amount of calories….. in what started out to be a healthy low calorie salad.

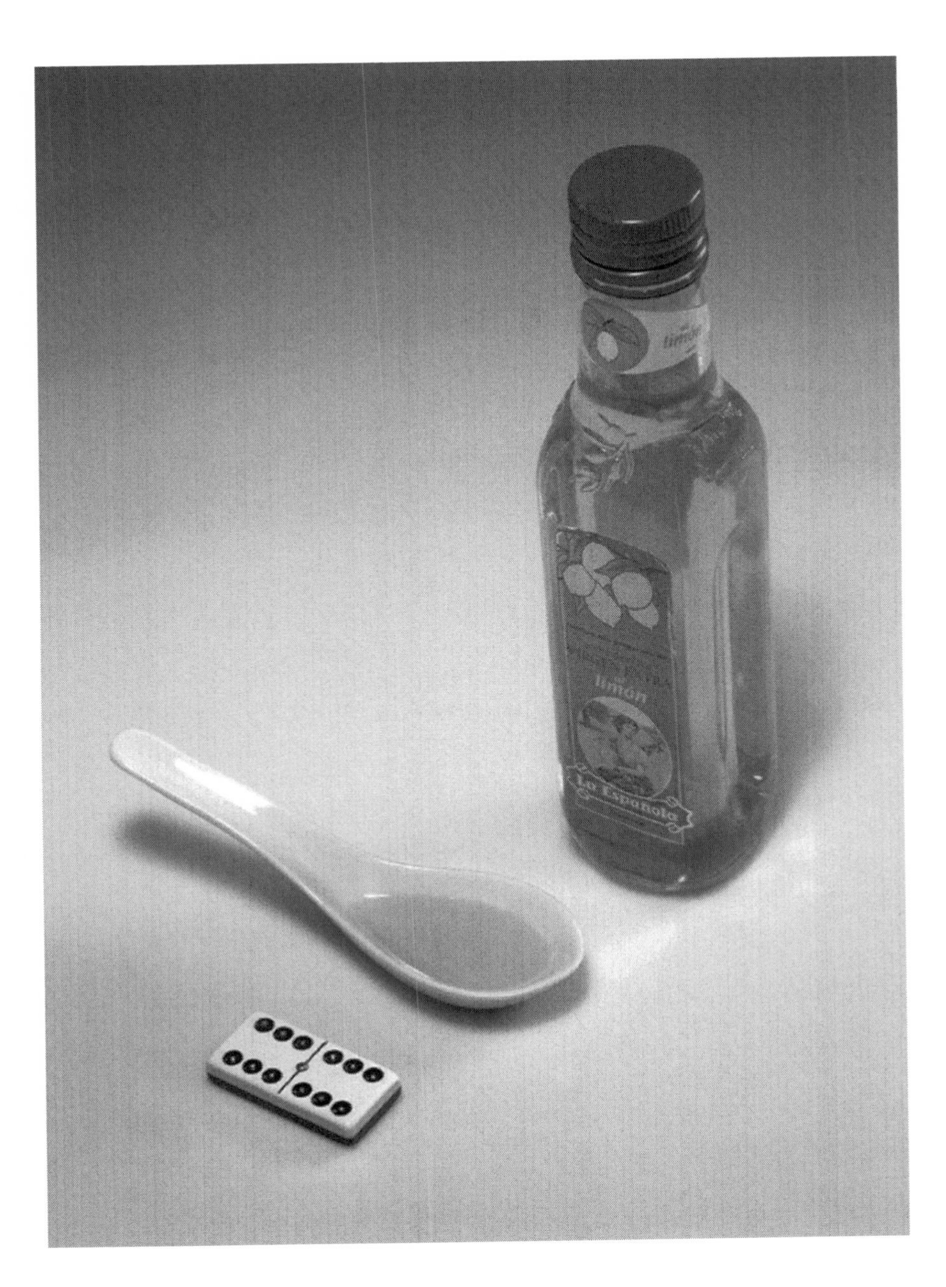

Just one extra tablespoon of oil every day amounts to a stone weight gain over a year!

People often make the mistake of thinking that because a certain food is healthy then that automatically means it doesn't count in their day's intake and they can therefore consume unlimited quantities of it. This concept, of course, is particularly unhelpful when it comes to weight reduction, as well as being totally unrealistic. So, although olive oil **is** very healthy and contains the right sort of fat, (mono-unsaturated) for our bodies, in the end, it **is** fat and therefore is also high in calories.

You can save yourself a lot of calories by easing off the oil in your dressing and adding balsamic vinegar – one tablespoon of vinegar equals just 16 calories.

½ cup = a child's fist, or a tennis ball

Ice cream. ½ cup of ice cream contains 150 calories, so 1 cup of ice cream adds a massive 300 calories onto your daily intake!

1 cup = a woman's fist

Pasta. 1 cup of cooked pasta contains around 250 calories. A typical restaurant serving of pasta can often be around 3 cups (i.e. 750 calories), not including the sauce.

A cup of spaghetti is about 64 strands. About 80g of dried pasta = 1 cup when cooked.

Meat and fish portions

A standard portion of meat is supposed to be around 3oz.

Ideally, you should aim to eat 2 to3 portions of protein per day. This can come from meat and fish, or alternative sources such as pulses; these include peas, beans and lentils. Other protein rich sources include nuts, seeds and eggs.

3oz of meat / chicken = the size of a pack of playing cards, or a woman's palm

3oz of chicken breast roasted without the skin = 140 calories

3oz of lean fillet steak = 170 calories

<u>A standard portion of fish is supposed to weight 4-5 oz, which is around the size of a cheque book.</u>

5oz of cod, hake or snapper baked or steamed = 130 calories

5oz of grilled swordfish = 215 calories

5oz of baked salmon or tuna = 250 calories

Other proteins:

2.8oz can of tuna = 103cal

1 egg = 90cal

½ cup cooked lentils = 120cal

½ cup cooked cannellini beans = 110cal

3½oz cooked chickpeas = 164cal

2 tablespoons nuts = 120 cal

Dairy Products:

1oz cheese = 110cal

1¾oz cottage cheese = 49cal

½pt whole milk = 70cal

½pt semi skimmed milk = 50cal

½pt skimmed milk = 38cal

yoghurt – 1 small pot (5oz) = 85cal

Fruits:

One average adult portion is considered to be 3oz.

1 banana = 112cal

1 apple = 62cal

1 peach/nectarine = 35cal

15 grapes = 45cal

2 plums = 50cal

6 strawberries = 18cal

2 satsumas = 58cal

2 kiwi fruit = 68cal

3 apricots = 90cal

6 lychees = 18cal

14 cherries = 34cal

half a grapefruit = 50cal

4½oz slice honeydew melon = 36cal

4½oz slice cantaloupe melon = 25cal

Carbohydrates:

Cereal, ready to eat, e.g. cornflakes -1oz (one cup) = 101cal

1 Baked potato, large (12oz), or two smaller potatoes = 278

Bread – one slice from a medium loaf, brown = 82cal

White= 100cal

Rice – white. A portion of ½cup dry rice swells during cooking to produce approximately a cup of cooked rice which serves two people and contains 380 cal.

Pasta – white. A portion of 5¾oz pasta (dry weight, all shapes) swells during cooking to produce enough to serve two people and contains 482cal.

Vegetables:

One average adult portion is considered to be 2¾oz.

Broccoli – 3½oz, cooked = 32cal

Carrots, 3½oz, cooked = 32cal

Sweetcorn, 3½oz, cooked = 24

Onion, 3½oz, cooked = 35

Cabbage – 3½oz, cooked = 24

Green beans – 3½oz, cooked = 25

Celery – 1 stalk = 6cal

Cucumber – 1 <u>whole</u> medium = 45cal

Pyramid, Pie Chart or Plateful?

One of the messages we are most keen for you to learn is that food is a fuel. It's not an emotional crutch, not something to fill a bored or boring life. It's just a fuel. Ideally, like you do for your car, you will choose the best fuel for the job – full of all the right nutrients to run your body healthily and efficiently (though a little of what you fancy can do you good..... in moderation!) This fuel, a bit like unleaded or diesel, is full of all sorts of ingredients. Unlike unleaded or diesel, however, it's not really possible to buy a perfectly nutritious diet in one fell swoop off a forecourt so it helps if you know the various bits you should be including, and in what proportions.

Often this is depicted as a pyramid, sometimes a pie chart, to indicate what foods you should eat least and most of. Maybe it's more realistic to see it as a plate full of food, in the way you'd look down at your own plate in front of you at a meal time. In the proportions shown, think of that plate as your day's requirements.... A health giving 'tankful'!

In quantity order, the plate should contain:

Mostly	Fruit and vegetables
Less	Bread, cereals and potatoes
Less again	Milk and dairy products
Even less	Meat, fish and protein alternatives
The smallest amount of	Foods containing saturated fats and refined sugars

✵

It's possible to look at fruit and vegetables as a **rainbow of nutrition** – do your best to include a good mix of colours at every meal. A very brief glimpse of some foods and some of their health benefits follows:

Red – e.g. Tomatoes, strawberries, raspberries, red onion, pomegranate….. help memory function, urinary tract health, heart health.

Orange – e.g. Carrots, pumpkin, mango, oranges……eyes, skin, protection against infection, boost immune system.

Yellow – e.g. Bananas, papaya, yellow pepper, pineapple, sweet corn…… teeth, gums, preventing inflammation, circulation, help cuts heal.

Green – e.g. Broccoli, lime, apples, lettuce, kiwi fruit…… vision, bones, teeth, circulation.

Blue/purple – e.g. Grapes, plums, aubergine, red cabbage, red lettuce……. Circulation, heart, memory function, urinary tract health.

White – e.g. Ginger, cauliflower, mushrooms, parsnips……. lowering cholesterol levels, joint health, prevention of cancer and heart disease.

Summary:

- **cooking too much is waste on your waist**
- **go easy on dressings & sauces**
- **good portion control = no forbidden foods**
- **learn to visualise portion sizes**

14

WATER

—

Hunger is just thirst in disguise!

—

While looking at portion control, let's not forget one vital ingredient in a healthy diet. Water. Water plays a sometimes muddled part in weight loss, not least because it is easy to confuse the body's signals for needing water as a sign of hunger - symptoms of dehydration include dizziness, headaches, fatigue, fuzzy short-term memory and the **sensation of extreme hunger**. So we often end up reaching for some food when all that was really needed was a drink – that hunger was just thirst in disguise!

Water is actually more important to us than food. Next to oxygen, water is the most essential element in our physiology. It is possible to survive for up to a month without food, but we can only live for a few days without water.

The human body consists of 70% water, and on a daily basis our bodies can lose up to 3 litres through both urine and perspiration. Even the simple act of breathing out causes us to lose precious amounts of water vapour. If you add in factors such as doing exercise, or living in a hot climate, water loss increases dramatically.

Water plays an important role in virtually every bodily function - the human body is designed to use it for many different vital processes, and lack of water leads to all kinds of problems. So it is vital for us to drink plenty of water each day in order for our bodies to function properly – the recommended daily intake is at least 2 litres per day. Drinking water will make you feel fitter and more energetic as well as reducing the likelihood of 'dehydration' headaches.

Dehydration can cause a dip in metabolic rate of up to 3%, so not only is drinking fresh calorie-free water good for your body full stop, it's also a good way of ensuring your body uses up those calories at the optimum rate.

Water is an essential part of our digestive system as it is found in gastric juices, pancreatic fluids and saliva and carries nutrients into the body's cells for absorption.

It dissolves and transports waste products from cells.

It makes up 80% of our blood, 73% of our brain, 73% of muscle, and 22% of bone.

It helps to metabolise fats.

It transports nutrients and waste products in the blood and lymphatic systems.

It is a component of sweat, helping the body maintain a constant temperature

It protects, cushions and lubricates organs, joints and the colon.

Did you know.....?

The reason you lose weight quickly in the first stages of a low carb diet is that the body stores sugar (glycogen) along with three times its weight in water. If you use up a lot of the glycogen stores, which is quite likely if food intake is cut dramatically or you're following a low carbohydrate diet, then the water is shed along with the glycogen. However if you return to old eating habits afterwards, the glycogen is likely to come back along with its water!
If you're losing weight sensibly, at 1-2lb a week, like with the Gastric *mind* Band, this is unlikely to happen.

We tend to think that we are getting our water intake by drinking any fluid that contains water, such as ***coffee, alcohol, and other manufactured beverages.*** However, whilst it's true that these beverages do contain water, what often happens in fact is that the other ingredients in these drinks ***deprive*** the body of more water than is contained in the beverage in the fist place, leaving you even more dehydrated. New research suggests that tea may actually be less 'guilty' than other beverages, and could even rehydrate nearly as well as water. The most effective way to replenish our water level is by drinking fresh water. Most fresh fruit and vegetables are made up of between 70 – 95% water, so eating plenty of these will help add to your daily intake of water.

If you keep a bottle of water with you, you can take regular sips continually throughout the day. If you wait until your mouth is dry, and you feel thirsty, that means you are already dehydrated, and this is the final signal that the body urgently needs water. A good sign that you are getting enough water is that your urine has either very little or no colour to it. If it is dark yellow you should drink more water. A good guide is that urine should be straw-coloured and odourless.

It makes it a lot easier for you psychologically to get through your day's water intake if you use a small bottle (say 33cl) – it's handy to keep with you at all times and much more portable than a big 1ltr bottle.

Every small step adds up to a big result in the end!

- ***Lack of water (not food!) is the number one cause of daytime fatigue.***
- ***Even mild dehydration can slow your metabolism down by as much as 3%.***
- ***A mere 2% drop in body water can cause fuzzy short-term memory, trouble with basic maths, and difficulty focussing on a computer screen or printed page.***
- ***If you drink a glass of water just before eating you will find that you actually eat less food, yet you will feel completely satisfied.***

- *Water has zero calories!*
- *Never forget tea and coffee are actually mild diuretics – and can affect absorption of vital iron into the body – so don't count them in your water consumption. However much you love your cuppa, pure fresh water is what you need most of!*

Summary:

- **Water should be your friend**
- **Hunger is just thirst in disguise**
- **Read the section again!**

15

OK – SO LET'S USE SOME CALORIES!

You'll hear it said that today's obese generation(s) could be forgiven for eating too much because they haven't been taught to consider that they do so much less exercise than their parents or grandparents, and that we move less than previous generations is so true. Not so many years ago we had to get up from the sofa and walk over to the TV to select a different channel. Now we have remote controls which can do just about everything except make the tea or coffee. Many of our mothers had push along carpet sweepers, now we not only have high powered vacuum cleaners, but some of us have even done away with the bag, as it uses **so** much energy, time and effort having to go out and buy and change the bags!

In the same way, no-one carries heavy suitcases any more; they now come with a minimum of two wheels – sometimes four. Our cars have power steering and electric windows. Some have electric wing mirrors. Some even have electric systems for moving the seat less than an inch! Long working hours allowing less time for physical exercise, greater use of household machinery, reliance on cars and public transport… all these may be factors in the (literally) ballooning nature of our obese population.

Many clients, when questioned about their eating habits, tell us that they do it because that was how they were taught or shown as a child. It was the norm. They tend to bring the habits forward with them in life. We try to get them to see the often 'selective memory' they are using; they don't believe in Santa Claus, the Easter Bunny, or the Tooth Fairy. They do, however, tend to stick with the nice 'supper before bedtime' just like we did with Mum and Dad. Convenient really!

However something has to happen, happen now, and if you are one of those prepared to take responsibility for your size, and do something about it, read on.

By now you know you've established:

- more or less how many calories you need to keep yourself alive
- how many you may be eating compared with how many you should be
- how many calories are in various foods so you can begin to change your eating habits
- what portions of foods will help you cut down that intake
- not to forget to drink water

Few people love it, many of us hate it, but we've all got to do more of it. Let's now take a look at how exercise can play a part in this journey.

If you like the gym, brilliant. But if you find gyms make you depressed about all the Lycra-clad folk around you, you have plenty of alternatives. You could walk around the block – that burns calories. Throw sticks for your dog in the park – it'll make both of you happy and burn calories. You could go to salsa class with your mates and have a good giggle (and burn calories). None of these means anything other than finding something you like that keeps you moving and gets your heart rate up! - Oh, and just because you try something then decide it's not for you after all, give it up by all means; just don't give up exercise. Find something else to do. So kickboxing wasn't for you? Try the tango!

To shed a pound a week you need to eat 500 calories a day less than your body needs for whatever activity level you lead. You can do this by eating less, by monitoring your food, but it will help if you include some exercise in your daily routine because this also increases your metabolism temporarily, meaning that during the exercise and for up to 24 hours afterwards, you're burning calories faster – but only very slightly. Some estimates suggest an average person might not burn more than an extra couple of dozen calories during that time, though an elite athlete could expect a much larger 'bonus'.

If you've not really been doing exercise at all, or used to and you've stopped, there's no point suddenly hoping to do loads of stuff you really don't enjoy. You can't get somebody to magically enjoy going to the gym if they hate and detest the idea of walking into a gym in the first place. It's important to find something you'd really enjoy and then decide what you plan to do to increase your level of exercise.

However much we want to achieve the mindset to exercise and exercise regularly, this doesn't happen without a bit of effort. You'll know from reading as far as you have that positive thinking achieves so much more than negativity. This applies to exercise too. Exercise will help speed up your weight loss process, and what better to do than start today? You may not have Halle Berry's flat abs nor Michelle Obama's toned arms next week, but you'll be a step closer, and what we do today affects how we feel tomorrow. Sooner rather than later those wobbly bits will be a bit less wobbly!

The trick is to go slowly – find something you like and go with it. Bit by bit you'll form a healthy habit to add to the healthy eating habits you're developing. It'll be your choice and your choice alone, to take control of the problem that's made you so uncomfortable and unhappy for so long.

Everyone burns calories at different speeds during exercise, as they do when at rest, and the heavier you are the more you use.... So actually the more excess weight you shift the harder you have to work to use up calories!

We know a pound of fat is 3,500 calories, and that to achieve a reduction of a pound a week you need to eat 500 calories a day less than your body requirements. So as an alternative, here's a suggestion for how to use up 500 calories:

Activity	Duration
Ski-ing	65 min
Brisk walk	100 min
Golf, table tennis, aquaerobics	125 min
General housework	150 min
Watching TV/relaxing	350 min

You can see it takes quite some time to 'burn' calories in some everyday activities, so by far the best way to achieve a long-term weight loss is to follow our suggested route of eating smaller, sensible quantities, only when you're hungry, and generally increasing your level of exercise.

Let's look at it another way: Every day try to incorporate one or more of the following:

They all use up 100 calories.........

Activity	Duration
Shopping	35 min
Brisk walk	15 min
Dancing	25 min
Yoga	25 min
Play with your children	30 min
Skipping/Jogging	6-7 min
Swimming	15 min
Squash	12 min
Housework	30 min
Light gardening	25 min
Aerobics	13 min

Cleaning out the garage	15 min
Washing the car	45-60min

—

Keep this is mind next time you are feeling tempted to reach for an unhealthy snack.....
You would have to power walk for almost an hour to work off the calories contained in a large portion of McDonald's fries!
It takes an hour of housework to burn the calories in just 1 Snickers bar!

—

We've been talking about all the elements you need to consider if you're going to change your relationship with food, and you'll probably find your attitudes, your choices, your ability to question each and every thing you are about to eat, will start to change overnight. It may not change enough immediately – it can take time to unlearn deep-held habits – but you'll likely see a start very quickly. It could easily be that way – you've been reading all these new ways of looking at things, and you've started focussing your subconscious on those elements you want and need to address and change.

You might find the next time you eat you'll only eat half what you ate before, or leave food on your plate for the very first time. Once you've done it once it'll be increasingly easy to keep doing it. You'll realise how pleased you can be with yourself, and knowing that feeling helps you to make the right choices again and again in the future.

Every time you eat a bit less, find you're comfortable without stuffing yourself overfull, it gets easier until it gradually becomes a habit. Then the old habits of mindlessly stuffing any old junk into your mouth until your plate was empty, they're gone. You don't need to go back to that – why would you?

Overweight people often leave their favourite food on a plate until last. Why do you do that? Why are you eating food you don't even like? You've been really looking forward to eating this meal, you've got food you like on the plate. Why don't you eat that first? Why get rid of all the horrible things first....then when you're feeling stuffed and really don't need any more food, you cram down the good things because they're what you really enjoy.

A slim person thinks – right, I don't like sprouts, I'll give them a miss, I like the look of the chicken, I think I'll have that. Chances are the chef will have put far too much on the plate anyway so you won't be eating everything, so eat your favourite things first because you should be enjoying it, not seeing it as a chore or a torture. Then if you've got any space left you could maybe eat a few of the things you're not so keen on.

So you'll end up leaving the restaurant having enjoyed your meal because you've eaten your favourite food and you haven't forced anything into your mouth that you weren't going to enjoy anyway and you've stopped at a comfortable level rather than forcing the whole lot in. It's just a completely different way of looking at things.

—

How about paying for your food in advance?..........

—

There is a certain school of thought, which involves an interesting approach to weight loss whereby you "pay for your food in advance". Basically this means you can eat whatever you want, so long as you choose some form of exercise to do first, in order to burn off the number of calories contained in whatever particular calorie-laden food item you want to eat. We touched on it just a few pages ago. Once you've done the exercise, then you can either allow yourself to have that tempting cheeseburger, chocolate bar, cake, whatever, knowing that it won't actually cause you to put on weight, **or, of course......** you could choose **not** to eat it, and as a result you will be really pleased with your efforts knowing that you have worked off those calories which will actually help you to achieve your desired outcome of getting slimmer.

If you're more muscular, you will use slightly more calories during exercise, and the heavier you are the more you use too. But of course that means that as you lose weight you gradually use fewer, and need fewer too.

There's yet another way of looking at how to use exercise to help lose excess weight. Say you've just had 'snack attack' and devoured a whole chocolate bar. Some 350 calories, all in one go. You could go for a brisk walk for an hour and twenty minutes – that'd get rid of it. OR you could go for that walk, for half an hour, and that would make it seem as if you'd only eaten a bit more than half the chocolate. As a famous British supermarket says, every little helps!

In case there's any doubt in your mind you've got to cut down on those high-fat, high-calorie junk and comfort foods, take a look at the exercise you'd have to do to 'get rid' of some of your favourites: (based on an 11½ stone person)

FOOD	CAL	EXERCISE TO BURN IT OFF
1 teaspoon sugar	15	2 minutes scrubbing floor on hands and knees
1 digestive biscuit	74	8 minutes walking upstairs
Ring doughnut	140	24 minutes gardening
330ml can coke	139	19 minutes playing tennis
1oz Pringles	155	12 minutes jogging at 6mph
Mini pork pie 2oz	196	43 minutes walking at 4.5 mph

Small portion takeaway fries	230	28 minutes moderate effort stationary cycling
1 Scotch egg	310	50 mins low impact aerobics
3oz bar milk chocolate	446	1hr 50min housework
Choc chip muffin	476	1 hour high impact aerobics
McDonald's Big Mac	490	45 mins moderate swimming

As with all these calorie-burning figures, always remember that the heavier you are the more calories you burn and conversely, as you shift the excess weight your use will drop so you need to do more exercise to achieve the same result.

Many people think gradual weight gain seems to be a fact of life. Well although it's often seen as some kind of joke, it's true that metabolism decreases about 2-3% per decade after the age of 30 – mainly due to losing muscle mass as our bodies age. So finding ways to maintain your muscle mass can help keep your metabolism working faster.

A pound of lean muscle burns between 2-4 times more calories than a pound of fat, so if two people are the same weight, but one person's body contains a lot of lean muscle and the other has a high percentage of fat, then the first person will be much more likely to have a higher RMR. If you lose body fat and replace it with muscle mass, you should see an increase in your metabolism.

People often use the expression 'muscle weighs more than fat', which is of course an illogical statement. The reason people have this idea is because muscle is about 30% more dense than fat so takes up less space in your body. The person with a higher percentage of muscle will not only have a faster metabolism than the person carrying a lot of body fat, but will also look more streamlined.

✵

The human body is very efficient and does not take much energy to maintain itself at rest. When exercising, it is amazingly frugal when it comes to turning food into movement.

At rest, for example, while sitting watching TV, the body only burns between 10-12 calories per pound of body weight per day. So if you weigh 150lb, that works out to:

150 x 12 = 1,800 calories per day

This number of calories is known as your ***Resting Metabolic Rate***, and this can account for up to 75% of the total number of calories you burn each day, depending on how active you are and how much exercise you do. Between 10 and 12 calories per pound per day is just a rough estimate – in fact everyone's ***RMR*** is unique to them.

Your RMR is the number of calories needed just to stay alive. These calories

- keep your heart beating and lungs breathing.
- keep your internal organs operating properly.
- keep your brain running.
- keep your body warm

Just thinking about sitting watching TV – which we all sadly do rather too much nowadays – let's look at the implications for a snacker. Say you watch one soap a week and during that one soap you nibble a packet of crisps – 5lb a year excess weight. A glass of wine to wash the crisps down? Another 2lb a year. And that's <u>one</u> soap a week equals half a stone at the end of the year.

—

(Basal Metabolic Rate is similar to RMR but is tested during sleep and is very slightly lower.)

—

In motion, the human body uses energy very efficiently. A person running a marathon (26 miles) only burns about 2,600 calories - about 100 calories per mile

A typical car achieves between 15 and 30 miles to the gallon

A gallon of petrol contains about 31,000 calories. That means that if a human being could drink petrol instead of eating food to take in calories, they could run 26 miles on only one-twelfth of a gallon of petrol).

In other words, a human being gets more than 300 miles per gallon!

(taken from www.howstuffworks.com)

We like to call 'junk' food, the type with generally lower nutrient contents, easy to eat, high fat, high sugar, quick fix type of food beloved by so many overweight people, ***'Beige Food'***. Avoid beige food and you'll not only be helping the process of losing weight but upping your vitamin and mineral intake. Beige food is food that is full of fat or highly refined and therefore mainly empty calories – e.g. crisps, chips, cake, biscuits, white bread, white rice and pasta are all typical 'beige foods'.

In comparison, foods that are healthy and unprocessed will often also be quite colourful – when you think about it, you don't see many 'beige' coloured fruit or veg, do you? The more vivid the colour, the more nutritious the food.

—

You should never restrict your food intake to extremes, such as 600 calories/day, without very close monitoring by a doctor

—

Ketones are produced when the body breaks down fat for energy. When the body needs to break down fat in this way, then ketones will be detected in blood and urine. This is likely to occur when carbohydrates are either in short supply or cannot be metabolised or made available for metabolism. This could happen, for example, after not eating for 12-18 hours.

Diabetic patients who detect high levels in their urine (maybe after high exercise levels or low carbs in their diet) should seek immediate medical help.

—

Another way of looking at food is to consider the amount of calories contained in relation to its weight, or what's sometimes known as energy density.* For example, a King Size Snickers bar, weighing about 4oz, has more calories than a main meal of 8oz grilled rump steak, new potatoes and broccoli

—

- *The more fibre and water a food contains, the lower its energy density, and as a result the more satisfying and filling it is. Most fruit and vegetables fall into the lowest energy density category, followed by whole grains, legumes (beans, peas, lentils) and lean meat. High energy dense foods are typically the 'empty calorie' foods such as sweets, biscuits, crisps, chocolate, etc.*

The 1lb Jar of Fat

If you want to give yourself a real shock, a visual aid to weight loss if ever there was one, go and find yourself two glass jars – one small, one larger, with screw top lids. Buy yourself a 1lb packet of lard. Soften (don't melt) the lard and put about half an ounce in the small jar and 1lb in the larger jar, and seal on the tops. You've just made yourself a reminder of what 1lb of fat looks like – that's 3500 calories; and the little one? That tiny quantity is 100 calories. Go on, carry it in your handbag or coat pocket. It's quite a wake-up call, now, isn't it! Each time you grab a packet of crisps – that's maybe a couple of handfuls if you're lucky – it's usually over 100 calories gone just like that. And if those 100 calories is on top of what your body needs, it'll become what you have in that tiny jar. Fat.

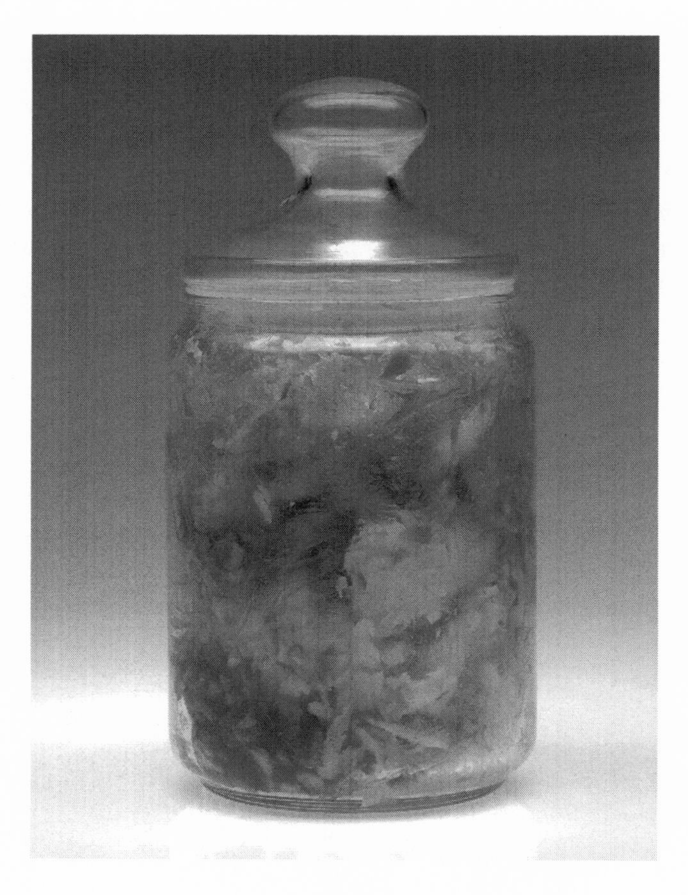

1. You can see how much space fat takes up and the scale of your problem

2. Remember there's 3,500 calories in there - if you break it down to 500 calories a day, you can see how just an extra bar of chocolate a day can make a difference to putting on weight and shifting excess weight.

3. You can look at it positively, because say you get on the scales and you're a pound lighter at the end of a week, and you're disappointed, just look at it in the jar and then you can say 'great! it's a pound of fat I've burned away. Another pound I'm not carrying around any more.'

4. Put it on the top shelf of your fridge.......you'll see it every time you go to reach in for something to eat!

So with that jar of fat fresh in your mind, stop and think about two arteries – one clear, from a healthy person, the other clogged with fatty deposits. What happens next in the clogged one? Well as the blood flow starts to become restricted, the heart has to work harder pumping it around the body and ultimately the strain can lead to a heart attack.

Because that's what it will be doing – maybe **is** doing – if you become and remain overweight. A clogged artery is a far from pretty sight. If you've ever looked at a furred up pipe, you'll have some idea what happens. What should be a clear route for your blood to course around your body carrying oxygen one way and carbon dioxide the other, becomes narrower and narrower as the fat deposits build up making the heart work unnecessarily hard. What comes next? Well, a heart attack's a distinct possibility. Death's not unknown. And there is only a slight chance of reversing the damage.

Think again – that gloopy marbled fat, creating harder and harder work for your poor heart. Not nice, and totally avoidable. Why do you do it?

Summary

- **Calorie counting is unnecessary and boring. An understanding of food values is vital.**
- **Knowing your Resting Metabolic Rate helps**
- **Try 'paying' for your food in advance**
- **Eat less, move more!**
- **Picture that jar of fat when you reach for junk food.....**

SESSION TWO
SELF HYPNOSIS

In the first self-hypnosis session we explained how, with the motivation for change, you can yourself provide a boost to the subconscious by relaxing yourself deeply. If you want to remind yourself before proceeding, you will find the section at the very end of Session One.

Please note that self-hypnosis should never be practiced when driving, operating machinery or carrying out any other activity that requires your full attention

Read your Positive Thoughts and make sure you feel completely focussed on what you are trying to achieve before you set about relaxing, so you don't have to 'wake up' to refer to notes or remind yourself what you meant to concentrate on. It's the subconscious you want to target, and that is best addressed when deeply relaxed.

Choose up to three suggestions from the list that are relevant and appropriate and read and revise them. You need to be able to repeat them silently to yourself at least three times. They are your messages to your subconscious to change your behaviour for life, starting now.

If there are more than three appropriate suggestions, then you can alternate and choose a different set each time you do this session.

Pick a spot (real or imaginary) on the wall or ceiling in front of you so you have to raise your eyes slightly in order to fix your gaze on it. Keep staring at the spot and mentally repeat to yourself at least three times "As I count from 5 down to 1, my eyelids are feeling heavier and heavier and when I get to 1 my eyes will close and I will completely relax."

Then slowly, mentally count down from 5 to 1, taking a deep breath in between each number. As you reach the number 1, close your eyes and allow yourself to let go and relax.

Now starting either with the tips of your toes, or the top of your head, focus your attention on each part of your body in turn, and gradually release all the stress and tension and relax every muscle one by one, while mentally repeating to yourself, "Relax", "Let go", "Deeper and deeper relaxed".

Then imagine a beautiful staircase with 10 steps leading down to a special place where you will feel totally safe, comfortable and relaxed. (It can be anywhere you want it to be, whether its a country garden, a tropical, deserted beach, or just your own bedroom).

Now count down from 10 to 1 and when you get to 1 picture yourself in your special, private, safe place. Spend a few moments allowing yourself to experience all the sensations, familiarising yourself with any sights, sounds, smells, feelings and tastes. The more senses you bring in to the visualisation, the stronger the experience will be.

As you are relaxing you are now confident that you are at last on the journey to conquering your bad relationship with food. Stop and think for a moment how good you feel that your figure no longer needs to be a constant worry. Feel good that you have taken the first step.

During the next few minutes you're going to take yourself on a mental journey to see just how much you have changed and will continue to change.

Picture yourself sitting down to eat a healthy, balanced meal. Think through the process of producing smaller meals, serving on smaller plates. Focus your attention on your food; eating slowly, mindfully; taking smaller mouthfuls, swallowing before you take another mouthful. Occasionally putting your fork down, and checking if you're really hungry before eating any more. Then picture yourself at target weight, focussing your attention on the positive feelings that go with being slim. If you find yourself reaching for food when you're not hungry, your subconscious mind will distract you to do something else - ....

Remind yourself by repeating your Positive Thoughts:

(choose at least three suggestions from this list for each hypnosis session)

- My stomach is much smaller and I feel completely satisfied eating less food
- I am choosing to eat healthily much more often now
- I eat slowly and mindfully and chew each mouthful thoroughly
- I am choosing to drink plenty of pure, fresh water every day
- I am choosing to drink less alcohol
- I only eat in response to physical hunger now and not for any other reason
- I stop eating as soon as I feel lightly satisfied
- I have no need or desire to eat until I feel stuffed full or my plate is empty
- I am in control of what I eat and how I eat
- I eat in order to live and food has no control over me
- I feel calm and relaxed about food and eating
- I love and respect my body and treat it with the love and respect it deserves
- My energy levels are increasing and I want to be more active
- I feel positive and confident that I can achieve and maintain my ideal weight

Now..... Count yourself up from 1-5 suggesting that you have enjoyed a wonderful relaxation and on 5 you will open your eyes, feeling refreshed and energised.

If you decide to do your self-hypnosis before going to sleep, you can suggest that on 5 you will move into a normal and natural sleep... until it is time for you to wake.

16

KAY's STORY

When Kay Lindley, a primary school head teacher, first came to visit Marion and Martin she weighed 22 stone 10lb and wore size 32 clothes. She was very clear in her mind about what was needed to sort her weight problem.

"When I lost weight in the past, it seemed as though a switch had flicked in my brain which made me able to restrict food intake, but over which I had no control. It had operated totally independently from my conscious thinking......I needed it to be 'magically' activated!"

Kay – a twice divorced mother of one – says she's had a weight problem all her life, her mother and sisters also struggling with 'pear shaped' weight issues. Having considered gastric band surgery but discounted it mainly on cost grounds, she came to Marion and Martin after seeing a web article about the Gastric *mind* Band. "It seemed like a possible alternative to surgery and at least I got a week's holiday in Spain at the same time" said Kay. "I toyed with the idea but became firmly confirmed against surgery when I was shown a band and then heard exactly what was involved in the surgical option."

Now 9 months down the line, 7 stone lighter and still losing, Kay is happy to explain her weight history. First let's let her give us an insight into her own wry way of looking at things:

Right let's get this straight from the beginning. I was a big baby, over 10½lb.... OK so it was 60 years ago, but it's my excuse and I'm sticking to it. I have plenty of other excuses too, so if you don't like that one, how about:

* Everyone in my mother's family has the same big bone structure and they are all pear shaped. It's in the genes and can't be changed.

* My mother was a City & Guilds teacher of domestic science at night school. She had to have three versions of every dish – a completed one, one part way through to finish off in class and one started from scratch in class and finished off later. Someone had to eat all these dishes. Most of her classes were about cakes and their decorations – coffee cream, chocolate icing, jam fillings – need I say more?

* Just after the war and with children starving around the world it was almost criminal to leave food uneaten on your plate – how dare you disrespect the poor starving children in this way?

* Need I go on? I can if you want – you see being obese isn't my fault. It is beyond my control and I am the innocent victim of this conspiracy......!

"I've had two periods in the past when I lost a significant amount of weight – in 1979-80 I lost 7 stone, and in about 1992 I lost 4-5 stone. Both times I ate a very small restricted and repetitive diet – e.g. a jacket potato with tuna mayo for tea every day!

"I've tried all sorts of diet programmes such as Weight Watchers, but always replaced anything I'd lost and more when I returned to my previous eating patterns. "I didn't eat because I was hungry. I ate as a treat, a reward, a comfort etc. etc. I didn't think that to suggest stopping eating when you feel full was going to work as I'd always felt full but kept on eating anyway and this seemed to be normal. Often I'd think how much can I cram inside, do I have even a tiny little space for something I fancy. I would also figure that if I waited half an hour I might have room for a bit more food!"She convinced herself that if she hadn't enjoyed something its calories didn't count and she could have something else to take away the taste.

"Food was a reward after a successful day. Food was a consolation after a less than successful day."
Kay Lindley, 2010

"The first time I felt that uncontrollable switch 'flick' in my brain was after the first time I lost a significant amount of weight. However I suppose it is a big excuse really - to say that it is beyond my control could mean that I don't actually have to do anything - but it is a very strong feeling. I think it is an extreme form of 'Que sera sera'!!"

"On my first visit to see Martin and Marion I wasn't the heaviest I've been – that's been as high as 24 stones in the past. I'm a Type 2 diabetic with arthritis in my hip, both knees and my hands. As I'm planning to retire next year and I would like to travel I was aware that my mobility problems would make this difficult. I want to be fit and active enough to enjoy the time I have.

"I knew this year at school would be physically as well as mentally challenging as we needed to reduce staff costs and I currently have no deputy nor any other senior leader I knew that I must lose some weight to make walking around the school possible and less painful."

So having made the decision to visit Elite Clinics, what's been Kay's experience so far? "I described to Marion the notion of a switch which needed to be activated to enable me to change my eating habits. I hoped that G*m*B would flick the switch for me and it seems to have done so.

"I started to lose weight the very first week, and a month later I had lost 26lb. I had lost 5½ stones in the first 7½ months.

"I was part of a Study Tour to China during October half term which was an exhausting experience", she explains. "We were walking what, for me, were long distances and climbing many stairs in multi-level schools. It was hard going but I did everything including climbing to the Great Wall and I would not have been able to do any of it had I not lost a good deal of weight before I went."

"I was at the stage of feeling tired of seeing myself as a victim – someone who couldn't do things rather than someone who could. Mobility was a very clear day to day example of this.

"I haven't even considered overriding the G*m*B," says Kay matter-of-factly. "I did have wine whilst on the Tour which I don't normally have now unless at a social event (I used to drink a bottle of wine per day). On my return I went straight back to a non alcohol regime unless in a social situation e.g. when we go out for our staff Christmas Dinner, I will have a drink then.

As for how to make it work in the real world, Kay took a hard line attitude that suits her. "I made sure that when I travelled to Spain for the first session, I had eaten up or thrown out all the 'old style' food I had in the house. When I came back I had a detailed shopping list to which I stuck. This only contained fruit, fish, salads, vegs, cottage cheese and rice cakes. I don't buy anything else.

"As I live alone it is easier for me to make sure I only stock the things that are good for me and I just don't buy what I shouldn't eat. Even when doing my shopping lists for Christmas I make sure I only list the things I can eat plus a very small amount of the things my family will eat on the day to ensure there are no leftovers. If there is anything left I know I will either send it home with them or bin it immediately."

"For me the most significant aspect of the whole treatment was more based on the CBT. None of what we discussed was new to me, but spending the time focussing on me and my thoughts was a luxury I rarely have.

"I felt that both Martin and Marion were very straight with me throughout the whole process. I knew very clearly all the things I was doing wrongly and had been doing for very many years. I tend to start slowly, treating myself because I have been so good! It takes a little while for the weight to start rising and so I make myself believe that eating these things is OK as I am not gaining much weight and

I can always lose the odd pound or two anyway. Of course that never happens and the weight does then start to go back on very quickly. Soon I am eating easily as much as before if not more. It was also a return to more choice in food rather than the very restricted choice previously.

"However, bringing all that thinking together and spending time focussing on my bad habits made a bigger impact than ever before."

The notion of hunger and fullness is a key part of G*m*B's detailed look at people's problems with food. Has it sunk in with Kay? "Yes, although I still try and eat at set times whilst at work because I can't have enough control over my diary to allow me to eat as and when I feel hungry."

The story didn't stop and as we write, hasn't stopped. Kay goes on: "After five months I visited Martin and Marion again. This time I needed braces for the clothes I had worn on my first visit. I've had a reduction in my diabetic medication because my sugar levels have regularly been much lower than before. I couldn't wait to get on the scales. When I did and Marion announced I'd lost a staggering five stones; it was hugs all round."

So....how does Kay feel looking to the future? "I think I feel much more confident now than before I lost some weight," she says. "Certainly this was my experience in the past on the two occasions I lost significant amounts. I remember years ago a 'friend' expressing great surprise when I said I could drive – she said "you don't expect fat people to be able to do things like the rest of us'. That sums up my belief that the general perception of overweight people is that they are lazy and thick. I think this has driven me to achieve more than I might otherwise have done just to prove them wrong. I work very long hours (6.30am to 6.00pm on a good day - often 9.00pm and every Saturday morning for Youth Club/Tuition and Sunday morning at the Cash & Carry) and this is almost every week of the year not taking holidays just to prove that I can do it and I am not lazy."

Kay is in a good position to see several sides to perceptions of overweight people. “Both in the case of me as a pupil and now as a teacher, I think that the impressions/assumption that people make about fat people permeates every aspect of life and so is totally intrinsic. I certainly feel that I constantly have to do more to prove myself whereas slim people are accepted at face value.”

Now buying standard size 22 trousers and 16-18 tops, Kay is enjoying the experience of selecting ‘off the peg’; “Imagine my excitement at being able to pick a top and trousers off a supermarket rail rather than trawling through catalogues full of clothes for fatties!”.

It’s not been downhill all the way, of course – she had a two week plateau after a few months, which she stuck through and the loss then resumed.

Kay feels that the ‘magical’ activation happened when Martin and Marion started their sessions with her. “I owe it to them to make sure I respond to it and that they would be the ones to turn it off should it ever happen. I know they will not do that and so, hopefully, it is permanently switched on!”

“This is still work in progress,” she concludes. “So far the progress has been very, very good and long may it continue. I could say you’ve nothing to lose if you contact Elite about G*m*B, but you have – a lot of weight.”

“Remember I had nearly 60 years of hard practice in becoming obese. If it can work for me then I think it can work for anyone.”

Kay has been featured on GMTV and in many national daily newspapers and magazines which were keen to cover her remarkable story.

Summary:

- **It takes hard work and lots of practice to become obese, but it can be overcome**
- **Shedding excess weight can reduce medication**
- **Food shouldn't be a reward or a consolation**

17

SESSION 3 – THOUGHTS, QUESTIONS, WANTS and DESIRES

So now you should have a good idea what level of calorie intake your body needs to keep you active and healthy. You really should, shouldn't you? Asking yourself the questions in Chapter 10, slowly and quietly, analysing your hopefully truthful answers, and reading the thoughts and results of past clients that have visited us at the clinic, should be helping you uncover the events in your life and other origins of your bad eating habits. This should help you identify what needs to be addressed in order for you to make the permanent changes that are required in order for you to arrive at your newly chosen destination.

What we need to do next is to help you find the tools and techniques which will guarantee you move forward to a healthier, slimmer, future with a clear understanding of just how you arrived at this place in your life and of course what you're going to do to change. From now on you'll have no need to cheat, partly because now you'll just be eating when you're hungry, but also (mainly!) because cheating hurts no-one but yourself.

If people could just learn to eat when they're hungry, not when they're bored, depressed or stressed, the problem of obesity would evaporate overnight, the Health Services of the world wouldn't be struggling under the huge load of excess weight problems, and the G*m*B therapy, and this book, wouldn't have been produced!

Martin Shirran

It's come up before, but it won't hurt to ask this question again: How do you manage to maintain all that excess weight? How do you **do** that? Because you do **maintain** it – in just the same way as a normal-weight person manages to maintain that far lower weight. It's taken dedication and effort to consume all those thousands upon thousands of extra calories. It's cost money and a great deal of your time. What do your family and friends think, say, and advise you to do about your problem? What would you say to someone in your position with excess weight to lose? Turn it back on yourself, like a mirror and see it from another's viewpoint.

A person who is, for example, six stone overweight, has had to consume and painstakingly maintain an excess intake of nearly 270,000 extra calories. That's a lot of packets of crisps, a lot of work and effort.

So now, instead of just thinking, wondering, dreaming, wishing about all the things that are going to happen between now and six months' time when you've got down to the weight and size you want to be, try taking some time out. Go somewhere quiet, warm and where you can really relax and daydream. Closing your eyes, use a bit of visualisation, go there now. Go there first and see what it's like, see yourself at your ideal size. See it, feel it, experience it. What's buying clothes going to feel like? Which shops will you go into? Will you still have to avoid public changing rooms? What will it be like to be able to put the tray down in front of you on your next holiday flight and see the strange little space between your belly and the tray? Feel confident you won't need a seat belt extension. Be assured it's a strange experience if you've never had it before.....

Going there first, seeing that picture clearly, and all the wonderful feelings and emotions that will be yours when you arrive at your goal weight, is a very important tool in your armoury. You will need it to help you make the right choices, now and in the future. The next time you're out having dinner with friends and you're not sure whether to have a starter or not, see the new you, take a moment to remember how good you're going to feel. Think about the energy and the new level of confidence. You'll have those positive feelings for the rest of your life. Alternatively, you can have the starter, which you probably don't need, and just get a little bit fatter. You decide.

Life will be a lot easier and more fun than right now, that's for sure. What's sex going to be like? Probably a whole lot easier and more fun, too!! What's your confidence going to be like? Will you still walk into a room full of people with your head down, desperate to be 'invisible'? Or will you do what you've wanted to do for so long, stride in proudly, head held high? Go there first and make sure it's what you really want.

That visual image of the new, confident you, will become a vital tool. A weapon that will help you time and again as much as anything else when you are forced – and you will be – to make different new, healthy food choices.

Successful people visualise in their minds what their ultimate goal looks like. They create an image so strong and real that it motivates them completely and literally draws them forward towards success. Top sports professionals always motivate themselves by visualising their success immediately before competing. You should practice visualising yourself as the new, confident you, until it becomes second nature.

Motivation, of course, is the key. Think about it. If you were offered £10,000 for every 10lb you lost (and some health authorities are actually starting to pay 'reward' money, which gives you some idea of the scale of the problem!) How many blocks of 10lb would you lose? Our 6st overweight person mentioned above would collect a tax-free sum in excess of £75,000 if he or she reached their target weight. Would that do it, or would it need to be a doctor telling them their likelihood of having a stroke was increasing daily?

Usually the answer to that will tell you that motivation is the reason your last diet didn't work. If you haven't succeeded it's quite likely it's because you're not sufficiently motivated, isn't it?

People say all they want in the world is to lose weight. So why does someone have to tell you how to do it? You're sitting there saying to yourself "More than anything else in the world, I want to lose weight. I want to be slim." There's every reason under the sun – marriage, sex, family, health issues – everything. More than anything else you just want to lose weight.

Smoking causes cancer, obesity causes diabetes

One of the questions we ask is 'if we could grant you one wish in life, anything, what would it be?' 'To be at my ideal weight is all I want in my life' is the most common answer we receive.

Well why don't you just eat less this afternoon, then? It's that simple. It's not rocket science is it – if you eat 500 calories a day less than your body needs, which isn't a big deal, every week you will lose a pound in weight. It's scientifically proven. There's no argument. There's no debate. Pretty much every single week you're going to drop a pound. You don't need this book. Just eat 500 calories a day less than you need and it'll shift.

When Martin started on the weight loss journey, he made a simple pact. A promise to himself. Every Monday from this day forward he would weigh a little less than the previous Monday. It mattered very little whether it was 2lb or 2oz as long as it was going down. You could start today if you wished. It's not hard.

Maybe you really should take a look at yourself, see yourself how others see you? How gross you look when the lights are on and you're getting ready for bed. How gross you feel when your thighs are chafing together when you walk, the sweat in your excess fleshy areas.

We have had many clients at the clinic who tell us they've caught reflections of themselves in a shop window. They've clearly seen themselves waddling down the road. They've told us about how they're aware that they were overflowing into the seat next to them on the flight over to Spain. We also often hear about the worst fear of all, the one that is dreaded by every seriously overweight person. Not being able to fit the seatbelt around their stomach on the plane and having to ask for an extension. Can you see the flight attendant, when you ask for a seatbelt extension: lighting the call button above your seat and shouting to a colleague at the front of the plane for all to hear, 'Can you bring an extension for the seatbelt for the lady in 32A please'.......

—

How much do you really want to do this? It really is so simple, is pain free and comes at no cost.

—

Just looking at smokers for a second, why do they do it? They'll give you a thousand reasons – they're bored, depressed, it relaxes them, but they'll never tell you they enjoy smoking. They'll tell you WHY they smoke, but do they actually enjoy the hot smoke going into their lungs, and the coughing? No. Do they enjoy the taste, what it does to their food? Do they enjoy the brown stuff on their tongue?

It's because there's a side issue with smoking. Why they do it is psychological. It's the same with food. Why do you eat too much? Is it stuffing so much food in until there's a stretched feeling in your stomach? Is it the lying awake at night with indigestion? Is it having to undo your jeans in the middle of a meal? Is that what you really like? Not very likely.....it's all part of a matrix.

If you go for a meal with friends, just picture what happens. You've just sat down and there's a bowl of freshly baked bread rolls and a bottle of wine on the table before you even get the menu...then you order your first course which is lovely, but often you'll find you're nearly full up by now because you've had the glass of wine, you've had the bread rolls.

Then you order the main course - if you haven't done so already. When it comes will it be like an oil rig worker's Desperate Dan dinner? Then you're sitting there perspiring, you've undone your trousers, your shirt's straining at the buttons; you've pushed your seat back from the table a little.......Next time you observe that scene, perhaps you should lean over and ask your friend quietly and calmly why they're looking at the dessert menu. If it's not because they're hungry, **why** are they doing it? At the end of a two-course meal which included bread and wine, it's probably medically impossible for anyone to order dessert because they're hungry. At that point, every membrane of their stomach will be stretched close to breaking point. They will push themselves back from the table .... And then they order the pud. Amazingly true. Truly amazing.

So why do we do it? Is it because we're pigs? Intimidated by the waiter? There's peer pressure from our friends? You need to have new thoughts dancing backwards and forwards, as many images as you think will help. You need that Pause Button.

> **To eat is a necessity, but to eat intelligently is an art.**
> La Rochefoucauld

There's a basic bit of psychology connected with overeating, the same as with addiction. The confusion of two words. **Want** and **Need**. I really really need a cheeseburger? No. You may want one but you need one as much as you need to experience a heart attack.

Next time you decide to put something in your mouth, stop for a second. Ask yourself the 'do you want it or do you need it?' question. Will putting this in my mouth move me closer to or further away from my goal weight?

There are other words you need to understand. **Try, could, should**. People who are determined to fail automatically pre-programme themselves with what we call 'licence to fail' words. Those words are just cop-outs. They don't mean anything. They're losers' words. There's no commitment, no determination. It sounds as though you've already got the seeds of doubt in your mind... 'Oh I'm going to try to do it but it might not actually work...' 'I should be able to do it', etc etc.....

If you put the book down are you going to eat 500 calories less than you need every day for the next week and lose a pound, or are you going to get fatter? If you ask yourself that and the answer is 'I'm going to try', don't bother because you're not determined or fully convinced to do it yet!

Can you do it? Stick to it for a month? 'I should be able to'. 'I could do'. How would you analyse those statements? The question asked for a straightforward yes or no answer. Not a could or a should or a try.

Is this going to work for you, having read so far in the book, all the planning, answering the questionnaire, learning about your bad food habits? If you say 'you know what, I'm really going to give this a try', well you're obviously setting yourself up to just go out and have a burger and chips. You can't analyse the word try. What does try mean? The question is: are you going to succeed? Yes or no? It's a cop out to say 'I'll try', or 'I should be able to'. Will you, yes or no? If you're still using the word try, some part of your motivation to succeed is missing.

Let's say you're a pork pie addict and the question is can you manage not to eat a pork pie for a week...that's a yes or no answer, surely. Where would try come from? How can you try? You either force it in your face and prepare for a heart attack, or you don't. The same as if you offer to do a friend a favour and pick them up from the airport – 'yes of course'. Until you know the flight time's 3am, so it's 'I should be able to'.... It went from yes to should. How does that work? Will you or won't you? Start to analyse your own internal dialogue that you have with yourself. Start to look for the coulds, shoulds and tries.

✵

Back to motivation – which do you want more? The pleasure of losing the weight you've been carrying around, or the pleasure of the profiterole in your hand? You can only have one thing here. You can drop a dress size or more by summer or you can have a plate of profiteroles, or chips, or cheese and get fatter still. Both things are in front of you. What turns you on the most? What motivates you the most? It's very simple. And of course you may be one of those who know a lot of what you need to do to deal with your weight problem, but still haven't done anything about it. That's down to motivation too.

Then think back to the question of the offer of £10,000 per 10lb. It's motivation. How can a pork pie compare to £75,000 tax-free? The whole £75k thing is interesting, don't you think? You see if you show someone £75,000 packed neatly in piles of £10 notes, shrink wrapped on a pallet, and say 'It's yours, guaranteed, tax free, and here's the paperwork to prove it, all you have to do is drop the weight over the next X months'. Would you? Would they? What's **your** motivation? If you wrote your list of priorities out earlier, get it out now and have a look. Are they in the right order?? Do you know your motivation now?

THE HUNGER QUESTION

Marion and I have some friends with a daughter at university and they were telling us that they asked what she'd like for her birthday. She asked if she and her Mum could have two EasyJet air tickets to fly from Luton to Prague for a girly weekend, as it was a city she'd always wanted to visit. Graham, her dad, told us he booked two tickets flying out of Luton on the Friday evening, arriving back after lunch on the Sunday. He told us he'd booked them into a nice hotel in the city centre on a room-only basis as he didn't think they'd want to be tied to particular mealtimes with them being there for less than two days.

Sarah's mother Rebecca told us "We arrived in Prague and took a cab to the hotel. We checked in at around 8pm, put our things in the room, and I said to Sarah 'your Dad's given me the money, let's go out and find a nice restaurant for dinner and look for somewhere to have breakfast in the morning'".

Sarah's comment back has been pivotal to many aspects of the G*m*B therapy. She said 'Mum: I've got a list of things I want to see in Prague, we're only here for a day and a half. If you think I'm going to spend my first and possibly my only Friday night in Prague sitting in a restaurant like a pig at a trough eating, and my only Saturday morning doing the same thing, you've got another think coming.

Let's go see Prague and we'll have something to eat at Luton with Dad when we get back on Sunday.'

Rebecca told us that other than a few coffees and a cheese roll, they did exactly that.

You see, the hunger question seldom gets asked. We certainly don't ask our children 'are you hungry?.... We just say 'It's 6 o'clock, come and have your dinner, and you're not leaving the table until you've cleared your plate.'. Maybe that's where the training starts.

Often this over-feeding is taken even further and children are encouraged to finish their dinner off so they can then be 'rewarded' with yet more food in the form of a sugar-laden dessert. Where exactly is the logic behind that idea? Eat as much as you can and the prize is..... more food!

A child, if left to its own devices, will actually eat when it's hungry. If you as a parent aren't instilling things like 'you've got to eat everything on your plate before you get down from the table', then the child will grow up as a normal eater......

We've all seen it – kids are playing, mum calls 'Come in for your dinner' and the kids say 'Yes coming in a minute', and they're jumping in and out of a paddling pool, or jumping on a trampoline, or whatever, and the mum says 10 minutes later 'Come on in, it's cold now' and they say 'Yes coming', then half an hour later she has to drag them in....because they're having fun, doing great things. Food gets in the way. What could be more boring than sitting at a table and having to stuff your face with food you're not sure you want?

As adults, we're sitting around filling our faces because we're so sad we've got no way of entertaining ourselves apart from eating. If you invite someone to your home, does it mean you'll go for a nice walk, look at some wonderful things? Watch a film, listen to some music or play cards? No it means food, food food. It's all we can do, hungry or not; it's as if entertaining using only our brains (rather than involving our stomachs) takes too much effort.

Kids are so often persuaded to eat by those parents who don't understand the idea of true hunger. How about allowing them to eat just kid-sized meals – what they want off a plate and nothing more. Why make them finish it if they say they're full? Then they wouldn't be conditioned the way their parents were, and they'd know it's not a crime to leave food on a plate if you've had enough. Their stomachs wouldn't be permanently stretched.

The UK government had an initiative in 2009 – identifying the principle of avoiding supersized meals for youngsters with the more obvious, and logical, catchline 'Me Size Meals'. Don't overfeed them, you'll do them a favour which could last for life.

Nowadays, diet food manufacturers, dieting pundits, advertisers, just about everyone seems to be saying 'use our method and you'll never have to feel hungry again'. Well why not? Why wouldn't you want to feel hungry? Do you want to feel full, stuffed the whole time? That's been the problem – no-one actually knows what or when to eat because they don't recognise true hunger nor do they recognise when they're full.

Gordon Gekko listen up – we don't say greed's good.
It's definitely not good.
Hunger's good.

It's crucial to recognise the differences between hunger desire and craving because a lot of people will respond to a craving, thinking that it's hunger or not caring if it's hunger or not. It's seeing the difference between hunger and appetite.

Differentiating between hunger, desire and cravings

- If you haven't eaten for a few hours and your stomach feels empty and is maybe rumbling, then this could be real **hunger**. The best way to check is to have a drink of water. If you're still feeling those empty feelings and rumblings in 5 or 10 minutes, you're definitely **hungry**.
- If you have just eaten a meal and feel that you still want more, this is simply a **desire** to eat, rather than actual hunger.
- If you have a really strong urge to eat a particular thing and you also experience feelings of tension then this is a **craving**.

Desire to eat might be the sort of situation when you're out for a meal, you've eaten, and you've enjoyed it so much you're going to continue eating even though you've actually had enough – there's seconds laid out in the middle of the table, and it was so nice you're going to have some more.

A lot of people who have struggled with their weight in the past have eaten food, responded to cravings and desire rather than hunger. There's also the low frustration tolerance....the I need that biscuit I've got to have it. But if it is a **craving** rather than hunger, it'll disappear. If you distract yourself, go and have a drink of water, remove yourself from the situation, send a couple of emails, for just a few minutes, you'll find the craving will have passed.

Absolutely everything, to do with eating - or anything else - starts with a thought. When it comes to food, it could be as simple as seeing that food advert on TV, or hearing that particular piece of music from that famous luxury food store....everything made to sound very sexy, with lovely voiceovers, beautiful photography to make the food inviting, appealing....

In fact you can actually get a dopamine rush merely from talking about, for example, chocolate followed up by the rush you get when you actually eat it.

So you see the ad, your mouth's actually watering as you are watching the ad. An overweight person in response to that visual trigger could easily go to the fridge and get something to eat, whereas a slim person would simply think 'oh that looks nice, next time I'm in there I might try that', or 'I'll try that recipe'…. then forget about it. The slim person wouldn't think 'oh I've seen some food on the television I'll go to the fridge and eat something'. How would that be logical? It wouldn't even occur to them to do that but an overweight person would be responding because the trigger activated a craving.

Have you ever seen an advert for food, the ones with the beautifully laid tables, and candles, with background music, and the open log fire, featuring a very very big rotund overweight person?

No you won't have. The people in the ad are slender, sexy even. They're never podgy. Probably, if you asked one of the models who acted in the ad, they would tell you they wouldn't touch the fat laden food with a bargepole. They do the ad simply because they're paid a small fortune to do so.

I was sitting at a coffee bar with a lady once; we were waiting for her sister to join us. I asked if she wanted something to eat. She said 'no thanks, I only eat when I'm hungry'. She had a perfect figure. We talked about it a lot. She said its how she has to be. She was very clear about it. She only eats when she's hungry and is amazed when people eat if they're not.

She explained her method: she fasts three times a day. Eats three meals a day, fasts between. No clutter, she knows exactly what she's doing. I learned a lot from that lady.

If you stop and think about it, recognising the difference between hunger and a craving requires one vital factor. You must be able to recognise hunger in the first place.

'Don't be silly, of course I know what it means to be hungry!', you say…. Really? Are you sure? When did you last go without food for long enough to check it out? That's something you should try (providing there are no medical reasons why you shouldn't, such as diabetes). Try fasting for a day, not forgetting to drink plenty of water.

How long does it take to know what hunger is?

If somebody is doing a fast they've got to keep up liquid intake. Try just missing out on one meal... or try getting up, having breakfast then not eating for the rest of the day and rate your feelings of hunger on a scale of 1-10 and every hour write down how you feel. If you go long enough, you find that your hunger will build up but then it will gradually drop off again.

Ask anyone who's had to go to hospital for tests requiring them to go nil by mouth or fast for 24 hours, just how they felt. However did they manage to go 24 hours without food? Surely it must be impossible?

What would really happen if you fasted for a day, other than losing weight? Detoxing a little and giving your stomach a break? Probably nothing.

If you actually try this, write down these feelings, maybe do it more than once, possibly for a few days, you stand a reasonable chance of learning to recognise what true hunger really is.

The flip side of course is that when you eat, you have to know, to be able to identify when you've had enough. For an overweight person who eats fast, that's a big ask because the stomach doesn't have time to tell the brain it doesn't need any more food. Furthermore, if when you sat down for the meal you weren't actually hungry in the first place then the signals will be totally confused. It's the same when people eat for emotional reasons, they might be eating continually but never ever feeling full. Because food will never solve the emotional problem because of which the person is eating.

A final point concerning fast eating that is worth giving a few moments thought to is taste; your total enjoyment of food is experienced courtesy of the 10,000 tastebuds on your tongue and the olfactory receptors in your nose. When you slowly chew food, not only do the tastebuds inform your brain about the wonderful food in your mouth, allowing you to distinguish between salty and sweet, bitter, sour (and now we're being told of the 'fifth taste', Umami) but the chemicals released travel up your nose, allowing you to gain additional pleasure and satisfaction. That's why taste is experienced less when you have a cold, or indeed when you smoke.

At the clinic, our own modest research/analysis of clients' data clearly shows an unquestionable correlation between fast eaters and being overweight. Overweight people eat as if the world is about to end. They hardly stop for air. They are always guaranteed to be one of the first to finish yet with the next breath they'll tell you how much they love food and the pleasure they gain from it.

Of course, once you have swallowed the food the experience has passed. Once the food's passed to your throat you may as well have been eating dog food for all you've actually appreciated it - so if you are eating something you enjoy, eat it slowly, and chew it well. Keep it in your mouth as long as possible. Of course if it's a foul tasting medicine knock it back quick.........

The final part of this equation is that the overweight person's definition of feeling full may be totally different from anyone else's. They'll have a big meal but won't feel they've eaten enough until they feel fit to burst. They actually enjoy that feeling of being really stuffed full. Or at least they think they do. Ideally you should only eat to the point of just feeling comfortable, a point at which you could actually eat a bit more but you are choosing not to because doing that would make you uncomfortable.

I remember being on a training course once and all the delegates were denied food for 72 hours. Three long days. There was an unlimited supply of fresh cool water, which we were actively encouraged to drink.

We were given cards with smiley faces on to record how we felt every three hours. We were even woken in the night to complete them as well. Funny, though - no-one died. A few suffered short term headaches but at the end we all went through a natural detox, lost a little weight and learned a quick lesson in what **real** hunger is all about.

Practise Tolerating Hunger – It really is possible!

Overweight people have a tendency to eat continually because they are anxious or afraid of feeling hungry. There's a brilliant tool in Judith Beck's book The Beck Diet Solution. To learn how to tolerate hunger you should choose a suitable day and try skipping one of your meals (unless you have diabetes or another medical condition which means you need to keep eating regularly). It is okay to feel hungry – it's actually no big deal – you really don't have to eat immediately as soon as you start to feel hunger pangs – in fact you will notice that after a time the hunger pangs eventually subside – it's not an emergency that needs to be dealt with immediately. You are no doubt aware of prisoners who survive for several weeks without food on a hunger strike – so long as you drink plenty of water, feeling hungry is not a life or death situation, so there's no need for you to feel anxious about it.

As you are going through the process of missing a meal, rate your hunger at various stages (every hour or so) on a discomfort level, using other experiences from your life to compare the level of discomfort – ie going to the dentist, doing an exam, making a speech etc etc. It helps to put the feelings of hunger into perspective.

Before you sit down to eat each meal really focus on how your stomach feels and rate your hunger on a scale of 0 –10. Then check in again with your stomach half way through the meal and rate your hunger again. Do the same thing immediately after you've finished eating and then finally 20 minutes after you've stopped eating. (Remember it takes up to 20 minutes for your brain to receive the "full" signal)

You chart your level of hunger, rating it on a scale from 0-10 , then as you eat rate your feelings of being satisfied and stop before you get to 10 because 10 is stuffed – stop at 5-6, because that's comfortable.

You can use this to make decisions when you're about to reach for some food, too. Before you do that, see where you are on the scale. If you're already at level 5, forget it you don't need the food. But if you're lower down the scale, then yes you're OK to eat. The key is picturing 10 as stuffed full, so anything between 5-10 is overeating.

Food is fuel for your body to give you energy, so ideally after you've finished eating a meal you should feel energised. If you feel as if you need to slob around and sleep it off, then you've seriously overeaten and all your energy is being taken up by your poor digestive system working hard to process all that extra food.

If you imagine going for a brisk walk, before you've eaten a meal; imagine how comfortable you would feel doing that. Then think what it would be like after a meal getting up and doing that same walk again, you should be able to do that without feeling desperately uncomfortable. That's the level of fullness you're aiming at. Often a big person will eat until they can't even move off the chair never mind go for a walk. That is way, way too much.

If you've eaten the perfect quantity at a meal, you should get up from the table **just** having had enough – if you get up and go phewwwww.... That's not good. Try leaving when you're no more than 80% full. Japanese culture says you should eat until no more than 70 or 80% full, the Chinese have similar patterns. Check out the Japanese obesity figures – in single figures - in comparison to the 20-plus% of Western nations.

Your body may well give you a clue: if you pay attention to your breathing, more than likely you will take a deeper breath a few minutes into the meal. Listen to your body, stop and take a drink of water. See whether or not you're still hungry a few minutes later.

We have a scale of fullness to help you learn not to eat too much – same idea as the scale of hunger, but this time keep a notebook to make notes of how you feel when you've eaten a couple of forkfuls, then a couple more, then a third of your plate, then half, and so on, and as you go mark yourself out of 10 on a scale of fullness. Once you've got the hang of this, the idea is to stop eating when you're no more than 6 or 7 out of 10. It's too easy to think you are hungry if you haven't tested your own levels of hunger/fullness.

If you really fancy a fillet steak, the first mouthful will be mind-blowing but if you really analyse it, with each following mouthful the taste and experience deteriorates. Why don't several pieces of excellent steak taste the same if you eat them one at a time blindfold? Because after a few mouthfuls you'll no longer be as hungry so the experience of the steak will deteriorate.

A client gave a brilliant analogy about overfilling your stomach: you know perfectly well if you put too much laundry in your washing machine that it won't work as well as it should. Why over-stuff your stomach and expect it to work perfectly, then?

The whole idea of suggesting a fast is to get you back in tune with your body. When you're a kid you get hunger pangs, you know what it's like. But a lot of big people say they've completely lost touch and don't actually know what it's like to experience hunger because they're almost afraid of it, almost as if it's a sudden life or death situation. Then of course if you never get hungry and never know when you're full it'll be because you're completely overriding your body's natural signals.

If you're only eating in response to hunger you get that signal from your body so you eat then you also get another signal, your stomach sends a signal to the hypothalamus in the brain and says 'OK full now hold off with the food' but it takes up to 20 minutes for that signal to arrive from the stomach to the brain so you've got that delay…

But then again if you're eating and you weren't actually hungry in the first place, you're never going to get that full signal anyway, so you're sort of completely turning the system on its head.

If you stop and think about it, you're not going to drop down dead just because you've skipped a meal. You won't necessarily be that healthy, but you'll still be alive as long as you've had water.

In extreme circumstances, say hunger strike conditions, a human being can theoretically go for several weeks without food. Two or three weeks – providing you have water – won't do you any great harm. If you can go weeks without food, **what** is the urgency **now**? What do you mean you've got to have something to eat? You've got a month. Why have you got to eat now? That urgency is a learned behaviour we've taught ourselves.

Martin's friend Gary – a slim person's experience.

My friend Gary would have a mug of coffee during his car journey from Northampton to Gatwick four days a week. One morning he visited, said yes he'd like a coffee but could he also have some toast, but didn't want to wait to have it with his coffee he wanted it there and then. It wasn't like him to be so blunt. He then explained: He'd gone to work the previous day, there was a motorway pileup and traffic jam, on the M25, and the journey took nearly four hours. He had meetings all day, no time for a lunch break, had a stopover at Heathrow to collect his son where he found the flight was delayed, dropped them off, got home at 10pm only to have to sort 40 emails, fell asleep on the sofa, got up, went to another meeting, arrived at Martin's flat not feeling too good and realised he'd forgotten to eat the previous day.

A big person will find that quite amazing – he'd just had a coffee in two days and it was only because he was so busy, so much going on. And he was quite happy with his life; pleased he was slim and healthy, his life was so full.....all he needed was to have something to eat and be off again.

When it comes to entertaining, dining out, food in general, quite often people's perceptions are wrong. If you go to a dinner party, are you a guest? Or are you a prisoner? Don't say you had to eat all that food. You weren't a prisoner, it's just how you see things. A cop-out, an excuse.

You'll see this example in many publications: because it's a good analogy - You were taught at school that the earth turns on its axis, and the sun staying still relative to the earth. You remember that? Accept it's true? So have you ever seen a sunrise? Or a sunset? If the sun actually stays still and the earth moves, how did you see the sun rise? It's a matter of perception. You can trick your mind to believe anything you want.

—

Remember: at the table you are either a guest or a prisoner.

—

Even though you know you've just eaten three bread rolls, a prawn cocktail, brown bread and butter, steak, chips, peas and onion rings, a bottle of red wine, you know it's impossible to be hungry but you're still looking a the dessert menu because the guy that owns the restaurant said 'desserts everybody?'..... Not 'do you want a dessert?' Even less 'do you need one'... It's a sales pitch. He's a terrorist. Very clever. When you go to a restaurant you're a guest, not a prisoner. So do not let them take control and 'force feed' you!

—

DEATH BY CHOCOLATE -
We've all seen it..
But what an amazing thing to put on a menu;
phone the paramedics so they're waiting outside with a defibrillator for you when you finish your meal.....

—

Have you ever given a thought to the portions in restaurants? When the meals come out from the kitchen, the waiters don't know whose is which by the size of the portions – if you're a smaller person you may well want to eat less so why are all the plates loaded with the same amount of food? Does the chef know how much everyone wants, does he know who's big and who's small, how many are male and how many are female? Of course not – they just do a standard portion as they've been trained to, and we go ahead like lemmings and eat it all even if we don't need it.

People usually clear the plate – why do we do that? No, don't just move on. Why do you do that? Is it because you've paid for it? You'd have paid if it was a smaller portion, wouldn't you – you didn't know how much was going to be on the plate, you just fancied that particular dish. You didn't plan to complain if it wasn't piled sky high, did you? Is it because of the clichés we're taught as children? They're illogical. Does it help any starving children if you eat all your mega-sized meal and feel overfull and get fat? How can we do that?

Eat that last piece of cake; it will only go to waste. Dead right it will, via the pedal bin direct to a landfill site, or alternatively via your toilet, the excess cake will always go to waste one way another. One way however, may kill you.

And what of waste? You must eat that last piece of cake or pork pie or it would only go to waste. Which would be such a shame. It's something we've all said or thought many times. But have we really thought it through in detail? Considered the scenarios? If you don't eat it it'll go in the bin, go to landfill, with a carbon footprint of x .... However what if you eat it? Well, whether your body needs it or not, it will, at least the majority of it, pass through your colon go down the toilet via the sewage treatment and possibly to landfill, once again with a carbon footprint of x. Is that what the word waste means?

Some people will by nature be less hungry than others, some will have smaller stomachs, some will have eaten lunch. Why do we eat everything put in front of us?

Why are you asked what you'd like for your main course when you've only just ordered your starter? Maybe if we were given the choice, or said we didn't want to order anything more than one course at a time, we'd end up only eating a starter.

> I had this idea of opening a G*m*B healthy restaurant. What would happen if the menu were laid out differently – not to favour the restaurant but to favour our hearts. What if the first item on the menu was the main course, the thing of course, that you wanted the most. The starters were positioned on the menu second, and maybe called fillers, for the piggies amongst us. Which they could have if they weren't completely full after the first course. I have a feeling that if the menus were laid out that way we'd all eat less – how many of us would have a starter, a mini portion, after we'd just finished our main portion? It's just a stupid thought, I know, but maybe it's one Jamie Oliver could give some thought to?
>
> *Martin Shirran 2010*

If you ask 1,000 people if they eat a bread roll before dinner at home, 999 will say no. So why do we go to a restaurant and pay handsomely for it? It's all very clever. We actually say thank you when the waitress gives it to us. Did we order it? Do we want or need it? Will it take the edge off our hunger? How wise is that.... Thank you for what? Making us fat? Giving us a carbohydrate addiction? Ensuring we don't enjoy the meal so much? Because once you start on carbohydrates you can get a craving quite fast, so if you have that bread roll before the meal, then when you're offered chips you'll want them, and sticky toffee pudding, the whole works. It's all pre-programmed by having the bread roll!

It's worth running your life on the basis that there are two types of meals. Meals that matter and meals that don't. The two evening meals Friday and Saturday might be special meals for you- whether you're at home with your partner or eating out. They can still be low fat and healthy, but you might decide or have a bottle of wine, or a dessert, and spoil yourselves.

The other five nights of the week are meals that are just not quite so important. They could be simple low-fat meals such as scrambled egg, or baked beans on toast. They're not special. You need to be aware, to tell yourself until you just can't overlook the message any more, that your body can't afford to carry on like this any longer.

If we were going out to a nice restaurant on Sunday with friends, we're going for the conversation, the atmosphere - we're going to get dressed up; that's a meal that matters. During the week when we get home late from work, we might have beans on toast or scrambled egg, or pasta with a simple pesto sauce. That meal doesn't matter. We like our weekends.....it's the time for friends and conversation. That's the time for meals that matter; it's like wine, we look forward to a glass of wine but we choose not to drink during the week. We save it for the weekend, for the meals that matter. It's special.

In a whole year you'll probably eat around 1000 meals. If you want to maintain your weight, actually relaxing and enjoying yourselves 100 times a year won't make much difference.

LAPSE vs RELAPSE

There's a huge difference between a lapse and a relapse. You'll eat 1000 meals a year on average. If you get it wrong say 10% of the time, that's about a meal every 10 days when you can be more relaxed as it will be nigh on impossible to undo the good you've done with the other 900.

So if you have a lapse, if you get it wrong occasionally, if you make a mistake, just think – I've made a mistake. That wasn't a good meal, I'm going to be better tomorrow and put that right. We have to understand the difference between lapses and relapses. If you have lapses, and can take knowledge and education from them, they can be good because you build up your knowledge bank. They're not going to make a difference to your long-term shifting of excess weight as long as you keep to the overall plan.

A lot of people get themselves worked up because they fear failure so much. Not just people trying to reduce their weight. They build failure up to be something they're really frightened of. But there's nothing wrong with failure. We all fail at something some of the time. Just prepare for it, learn from it. Make it a sort of education. Accept that you will do it. After all, nobody can be perfect all of the time.

If you're trying to shift some excess weight and you go on a week's holiday and have a little lapse? That's OK: you can put it right afterwards. Don't fear failure. Failure doesn't have to be forever.

—

Past failures have zero effect on future success, however a smart person always learns, so as not to make the same mistake twice. Anyway it's not wise to fear failure; after all it's unlikely you will get everything right the first time. Learn from the mistake and get back on the bike straight away.

—

Will you spare us a week?

The way to look at it with long-term weight loss, this permanent change in your eating habits, is to see it as 'chunking' – looking at each little success as valuable in its own right. If you've got 6 stone to lose, you won't be able to do it in a fortnight. It could take you 42 weeks – 10 months or so – probably a bit longer.

See it as a journey. It's possible to enjoy travelling just as much as arriving. Enjoy the whole experience – booking the holiday, packing the cases, getting to the airport, at the airport, getting on the plane… enjoy getting to your destination as much as the destination itself. Do it a bit at a time.

Someone who has to lose, say, 68lb, will take the best part of a year, and all they see is getting to a size 12. So we say where in the world do you really want to go? You might say San Francisco…. So we suggest they see it as a 12 month round the world cruise, taking in all these wonderful places – Ireland, France, Gibraltar, Portugal, Africa – you're going to enjoy all those places on the way to San Francisco. It'll be brilliant when you get there, but the journey's wonderful too. If you're 15st 11lb and want to be 9st 7lb, enjoy being 15st. It's wonderful compared to 15st 11lb, isn't it? Treat yourself and look forward to the next stop on the cruise, which may be 14st 7lb or 14st 2lb. Enjoy that and then do the next bit. Don't say 'I'm not going to relax, not going to reward myself until I get to 9st 7lb, visualise it as a long-term project, because at some point your weight will plateau.

Martin did extra exercise, was weighed at the end of the week and had put on a pound – 'how could that be possible?' he wailed. But you have to go through that – there are reasons. Your metabolism is adjusting, you need slightly less food the less you weigh, and if you are doing quite a bit of exercise you may not have altered on the scales but your body shape and composition may be changing.

If you say to yourself 'I *need to drop 6st 9lb over the next 8 months before I get down to my target weight'* – it makes it all sound very difficult and long term, like having a huge mountain to climb, so it's harder to stay motivated – but if you think in small steps and just say *'I'm aiming to be a pound lighter by the end of this week',* it sounds so much easier, and you will also see those smaller, shorter term results, which are part of the long term journey, very quickly.

Celebrate a bit all the way along the line. Don't wait until you get to the end of that 6st 9lb. Try changing your eating habits just for five days. Weigh yourself now and start the process, the eating mindfully, thinking before you eat anything, checking if you're actually hungry or just thirsty, do it religiously for a week.

Will you spare us a week? It's a question of being able to commit to it. Think 'I'm over 18, no-one controls me. No-one can make up my mind for me. This will be my decision and my decision only. If I want to change my life for a week, I will. If I want to do it for longer, I will be the one to decide that too.' So embrace this new way of living for one week and one week only, and in a week sit down and think, maybe write down how you feel, maybe weigh yourself and then decide whether to go on or not.

If we asked you to say you would do it for six months, you wouldn't. It would seem too big a commitment. So all we ask is a week. Of course we're sure you'll get through it – you'll feel quite nice, maybe have detoxed a little, dropped a couple of pounds. Then you'll realise that wasn't so bad, and try another week, and work it from there.

Nobody's got a gun to your head. Nobody can make you do this. If somebody said to me you can't drink red wine for the rest of your life, it may frighten me. If somebody said I couldn't' drink red wine for a week it wouldn't worry me at all. If at the end of that week I got on the scales and I'd lost a couple of pounds, I might think 'do you know what that wasn't so bad I might do it for another week'.... of course every week, and every couple of pounds down, you realise how worthwhile those changes have been.

Something to think about:

Everything starts as a thought. Nothing can happen in your body, not a thing you do in your whole life, without it starting as a thought.

For example you're walking past a baker's shop. There's that lovely smell coming out. It could remind you of happy schooldays, or your Mum's cooking, everyone will be different. This thought can then create a desire, and at that point an action will take place. It could be to buy a dozen doughnuts, or it could be to walk past and enjoy the moment. But as long as you are aware that everything starts with a thought first, and how that process is going to run, you'll be OK.

People often say that they're OK as long as they don't go out with a particular friend because they always go to the same place and have the same foods. Well you have to identify for yourself what those people, places and things are that combine together to give you food choice headaches, and work out some avoidance techniques. Maybe if you were having a particularly healthy week, you'd go to a Japanese restaurant rather than an Italian, or make it a week when you didn't see the friend who loves a couple of bottles of red wine...

Here's another little theory......... maybe fat people think too slowly. Maybe normal weight people are faster thinkers - in as much as you're at a buffet, they're coming round with a pack of junk sausage rolls, a thin person thinks 'full of fat, no taste, don't want it,' and ignores it. Maybe the fat person's not quite there yet: has it and thinks - probably regrets - afterwards. Maybe the slim person's trained themselves to think faster, and the fat person hasn't yet learned to walk away for five minutes and work out what to do if they're faced with a food choice they're finding hard. Because just as with anger, if you can take a 'time out' it often defuses the situation, gives you a breathing space.

Marion uses the idea of a 'pause button' in her sessions in the clinic. (more detail later in this chapter) She convinces clients to imagine they have a pause button in their head, that at any time in any situation they can press and stop the film, the activity. Stop, pause the situation and take a minute or two to think about your choices, your decisions and the long term effects of what you're about to order to put in your mouth.

TLE stands for a 'Time Limited Experience'. That's what the feeling is that the majority of people call hunger. It's time-limited: leave it alone for a while, press the pause button; it will normally pass.

Breaking Habits

Much of what lies behind the Gastric *mind* Band, the hours of work you and we put in before and after the hypnotherapy, is to do with getting rid of your existing bad food habits and replacing them with new, healthier ones.

Habits and skills can be learned a lot quicker if they're attractive enough to you. Some people will tell you it takes 21 days to learn a new habit or a new skill, others consider it's six weeks. It's really down to motivation. You often find it hard to remember phone numbers? Many of us need to keep a note of PIN numbers. Then you meet a stunning girl in the street or guy at the frozen food counter, they say their phone number and lo and behold you remember it! If something is positive, it's easy to learn quickly. The things you don't want to adopt you find harder to pick up. It's something you need to be aware of.

The way we develop habits is an indication of the way we 'unlearn' bad ones and learn new ones..... we have neural pathways in the brain, which carry the signals. If you imagine it like a physical pathway we can develop the thought process from there. See the habit as a path you're going to walk along; when it's a new habit the pathway might be quite narrow, hard to find your way along through the weeds. This is how you'll feel when learning to eat less, not to reach for a bun or a doughnut or a curry. You'll have to work quite hard to make your own pathway through. But the more often you do this action, this habit, or behaviour, the more you'll make the path wider, the route easier. In the end it'll be like an elevated three-lane asphalt highway.

That's exactly the way the signals and pathways work in the brain. New habits that we're only just starting on are not that strong in our mind but once you've repeated a habit over and over enough times it becomes very strong in your mind and you will do that behaviour almost on automatic pilot.

Which is of course what you've done with your current eating habits. Eating for the wrong reasons is so ingrained in your mind it is something you do automatically. But to change these habits, create new ones, leave the old ones behind, you have to create new neural pathways just like the path through the undergrowth. It'll be a bit harder to follow to begin with but you'll trample it down, build up the new way and bit by bit the old habit, the old pathway, will fall into disuse and the weeds will grow over it, it'll fall into disuse and eventually it'll disappear completely and you'll only be able to go down the new way. So once you've created the new habit there's no reason to go back to the old way. However if it does happen, see it as what it is. It's a lapse, not a relapse. Get back on the bike, take control. Learn from your mistakes, take knowledge from it.

Habits are created for us to make our lives easier - walking, talking, driving, shaving, etc., if you had to re-learn how to clean your teeth on a daily basis life would become a chore and it would all take a very long time. When you're starting on a new habit you have to consciously make the effort to do this behaviour, whatever it is – it will initially be unnatural. Driving a car, walking, talking, riding a bike, you have to do it over and over, practise, consciously think about it and try hard to do it and then eventually when you've done it often enough you get to the point where your conscious mind doesn't need to concentrate on it any more and that's when your subconscious takes over because your subconscious controls all your habits.

When you first start driving there are so many elements to think of: brakes, gears, mirrors, synchronizing indicators, clutch, it's all quite hard work. But when you've passed your test and you're an accomplished driver, you know that when you get in, start the engine and drive from A to B often you'll find you've no idea how many cars you've overtaken, how many times you've changed gear, etc., because it's become a habit, your subconscious has taken over and it knows exactly what to do in that situation without you actually thinking about it. The same goes for a person's eating habits. If you reach for a bar of chocolate every time you feel stressed, then eventually you get to a point where your subconscious takes over and thinks OK this is a habit, this is what we do now.

But our subconscious doesn't recognise logic at all, what is a good habit and what's a bad habit. All it does is what it's programmed to do. It's like a computer – takes in all the information that we give it then churns it out exactly as it's been programmed to do. So if you've programmed your subconscious that every time you're stressed you reach for a bar of chocolate, then it thinks it's helping you by throwing out that behaviour every time you're in that situation. Once you've repeated it often enough then it's strongly ingrained in your subconscious mind. That's why when somebody goes on a diet they'll see it in their mind as a temporary thing because it'll be for x number of weeks, you know in advance it'll be hard work, or at least you think it will be; it'll be frustrating, you'll be going against all your usual habits; however you're not addressing what those habits are – you're setting yourself up for a short period but when you get to the end of it you think OK you've lost the weight you'll go back to your normal eating habits....but of course the problem is your normal eating habits are to over eat, eat the wrong things, and so on....

W HO'S IN THE DRIVING SEAT?
ANOTHER CAR STORY:

Picture yourself as the sort of car you would love to own - one that would be your pride and joy. Your body is the vehicle that takes you on your journey through life, so you ought to treat your body with the same respect as you treat your car, if not more. After all, when your car wears out, you can always buy another one to replace it, but you only have one body to get you through the whole of your life. If your car runs on petrol, for instance, then you wouldn't dream of filling it with diesel instead, because you know that the engine is designed to only use petrol. In the same way, you are aware that your body functions best when you eat healthy, nutritious foods, so you shouldn't expect to be able to consume large quantities of highly processed foods that are full of refined carbohydrates (and so lacking in nutritional value) and still maintain a healthy weight.

To continue the analogy, your car's fuel tank has a warning buzzer or light to let you know when it's close to empty and this serves as a reminder for you to fill up – similarly, your body sends out hunger pangs as a signal that your stomach is empty, and this is your reminder to "re-fuel" (eat). It wouldn't occur to you to pull in at every service station you pass just to try and squeeze some more fuel into the tank before the fuel level has moved very far. You would think it was wasteful to allow excess fuel to spill out all over the forecourt; yet overweight people are doing exactly that with their own bodies when they eat excess food unnecessarily for emotional reasons rather than to satisfy real hunger.

Bad programming = bad habits

If there is ever conflict between your conscious and your subconscious, such as happens when you're trying to break a habit, the much more powerful subconscious will always win in the end, eventually causing you to go back to whatever habits (including eating habits) your subconscious mind considers 'normal' for you.

In order to make permanent changes in your life it is necessary to get your subconscious in agreement with what you want to accomplish consciously – rather than fighting and struggling to work against it. This is why diets, which rely solely on 'willpower', are very rarely successful. It has nothing to do with being weak willed, you're actually doing exactly what you really want to do – a perfect demonstration of just how powerful the human mind is.

—

To create a new habit does require a bit of effort because the easiest thing to do is to do what you've been doing for years!

—

Will you need loads of willpower – Does willpower actually exist?

There are people who say willpower is just a word we use when we haven't got another explanation for why we can't do something. It's arguable if it exists. How would you define it? Doing something you don't want to do – is that willpower? Others say it's stopping yourself doing something you don't want to do.

Another example: Imagine a young couple with a small child, on their first overseas holiday. In a hire car, they're following a map from Malaga airport, it's the first time dad's driven on the right hand side of the road in his life. It's the first time he's driven around a roundabout 'backwards', he will of course be changing gear with the hand he's been opening the window with and opening the window with the hand he's been changing gear with for years. Will he get from Malaga to Marbella through willpower? Or will it be concentration? It's doing something that's against his norm. And it's the same for the person trying to lose weight. That's concentration. So is deciding not to have a chocolate cake. Does that need willpower or does that need concentration?

Ultimately it all comes down to the power of the subconscious mind. Your subconscious is programmed to do what you've been programming it to do for years and years – to reach for the chocolate when you're stressed, or buy a cake because you're passing the bakers. So it's still churning away in the background, and is a lot stronger than your conscious mind. So you can only act against your subconscious for a short time. You can win short battles with your conscious mind. But the war will always be won by the subconscious because it will revert to its programming. The only solution is to re-programme.

Diets rarely work as a permanent solution because you follow a diet using your conscious mind. The diet doesn't touch the subconscious at all, and it remains there fighting away in the background. Then as soon as you reach a blip in the diet, or you decide you've lost enough weight, your subconscious will drag you right back to where it's always been taking you. But it doesn't have to be that way.

—

To achieve a change in your relationship with food you've got to change your subconscious attitude to it, and you can only achieve that by spending a dedicated period of time re-training it.

—

Hopefully you now realise that to achieve the weight loss you've been wanting, you need to re-train your subconscious. In order to do this, you must first acknowledge what triggers you to eat and how simply recognising that is your first step to dealing with the same situation differently next time.

Do you know what triggers you to eat?

- Biological – hunger pangs, (stomach rumbling), thirst
- Environmental – seeing or smelling food, watching a cookery programme or advert
- Mental – simply thinking about food or maybe reading a recipe or remembering something you ate in the past
- Emotional – stress, boredom, loneliness, celebrating, commiserating, etc. etc

- Social – being offered food by someone or being around other people who are eating

Whichever type of trigger it is, it has three components.

Situation – which creates **Desire** – which creates **Action**

Triggers don't automatically lead to eating – it is your own thoughts in response to the trigger that determines whether or not you actually go ahead and eat something. CBT teaches you how to recognise sabotaging thoughts, which lead to inappropriate eating, and turn them into more helpful thoughts instead.

Everyone is exposed to exactly the same triggers, but slim people respond differently, and tend to only eat in response to biological triggers. For example if a slim person passes by a baker's not long after eating they will certainly enjoy and appreciate the lovely smell of freshly baked bread, but it wouldn't occur to them to actually go inside the shop and buy something there and then to eat, just because it smelled nice – after all they are still full from their lunch.

On the other hand, if you put a person who tends to struggle with their weight in the same situation, they will probably be in the shop in a flash, buying a selection of bread, croissants and maybe a cream cake too, while they're in there, as they think that because they've caught a whiff of something tasty then they 'can't possibly resist it and absolutely have to have it', regardless of having just eaten a meal only half an hour beforehand.

Dr Judith Beck (daughter of CBT founder Dr Aaron Beck) gives a helpful description to convey the idea of the two different ways of reacting to these triggers – she refers to two 'muscles' – your 'resistance' muscle and your 'giving in' muscle. If you always eat in response to triggers, then you are establishing a certain pattern of behaviour (strengthening your giving in muscle), but if you recognise that triggers are not commands that have to be obeyed and you resist the temptation to eat unnecessarily, then you are establishing a more positive and helpful pattern of behaviour, (or strengthening your resistance muscle). The more often you repeat a certain action, the easier it is for that behaviour to become a natural reaction for you.

For example: Say you've got this cream cake sitting there, you've just had your dinner, you're not actually hungry, but you're tempted by it. If you resist that cream cake, think 'no I'm full. I don't need it. I'm just going to walk away from it', you can imagine that as flexing your **resistance** muscle – and every time you flex a muscle it gets stronger. The next time you're presented with a temptation of some sort, you can say to yourself 'well I managed to resist it last time, this time it's going to be easier'. So every time you do it you're reinforcing that positive behaviour.

Conversely, if you give in and eat it, you're flexing that **giving in** muscle, and strengthening that. So next time you're faced with temptation it'll be that much easier to give in.

People with weight problems often share certain traits that sabotage their efforts to shed excess weight.

1. **Confusing** hunger with the desire to eat (as in the baker's shop)
2. **Low frustration tolerance** to cravings – ie seeing a craving as a life or death that needs to be dealt with immediately – 'I really fancy 'x' and I need to have it now'. A more helpful response is to say to yourself 'This is just a craving, which is just a thought, that's all – I don't have to take any notice of it. If I concentrate on something else for just a few minutes I'll forget all about it and I'll be really pleased with myself that I didn't eat something I didn't need'.
3. **Enjoying feeling full**. Slim people usually stop eating when they feel comfortably satisfied, whereas an overweight person tends to keep going until they feel really stuffed full. Every time you eat less food than previously, make sure you congratulate yourself and you will soon start feeling glad that you didn't overeat. Can you honestly say you've enjoyed every single mouthful of a meal? This should be the case when you stop eating at the point of feeling satisfied, rather than stuffed. Go ahead and try it!

4. **Being unrealistic about exactly how much you eat**. Slim people are more aware of how much they eat, and if they overindulge occasionally they naturally eat less at the following couple of meals to balance it out. An overweight person often deludes themselves about how much they eat. For example, telling themselves that all those extra bits and pieces don't count because nobody saw them eating them and it wasn't a proper meal anyway. Now it's time to be really honest with yourself because the only person getting hurt and losing out in the end is you. So make sure that 'spoonful' of ice cream that you ate straight from the tub really was just one spoonful and not half a litre!

Eating for emotional reasons. Using food to feed an emotional void never works as a solution – for example if you eat when you really need to cry then you may feel better momentarily, but as soon as the food has gone your original problem is still there and you will still need to cry anyway and on top of that you feel even worse than you did before you ate the food.

5. **Getting things out of perspective when you hit a plateau or even gaining weight.** When an overweight person gets on the scales and they weigh more than they expected they think it's a complete disaster and probably end up spending the rest of the day (or week) eating everything in sight. A slim person puts it all in perspective, and simply adjusts their eating/exercise for a few days until they get back on track. You must focus on the positive – if you've reached a plateau in your weight (which will definitely happen at some point) then use it as a learning curve – you just need to readjust your eating plan and aim to increase the amount of exercise you do this week to get you back on track. Remind yourself that it is not a catastrophe – you are still lighter than you were a few weeks ago, which is something to feel proud of.

6. **Matters of unfairness.** Overweight people often think that life hasn't been fair to them and wonder why they should have to watch and restrict what they eat. In actual fact slim people do exactly the same but them it's a way of life that they don't even think about. **It's no big deal.**

From data gathered at our clinic, we can add a few more you may recognise:

- Overweight people are often fast eaters
- Most overweight people don't eat breakfast, or if they do, then only infrequently
- People with an unhealthy attitude to food are constantly thinking about their next meal.
- Overweight people usually clear their plate

The following table shows the essence of the CBT element of The Gastric *mind* Band – all your bad food decisions, poor choices, that flawed relationship with eating, is all in here. It comes down to what are known as Sabotaging or Negative Automatic Thoughts.

Automatic Thought	Details	Example	Rational Response
Confusing wants with needs	You fancy some food therefore your body must need it	The bread smells wonderful. I want some; I probably need it anyway	It does smell wonderful, but I ate an hour or so ago so I don't need to eat now
Negative thinking	You always see the negative first; sometimes that's all you see	I have tried every diet in the book. They all failed. How can this one be any different?	I have read of other people who have been successful on this diet. I will be positive and really give it my best shot.

Fortune telling	You predict your own view on a future event or experience regardless of your degree of knowledge	I know there will be no low calorie foods at the party. I'll put back on all the weight I lost over the last two weeks	Until I get to the party I don't know what food will be available and anyway, as long as I am not silly, one night won't hurt
Discounting the positive	You put yourself down by disregarding any positive qualities or achievements	I've only lost a pound this week. I've such a long way to go in order to reach my target weight	I deserve credit. Every small achievement counts towards overall success
Labelling	You label people, including yourself, in a negative way	I'm really bad because I've eaten too much today	I'm not a bad person. I just ate more than I intended to
Mind-reading	You start to believe that you know what others are thinking	My friends are laughing at me behind my back because of my past dieting failures	I do not know what others think of me and maybe it is not that important anyway
Self-deluding thinking	You convince yourself to believe illogical thoughts	If I eat standing up or if no-one sees me eating then it doesn't matter	Everything I consume counts towards my daily intake of food

Illogical rules	You have set ideas about what you should or should not do	I have to eat everything on my plate because I can't waste food	It's better to waste food by putting it in the bin than end up wearing it on my own waist!
Irrelevance	You make an irrational link between two completely unrelated concepts	I need this bar of chocolate because I've had a bad day	Emotional eating is never the solution. I need to solve the problem without turning to food.
Exaggeration. All or nothing thinking	You make a sweeping statement based on a small amount of information	I ate a biscuit so I may as well go ahead and eat the whole packet now that I've blown it completely	I ate some food I didn't plan to, but I can get back on track again right now.

Dealing with Automatic Thoughts

Work through the steps below whenever you catch yourself being bothered by a sabotaging thought - as originally suggested in Judith Beck's book -

a) What is wrong with my thinking?

   I am going to Liz's dinner party this evening. I know she won't have any low calorie – low fat foods available. My diet will fall apart, I just know it, now I'm depressed before I even get there. I bet I put on two pounds tonight, shame.

   Thinking this way is called - **Fortune Telling....**

b) What evidence do I have that this is true or false? – (Imagine standing up in court presenting evidence for and against)

   To tell the truth I don't have any evidence, I suppose it could be possible that Ruth is now dieting as well, she may have prepared a number of low calorie alternatives, if I am careful maybe I won't put on any weight after all.

c) Is there another way to look at the situation?

   This is the first time I have been out for weeks, it is important to maintain a social life, and I remember being told that we eat over a thousand meals a year, a dozen slip ups will have virtually no effect in the long run.

d) What is the most likely thing to happen in the end?

   It is possible that I will consume a few more calories this evening, but I will enjoy myself, and look at it as a reward for my recent efforts. If I get straight back on track tomorrow I will still have lost weight by the end of the week.

e) What does believing this thought achieve and what could happen if I change my thinking?

   By Fortune Telling and only seeing negative outcomes I make myself depressed and prepare myself for failure. If I stop this way of thinking I will become more optimistic, I will start to believe in positive outcomes I will be generally happier and more able to stick with my healthy eating plan.

6. What advice would I give to someone I care about in the same situation?

   Stop trying to guess future outcomes, statistically you will be wrong at least half the time anyway, and if you are prone to negative thinking maybe more, try something new like always thinking and looking for the positive. Remember "You usually don't get what you want in life, but you do tend to get what you expect" - so, predict a happy ending and guess what you're likely to receive... you guessed it!

7. What is the next step?

   Enjoy yourself, and look forward to spending many happy years with the new, happy and slim you....

Do you really think that a craving is a command that absolutely must be obeyed otherwise you'll simply collapse in a heap and die on the spot? Well here's the good news... it's **not** and you **won't!** A craving is simply a thought and it will only take up as much space in your head as you allow it to. You can control your thoughts and squash all unhelpful thoughts before they make you react in a negative way.

There are various mindset techniques and behavioural techniques you can use to help you deal with and resist cravings. At first they may be quite difficult to employ, but the more often you put them into practice the easier they will become.

Mindset Techniques

A) Be strict with yourself. Remind yourself there's no emergency – tell yourself it's just a craving. It will go away. You don't **need** the food, you're not **hungry** – you just **want** it.

B) Picture yourself at the fork in the road.... Remind yourself that you have no choice apart from the choice you've already made by deciding to head up the right road and getting rid of the excess weight. You can either give in to the craving or you can slim down to your goal weight. But you can't have both. It's your choice. Nothing terrible or earth shattering will happen if you resist that craving. Tell yourself how proud you will be when you've resisted. Don't argue with yourself – remind yourself you have no choice. You just don't eat if you're not hungry. Simple as that.

C) Keep reminding yourself of your motivation – why do you want to get rid of the excess weight? Read through your list of what is important to you to refresh your memory. As long as those reasons are important enough to you this quick reminder will stop you from eating unnecessarily.

D) Remind yourself to be clear in your mind what is more important to you – that quick fix or the long-term benefits to your appearance, self esteem and health if you lose excess weight and achieve a slimmer you.

Behavioural techniques

If you still feel tempted to give in to your cravings after using the mindset techniques, then you can also work your way through the behavioural techniques to help you.

A) Physically distance yourself from whatever it is you are craving – either by removing the food, or throwing it away in the bin, or by removing yourself from the same place as the food – going into another room, or going outside, etc.

B) Get yourself a drink of water – remember that you may think you are hungry when you are in fact just thirsty.

C) Try a relaxation technique such as focussing on your breathing for a few minutes. Take long, slow, deep breaths through your nose – count to four as you inhale and again as you exhale. Keep it up for at least 2 minutes, and you should feel much more relaxed and in control afterwards and the craving will probably have disappeared by then anyway.

D) Focus your attention on something else entirely and distract yourself for a few minutes until the craving has passed. For example, you could make a quick phone call or send an email, or go for a stroll.

You may be one of the people who say they don't have a chance to question, to stop themselves every time before putting food in their mouth. It's in before they've realised it.

Everything Begins with a Thought (Yes, we've said it before)

BUT – there's always that split second when you have the thought before you go ahead with the action. That's because as we've said, and we'll keep saying, everything starts with an idea, a thought. It might only be a split second but it's a thought that passes through your mind and then you react to it. But of course in the past you've been so used to reaching for food every time you're bored or down or a bit stressed or whatever, and you've got into that pattern and don't even notice the thought.

The thought might be 'I feel upset, or 'some chocolate will make me feel better', or 'I'll have one of those biscuits'; anything like that. Nothing to do with hunger. It's a thought simply relating to the food being there, or to the emotion of wanting to feel better and associating that with food. It gets to the point where you're not actually even noticing the thought, you think you're reaching for the food and simply can't stop yourself. But if you put the whole episode into slow motion you will realise the thought **is** there, the key is to recognise it and then stop yourself acting on it by not following through and putting the food in your mouth.

Make it a comedy moment in your mind if it would help – the long drawn out slow motion with silly sound effects…. STTOOOOPPPP!!!!

Take the analogy one step further….. we dub it 'The Pause Button'.

This is a really effective technique you can use for times when you are feeling tempted to eat something that you know fine well you don't actually need.

In CBT they call it suffering from "low frustration tolerance" – what it means basically is that you can be perfectly controlled and self-disciplined in various other areas of your life – maybe you don't smoke or drink, or take drugs etc etc, but when you are faced with this one particular thing (in this case food), you suddenly feel as if you are completely helpless and powerless – it's as if this thing has some sort of a hold over you and you have absolutely no will power against it – almost as if it is consuming your whole being and turning you into a quivering wreck – and you even feel that the urge is so strong that if you don't go ahead and give in to it then you will literally just about collapse in a heap and die. (Does this sound familiar at all?)

So, whenever you find yourself in this - seemingly hopeless - situation, this is the perfect time to employ the Pause Button. All you need to do is imagine that you have a remote control for your life (similar to the one for your TV/DVD player etc), so you can pause/fast forward/rewind etc as and when necessary.

<u>PRESS PAUSE</u>

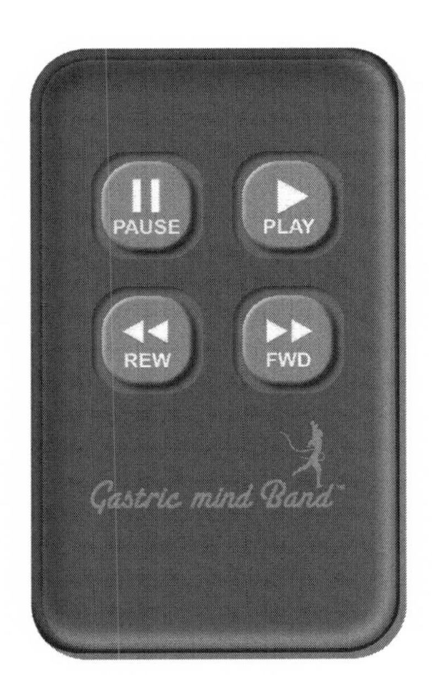

Picture yourself there – your greatest weakness (chocolate, crisps, biscuits etc etc) is sitting there right in front of you and you are starting to feel weak and about to reach out and gulp it down on the spot.

Quick as a flash you must hit your ***pause button*** *to freeze-frame yourself physically for the next few seconds. Now, while you are on pause physically, just spend the next few seconds running through the whole scenario mentally in your head and see yourself going ahead and eating whatever it is that you're feeling tempted with and enjoying (or maybe not even enjoying!) a few quick seconds of instant gratification from it. Then you need to fast forward (mentally) to 5 minutes after you've finished eating and think about how you are feeling now and what you're thinking – I bet you're going through the usual routine of feeling guilty and beating yourself up (yet again!!!), telling yourself you've been stupid for scoffing all of that unnecessary food – Why on earth have I done this to myself yet again when I promised myself I wouldn't? etc etc*

So, now you've reminded yourself of exactly how bad you're going to feel if you DO go ahead and eat this, now you can mentally rewind back to the present and then spend a few moments playing through the scenario once more, but this time add in the nice happy ending, and see yourself recognising that you're not actually hungry and you certainly don't need this food, no matter how much you think you want it – it's just a craving, which is no more than a thought that starts in your head, and you are completely in control of your own thoughts if you choose to be.

So you see yourself deciding to walk away from the food and then fast forward to 5 minutes afterwards. Now how are you feeling? You are going to be feeling so virtuous and self-righteous, strong and positive etc etc, because you know that you've reacted in the right way and you've actually done the right thing at last!

In the end a thought can only take up as much space in your head as you allow it to, so if you recognise a sabotaging thought as such, then you have the power and control to stop it in its tracks right there and then if you want to, or you can choose to allow it to build up out of all proportion. So whatever the outcome is really is your own choice. Notice how we use the words power and control and choice – this is all about empowerment and getting you to recognise that you are the one who is in control and you can decide what the outcome is going to be, depending on how you react to a situation or stimulus.

Now you can rewind mentally back to the present. You have now shown yourself the possible options and two totally different outcomes to this situation, and it's up to you choose the path you're going to take.

The next step is to take yourself off pause and make your choice – are you going to go down that same old road by eating that unnecessary food and putting up with all the negative consequences that follow, or are you going to take a more positive route and not eat the food, which will mean you will be taking a step towards achieving your target weight. The choice is yours!

You can hit your pause button whenever you need to give yourself a few seconds to take time out and think through a situation and remind yourself of the possible consequences, rather than just carrying on regardless and only facing the fallout after the event.

We give our clinic clients a credit card sized Pause Button to take home with them to help remind them when they need a 'freeze frame' moment. You might like to photocopy the image from the book to put in your own purse or wallet!?

Some eating and drinking is by way of a habit – it's 7pm so you have a glass of wine and some crisps. It's actually the same thing, though – the thought process is there and you're reacting to the thought that's set up the habit in the first place. On top of which, we're talking about avoiding extremes. Without a moment's thought, in the bowl the overweight person's hand goes and as if by magic 500 unnecessary calories go around their waist, all in a heartbeat. A 'normal' eater would with barely a thought, handle it differently. 'I'll be eating in 10 minutes, it'll spoil my appetite', they think, or 'I'm not stupid – they contain more calories than the entire meal. I'll leave them to the other sad guests'.

A slim person might eat quite a few things but it'll be a banana, or five grapes, or a couple of green olives. Having a glass of wine? How many peanuts or crisps would you have? Honestly? A slim person might have four peanuts or of course none.

Once you've got into the habit of stopping yourself before you start to eat, to ask the question, you should find it will become easy to develop it into an automatic process. Not before every forkful, just at the beginning of every 'eating episode'. Then as you go through the meal you need to learn to recognise the feelings that hunger is subsiding and you're beginning to feel satisfied and stop at that point.

Every time you eat to normal fullness, give yourself credit for it – tell yourself you're exercising and so strengthening your 'resistance muscle'.

A lot of people who are overweight have got into the routine of bypassing the body's signals, and overriding and ignoring them and continuing to eat until they feel stuffed rather than comfortably full.

—

You'll find you latch on to a few of these ideas more than others, but together they'll give you the clues as to how you can start thinking like a slim person. And you will.

—

So you've redefined your levels of feeling full, or you're starting to. That's just one piece of the jigsaw, even if it is a critical one. There are many elements you can put together to change your attitude to food and your method of making choices.

If you can't even get out of the chair at the end of the meal, if you've had to push your seat back and undo your belt one notch, at that stage you've definitely overeaten. A lot of people will do that at every meal. So they need to back off from that and redefine their levels of feeling full.

Everybody's different. Some people will be having a big plateful at mealtimes, and never eat between meals. Others will eat normally in front of other people then bring out a packet of biscuits, for example, permanently grazing between meals yet make out they don't eat much.

In CBT terms that's one of the negative automatic thoughts, sabotaging thoughts, seen as it can relate to food and eating… people will say to themselves 'oh that packet of biscuits doesn't count because I'm not sitting down to a meal.' They delude themselves into believing something that's completely illogical. They tell themselves these things because they're making excuses. You can believe all sorts of illogical concepts if you choose to in order to justify your actions.

Once you start looking for them, you'll almost certainly find you have these thoughts throughout the day – now you need to recognise helpful, positive ones, as well as vitally spotting when you have negative, unhelpful, sabotaging thoughts. If you respond to those ones, they won't help you to achieve what you want to achieve; to move closer to your goals.

Irrelevance: I've had a stressful day so I deserve to eat this whole family size trifle because it'll make me feel better. Putting two completely different concepts together that shouldn't really go together… why do you deserve to have this trifle? Just because you've had a bad day? How is it going to make you feel better? Because it isn't. It will of course actually make you feel worse.

There are different types of negative automatic thoughts, we've listed them already, and here is a closer look. You might recognise yourself in here…..

All or Nothing Thinking (being a perfectionist): Making yourself jump through unnecessary hoops and setting yourself up for failure: you shouldn't expect to be perfect. In the situation of somebody who's been on a diet in the past, they've had a programme of food they can or can't eat, and one day they end up having one of these forbidden foods and so straight away they see this as failing completely because they haven't stuck to the list. They blow it up out of all proportion and figure what the heck; I may as well eat a load more…. I've completely stuffed it up. Whereas that one slip is neither here nor there so you need to put it in perspective, take a step back and say for example is one biscuit such a disaster? In terms of what you're going to eat over a whole day? - No, it isn't. Maybe you didn't need it, maybe you shouldn't have had it. But you stopped yourself after one biscuit. That's the thing to do – get a grip, say never mind I'll get back on track.

What would make a difference is it you went ahead and had the whole packet of biscuits, then a couple of croissants, cakes, go mad, have a bar of chocolate – that would be a bit of a disaster! But one biscuit isn't. It's black and white thinking from a perfectionist. All or nothing – but in reality there are grey areas. You just have to see it in perspective. A setback. One biscuit, one whatever.... Get back on track again straight away. Now. You can avert disaster!

That 'One Biscuit' Thing – No, you haven't stuffed up!

It's a very typical thing, especially for people who've been on many diets – so many are very restrictive, you have this whole list of things you can and can't eat, and is it a red day or a green day, how many points is this, and I'm not allowed that and I'm sorry I can't go out for dinner because I'm on a slimming shake, and it's all been very difficult and regimented in the past – black and white, this is what you can and can't do.

You get kind of pre-programmed that diets are difficult and there are certain forbidden foods – could be all your favourite foods of course - biscuits, ice cream, cakes, whatever... so if you slip up, make a slight mistake and you have a biscuit with your cup of coffee that wasn't on the diet plan, you then say to yourself oh god I've had a biscuit, I've blown it now, I've stuffed up the whole day. It wasn't on the diet plan. I wasn't supposed to have it. That's it, stuff it. I may as well have the whole packet now.

How is that logical?! In the overall scheme of things one biscuit isn't a disaster, it isn't a catastrophe. It's not a slip up. It's only 75 calories and in your overall daily intake it's nothing really. Maybe you shouldn't have had it but you fancied it, you had it. That's it. It's done now. Draw a line under it. Put the rest of the packet in the bin if you want or give it to your friend or next door neighbour or someone.... If you do go on and eat the whole packet then it will be more of a catastrophe, and you will have stuffed up at that stage.

But after that **one biscuit** you **haven't** stuffed the whole thing up.

Marion Shirran

A really effective way to determine whether what you are about to do (or have just done) is a logical reaction to a particular thought is to imagine that you have to present a case defending your behaviour in court in front of a judge and jury. Go ahead and see whether it would be endorsed or simply laughed out of court!

—

Forget past failures.
They have no connection with future successes.

—

Discounting the Positives - You discount all the positive aspects and only focus on the negative things, such as getting on the scales one day and the numbers haven't gone down, you've stayed the same. So the negative way would be to focus and say that's it, I haven't achieved anything this week at all. My weight's exactly the same. It's not working for me. I'll stop right now. Whereas you should focus on the positive, and say OK, my weight hasn't gone down this week - but I still weigh less than I did two weeks ago. And that's good, isn't it.... Really focus on the positive side of things. Also recognise that with exercise, you may be burning off fat but replacing it with muscle so your shape may be different even though your weight hasn't dropped.

Fortune telling – predicting what's going to happen, often in a negative way. For example if you're invited to a dinner party you get it into your mind that it's going to be a complete disaster, loads of fattening foods, you won't be able to eat anything healthy so if you're going to the dinner party, you might as well give up right now. Whereas you might find there's healthy food to eat and anyway nobody's going to force the food down your neck. It's still your decision how much you eat and what choices you make. Instead of thinking you won't be able to resist the dessert because you've never been able to in the past, you shouldn't base it on past experiences because you've decided now that losing weight is more important to you than putting everything into your mouth that's on offer.

Mind Reading - Putting thoughts into other people's heads. Thinking you're going to offend the host by turning down this beautiful dessert that they've spent all afternoon preparing, whereas the friend might not even notice that you don't have a dessert or might momentarily think, oh you didn't like that.... but she probably won't even remember the next day, and she's not going to hold it against you just because you didn't eat this dessert..... and in the end if she's any sort of friend she'll be happy for you that you're finally getting a grip on your weight.... and she'll feel happier that you're happier with yourself rather than trying not to offend her, which she probably wouldn't even notice anyway!

There are still different viewpoints to help you see the ways you can begin to change. NLP is often used in tandem with the hypnotherapy element – it's about learning to see yourself from a different perspective. An example of NLP would be 'going there first', e.g. if you're a size 16, 20, whatever, close your eyes and imagine yourself on Christmas Eve or some similar date in the future as a size 10. Try and recognise in detail what you'll smell like, feel like, how much confidence you'd have, how much energy you'd have, the acknowledgement you'd be getting from others, where you'd be going that evening, what you would be eating, what your friends would say to you, how happy you'd feel etc. Another example would be to look at the difference between yourself and someone who has the correct relationship with food and try to model yourself on that person. What does that person do with food that is different?

So. Imagine yourself in jeans or a top you haven't been able to wear .... If you really imagine yourself, see yourself in the jeans in your mind's eye, visualise how you will look walking into a party in that fashionable outfit, it is a positive image. It's all to do with feeling better about yourself.

You'll see how you feel with improved self esteem, self image. Instead of all the negative feedback you've been pouring on yourself, you can project yourself into a better, slimmer future. You can see yourself standing in front of the mirror feeling really good about yourself in that dress or those jeans, really focus on the positive.

Still thinking about visualisation, it is possible, though it sounds a bit odd, to acknowledge your internal voices, the ones you've seen as critical. If you make friends with them, filter out criticism and listen to support and encouragement, it can help you achieve inner harmony.

Everyone tends to see things with their own 'filters' based on their experiences; now is the time to start removing those filters, boosting the positive. For example, two women walking along a pavement see two men walking towards them. One man's wearing a baseball cap; one of the women had a bad experience as a kid seeing a film in which the baddie wore a baseball cap so she's got this idea that anyone wearing a baseball cap is a bad thing.... and she starts having a panic attack. The other woman walks up to the men and simply says a normal friendly hello. In fact the guy in the baseball cap is an off duty policeman, and is the other woman's cousin – so there are completely different filters from both of them according to their past experiences.

If when you look in the mirror you continually criticise the way you look, say negative things like 'I'm frumpy', 'I can't wear nice clothes', 'I'm ugly', you're putting your own filters on your image. You'd find your other half loves you to bits because of who you are, they don't see you as overweight and frumpy at all. It's all been down to your negative filter.

‘As I see it’.....
this is Martin speaking directly to you!

Do you normally wear a seatbelt? Most of us do. Why do you wear it? Most overweight clients we ask give their reason as accidents – going through the windscreen, etc. Sometimes we ask if the car’s got airbags as well. Normally they say yes. Then we remind them how bizarre it is that they sit in the car with their seatbelt on, surrounded by airbags, driving along eating a pork pie. Only about 2,900 people die in road traffic accidents in a year, yet some 68,000 die from obesity-related illnesses. How illogical is that behaviour?

Do you accept responsibility for your situation and for all the consequences of your actions? If like many clients you believe you do, you need to start thinking about why you are fat and why you’ve done nothing about it. Why have you failed to take control of your reaction to the stimulus of food?

How do you manage to do it? Do what, you may wonder..... how do you manage to stay overweight! Well how do you? This question surprises many people, but in the same way as many people have to work to stay slim, we work on the assumption that fat or overweight people have to put a lot of effort in to maintain their size.

Would it destabilise you, mess your head a bit if we asked how you managed to get so large? How you manage to maintain it? Do you think it’s a weird question? You’ve probably not been asked before. So how did you manage? It must be such hard work – in the same way as a slim person grafts her butt off to always be a size 8, how do you manage to stay a size 16, 18, 24, 32? It must take so much effort, you must write a shopping list on a spreadsheet on the computer. Wouldn’t it be better to put in a bit of effort to become slimmer and maintain **that** size?

What do you really want, dream of? Can you see the end result if you close your eyes?

Now is the time to start 'going there first', seeing the end result of your efforts to shift that excess weight. Smell it, feel it, taste it, live it. What will it be like?

What would it take for you to lose weight? What is your motivation – would it be money? If someone paid you enough? Would it be the thought of having a stroke if you continue eating the way you are? Would it be to improve your relationship? We'd suggest you sit back in an armchair, close your eyes and try to think of the scenario of having a stroke last night and losing the use of an arm and a leg and never being able to go to the toilet alone for the rest of your life. If that had happened yesterday, would you need to be here today? Is that the wake up call you need?

If you went to the beach on Friday and saw a big sign up saying very strong undercurrents, risk of drowning, do not swim in this water – you wouldn't go in. But the fat person would go and have a cheeseburger and chips. What's the difference? Just because that one cheeseburger and chips isn't going to kill him? So what we're saying is let's go to the zebra crossing, put a blindfold on you and say go on walk across there and you get to the other side and say 'yeah I've done it!' .... Then make you come back because you managed it the first time? What a dozy attitude! Because that one cheeseburger didn't kill you doesn't mean you can carry on as often as you like, because chances are one day one of them will. Because they probably will. They may think they're safe but that's because they're using here and now thinking - and that's why a lot of this is education about healthy eating.

Often people will cherry-pick the advice they're willing to believe.... You may have heard years ago that an aspirin a day helps keep your blood thin, so you might avoid stroke, or DVT, or whatever. So you've done that for nine years. But the same newspapers where you read that have been saying monthly, weekly, maybe even daily, that you should try to keep your BMI below 25. Did you follow that piece of advice? Or was it too much like hard work? You had to make an effort.

We encourage our clinic clients to try our walking frame (Zimmer frame) to make their way around our therapy suites. You may have an elderly or disabled friend or relative you could borrow one from – go on, give it a try. You may find it funny but if you carry on your poor eating habits, it'll be anything but funny. You could need to get used to it for real. Yet overeating, which has got you here, is simply a learned behaviour, like reciting the alphabet or being able to drive. And you can unlearn it!

So why do you eat? Many people say it's because they're bored, depressed or lonely, like a lot of smokers. Whoever taught them (or you?) that burgers, or cream buns, or chicken curry, can be used much like a pharmaceutical drug to overcome these emotions?

Isn't it sad that the only thing we've got to do is put more food into our mouth.

Can't listen to music, can't read a book, can't go and look at the scenery, can't write a letter, can't paint a picture, it's all we can do we're that sad, that dim. There's nothing else we can do in our life but get fat and shorten our lives and become a burden on society. Wakey wakey.

All feelings and emotions are constructive. Even if they're painful, they are there to tell us something, whether good or bad – but the correct action should be taken. When the temperature light comes on on the dashboard of your car, you don't fill up with fuel. When the petrol light comes on, no-one pulls into a garage and tops up with oil. So why, when you're bored, would you even consider eating a pork pie? Wouldn't a book, or a walk, or a cinema ticket, be more appropriate?

Do you know any terrorists? Of course not, you shout. Well I bet you do! I believe the friends, family, etc., who invite you to dinner and feed you four courses plus nibbles to start with, wine with every course, cheese after, chocolates with the coffee….. these are terrorists, anarchists, causing chaos with your food choices. Terrorists, anarchists and chaos are simply little terminologies we use to identify people screwing up you and your eating habits. Who's going to set you up?

I know a Mum who will have Shepherd's Pie, Yorkshire pudding, cheesecake and the whole works ready when family arrive – she wants to feed them up, but it might give them a heart attack..... she's a diet terrorist but doesn't know it.

The terrorists are clever. They can, and often do, take on many guises. They can even disguise themselves as situations or events. I remember going back to the UK to visit my mum I'd got to the airport early. Once airside I realised I'd forgotten my glasses, just as an announcement came over the tannoy stating that the flight had been delayed for two hours. I now had three hours to kill. I was alone, with no reading glasses. At that moment I was sitting outside a bar serving drinks and snacks and in that instance the terrorists won.

If you think a dinner party you've been to was a disaster because you overate, stop and ask yourself were you there as a guest or a prisoner? Did they force you to eat? Couldn't you have said no? Would they have stopped being friends with you because you turned down their pudding? Would they shun you for not having seconds? Are they friends or just an excuse to get fat?

You go to friends for dinner and they load you up with booze, peanuts, pickles, hors d'oeuvres, canapés, crisps – all this food before you're even seated at the table. Haven't had the first course and you've undone a notch on your belt. Then they come to yours and of course guess what happens you produce twice as much, twice as fancy – the competition sets in. You've got a pound of peanuts yet you top the bowl up before it goes down too far, two litres of dip; you're scared you're not going to have enough – laden with cholesterol, recipe for a heart attack. Why do we do it?

Have you ever questioned why you have a pudding at a restaurant? No-one has two courses then orders a pudding because they're hungry. It's impossible. They may have a dessert because they're a pig, or because they want to get fat, or maybe they want to get some of their money back on their medical insurance when they have a cardiac arrest. But hunger's definitely not the issue. Do you wake in the morning starving? Why not? After 14 hours without food you should.

If you're faced with choices and struggling, ...Just walk outside and think 'do I actually want chips and roast potatoes and Yorkshire pudding', do anything just to slow the situation down..... go outside and think about it, press the pause button, then go back in....

Addicts, which is what many overweight people are, confuse thoughts like Want vs Need. They will say they really really need a pork pie. Really, they need a pork pie about as much as they need terminal lung cancer. They may want the pork pie, but they certainly don't need it. They (you?) think in the here and now, use words like could, should, try. All these words are just licences to fail.

What do you think motivates you more? The pleasure of losing weight, or the pleasure of eating the chocolate cake? The decision may be made in a split second. The pleasure of the chocolate cake will last a couple of minutes at most; being slimmer will last for ever. Eating the chocolate cake is a TLE – a Time Limited Experience.

What tastes do you really like? Maybe you think it's a strange question, but it really interests me. Let me explain. You see I really like red wine. Ask anyone who knows me – they'll confirm! Then a doctor friend of mine arranged a little test which made me question my tastes. He opened a bottle of my favourite red to have with dinner which was excellent. Then the next morning at breakfast he gave me a large glass of the same wine. Not a very pleasant experience at all. We talked about why red wine could taste excellent at 7pm and awful at 7am – what if anything changed?

We then went to a wonderful Italian restaurant for lunch. He asked me if I liked pasta – 'Yes', I replied. I ordered a pasta dish with a Bolognese sauce. That evening when back at his house he cooked a cupful of pasta in clean boiling water and served it to me for dinner. Just pasta cooked in water. Not that nice really; try it sometime. His view was that very few people actually like pasta per se, most people love the small serving of sauce that is with it. So why not just eat the sauce he said – no starch that way, he figured.......

Summary

- Meals that matter and meals that don't
- You have to re-train the subconscious over a period of time
- Everything starts with a thought.
- Food is better wasted in the bin than added to your waist
- Watch out for terrorists and anarchists
- Use your Pause Button

18

JOH'S STORY

A personable and articulate bilingual legal assistant, Joh lives with her husband and 5 year old son. She last lost weight in the run-up to her wedding nearly eight years ago.

"In the last ten years or so, I think that I have been around a size 14/16", she says, "and at 5´3" it was too much for my liking. So I was pretty much always on/falling off a diet of some sort. I could yo yo anywhere between 10 and 13 stone. As long as I can remember I have been the biggest in my group of friends..... quite sporty at school but I still felt big.

"When I got married in 2002, I decided to do something about my weight and lost 2 stone doing a horrid Atkins type diet.... it worked very effectively to get the weight off but as soon as the wedding was over, weight crept back on, then there was pregnancy then it felt out of control again. Last summer I reached 13 stone and wasn't fitting into anything so I'd reached desperation point again, and that was when I heard about Martin and Marion, and the G*m*B therapy.

She explains the common feeling so many overweight people have – almost a terror - about cameras: "I realised that I wasn't in any family photos with my son and had the awful dread that one day he'd say 'Where were you?' I couldn't come up with any before photographs with the family because I would say 'no, delete it' and so my poor son is going to wonder where his mother was for the first five years of his life. There's one 'permissible' photo at his christening; that's about it. They're either of my husband and son, or my son on his own.

"I was so self conscious that I hated being photographed and days out at the beach, pool etc were horrendous. Being in Spain didn't help..... it's difficult to buy bigger sizes and most of the women I know are tiny so I constantly felt like I was the odd one out and it really got me down..... I then went out less, and made excuses all the time to avoid big occasions...... weddings were the worst! I felt ugly and unattractive."

Joh's contact with Martin and Marion came about by chance. "A family member was having treatment", she explains. "I contacted Martin about something, and he then told me about the Gastric *mind* Band treatment."

"I never actually considered the surgical gastric band, but although this wasn't really a last resort, I think that I would have just carried on in denial and got more unhappy...... but I wanted to change desperately.... I just felt that I needed an outside helping hand! - If that makes sense?"

She describes her small group of closest girlfriends as classic yo-yo dieters. "I was on holiday with them at the time the biggest I'd ever been, feeling quite uncomfortable, and they said G*m*B's too good to be true" she explains. "At the same time I knew I was completely out of control with my eating at the time – I was actually eating more on that holiday. My best friend later said to me if I hadn't done something about it she would have said something to me – she said I was almost in an eating contest with myself at the time.

There was nothing particularly to make me be like that – maybe I was just ready for a change. So I made the decision to come and find out about it; I was still quite sceptical.

"My husband's been very supportive. He's made it very clear it doesn't bother him. I think it would bother him if I got extremely large, but even at a 16 I still had a shape. It didn't affect us personally my weight going up and down – though it affected my confidence. I'd spend 10 times as long getting ready to go out, sometimes throw a strop or whatever.

Going through Gastric *mind* Band therapy wasn't an easy financial decision. My husband and I spoke about it and it feels like a frivolous expenditure – part of you knows if you put less food in your mouth you won't be overweight. But I'd got to the point where I couldn't do it by myself. I don't know why, because normally I'm quite a controlled person. In many of my areas of my life I'm very good at that. I smoked for a while but then decided to stop and one day I stopped.

"Thinking about it since then – you don't have to smoke ever again if you don't want to. Nor drink nor take drugs. But with food you still have to eat so you have to learn to make good choices three times a day for the rest of your life. I know I can be very wilful and very controlled – I'd done diets where you're practically allowed nothing for weeks on end and the weight dropped off me; but of course it had an end. Either I'd gone to that wedding, that event, got into that dress – as soon as that event was over, the weight was straight back on again and more.

So how has the therapy worked for Joh? She's no doubt about that: "Absolutely it's worked," she says "..... I've lost 42lb to date and I'm still losing", says Joh.... and she is quite adamant that the Gastric *mind* Band element played a part in the success of the treatment. "It is a big part in the beginning as a kick start of the mental process", she says, "but surprisingly I have found the counselling is the thing that has kept me motivated. I think that people who would have the actual gastric band operation would lose weight as a result of a physical restriction but I am thrilled that I have lost and am maintaining the weight loss as a result of a mental restriction....it gives me a feeling that I have never had before... that I am not scared to eat or be around food as I can control it."

Martin, as we know, is quite blunt in his approach to obesity and weight management. We asked if that came across in therapy. "Very much so....." Joh laughed, "But I think that I respond better to straight talking, and it also helped that he had had a problem with food too."

So does she think the process has changed her? "I am more confident, less defensive, less defeatist.... before when I dieted I had no doubt that I could lose the weight but always felt it was temporary... like

I knew that I would always let myself down later and put it back on...... this time I feel different. I don't have that dread."

Has the weight loss process been hard? Easy? Joh explains: "My first weigh in was a small loss, then it gathered momentum and I started to lose more and more ..... the weight loss gave me motivation to lose more.

"It's been fairly consistent. I'm happy with the way that it has come off; before I always wanted the quick fix and this time, as a result of the treatment, I have been happier to be on a longer road moving in the right direction..... I have plateaued, but as long as I have been moving forward that's been OK...... before, a plateau would have been an excuse to go eat some biscuits!!!! I've passed my target weight now and am still losing although much more slowly now... but that's OK...... because I don't feel restricted or 'on a diet'..... "

If she'd wanted to, would she have been able to 'override' the Gastric *mind* Band? "I think it's possible..... I have been in bad moods and thought 'sod it' and tried to overeat and managed to eat a bit more than I would normally since the treatment, but I end up feeling rotten (physically) and thinking 'That really wasn't worth it, was it?'..... stupid really.

"For me, getting back on track without a problem has been the best part of the treatment! Every time I've been on a diet before I have had one bad day, that led to a week and then the scales either don't show a drop or actually show a slight increase and I'd think 'that's that, I've ruined it'......

"This time if I feel I've overdone it a bit (and my husband says that I never overeat like I used to even when I feel like I've really pigged out), I just know that I have to even things up...... sounds ridiculously obvious doesn't it? Before I would have just kept overdoing things ... now I know that if I eat less the next day or up my exercise that I have no reason to gain weight for one night out...... it's a revelation to me!!!!

"Joking aside....... I can do it now....... I just couldn't before."

We asked Joh if she thought her eating patterns had changed from the way they were before? "They were pretty standard before, I think" she says. "I ate when I was bored at home, I ate when I was stressed. I thought that I was fat and almost too far gone to bother... the yo-yoing was so utterly depressing and so not to run the risk of gaining weight again...I didn't bother trying, even though that doesn't make sense.

"The change for me came in a session with Martin when he said 'You just concentrate on losing it and I will take the responsibility of making sure that you don't put it back on...it's not something you have to worry about'... It's weird but with that "weight" off my shoulders, I thought 'I'll do it again and we'll see' ..... I wasn't sure that I believed it but I have to say that all this way down the line, he seems to be right!"

And what did Joh make of the actual Gastric *mind* Band part of the therapy? "It's odd. Honestly, in my mind, I know that I have not had the gastric band fitted..... but I cannot act like before even if I want to.

"I didn't wake and believe that I had been operated on to the extent that I was checking my stomach etc..... but the results speak for themselves. I might not have believed it in my conscious mind but something has definitely changed in my subconscious I guess...... my feeling now is that it doesn't matter whether you believe in the operation or not.... the results happen anyway.

—

I'm not scared to be around food any more – it doesn't control me, I control it

—

"I was a generous 14, maybe a 16. I'm now below target. My target was 10st 4lb, and I'm now 9st 6lb. I had a target, that was what I was the day I got married. I had it in my head – I was very happy with myself, it was a very happy memory that I had and I didn't have any kind of crisis about what I put on at that time in my life. I thought if I could try to get back to that it would be ideal for me. But when I got to 10st 4lb, because of the lifestyle change that I've now got, the weight was still coming off without me having to do too much so I thought maybe that isn't the natural weight that my body would be happy with.

"As an adult I'd never been below 10st 4lb. When I was still living at home with my parents, 16 or 17, I was up around 11st, 11st 5lb, and I can remember being at that weight for quite a while then when I got married it was the slimmest I'd been in my adult life. Now – my weight's never been this low in my adult life at all.

"Not that I'm desperate to lose a lot more weight, because I'm perfectly happy with the way things are at the moment. It's just that I'm probably even more conscious of my size now, if that's possible. I think when you're a bigger person, and you've been that way most of your adult life you think you'll be perfectly happy just to get into a size 12 or whatever, or be a particular weight that from where you are, you think is really low.... But when you get there it becomes more realistic to think it wouldn't hurt to lose a bit more."

Joh's experienced the sense of weight discrimination in her professional life: "When I worked as an actress, being a bigger person was part of my character" she says. "I never got the leading lady stuff, I was always the friend, or whatever. You sort of accept who you are. And it's not that I was 100% happy, or confident, being bigger.... Now that I'm slimmer I've changed my sphere of reference. Someone called me small recently, and I've never been called small. People don't directly say you're overweight, do they – they might say you've got a round face, or you look well, or that's a nice handbag, or talk about other things not directly related to your weight so as to avoid it.

"At drama college, they kind of make you believe that everything's possible – you can be Lady Macbeth if you really want it. And that you can be the leading lady. But when you get out looking for work, doing auditions day in day out, you know after a while they go 'no' and it's absolutely on physical appearance. But I worked that to my advantage. I worked in comedy....

"I did theatre work and a lot of touring work, and I did most of my comedy work on cruise ships, that and presenting, which was great. I was able to get away with being a bit more risqué with the kind of comedy I was doing because people weren't threatened by me physically. You've got Dawn French, Jo Brand, Victoria Wood, all of those people were my heroes when I was growing up – of course I admired them for their talent but also maybe I wonder if I had some aspiration to be like them because they were accepted as they were because they were larger."

Brutally honest about her battle with her weight, Joh considers there's always doubt about the future. "I think when you've had a problem with weight it's very difficult; I'd love to have 100% confidence and say I'll never go back again. But there's a little part of me that worries - because I've always put the weight back on before. But it's been a completely different scenario this time. I've lost the weight more slowly this time, and a lot more healthily. Before where I would have found it frustrating losing weight slowly, this time I've thought 'OK it's only a pound, but I'm a pound lighter than last week.'

"Now I realise I had a lot of sabotaging thoughts before – I'd eat more when friends visited then be unable to stop when they went back, and be furious with myself. Since then I've had friends visiting and I can still go out and have a nice time, and try everything but it's the amount. I don't even eat a quarter of the amount."

Her new understanding of portion control has definitely helped, she says. "In the beginning I didn't quite trust myself with portion control – though it's essentially common sense. But with the pictures of portion sizes it's much easier. Now I don't need to do that. I don't eat when I'm not hungry and I eat until I'm full and no more. If I overeat I know I have to maybe eat less the following day, or even – and this was unheard of before – if I know I've got an event coming up when I might possibly eat more than I would on a daily basis, I will be careful a few days before. And that's not me at all!

"The motivation has definitely crept up on me….of course since I knew the amount of calories I needed to consume every day to lose weight, Marion also pointed out that if I did exercise, either I could eat more or I'd lose weight faster!"

So she was someone who chose to increase her calorie use as well as keep an eye on her intake? "To start with I preferred the thought of eating less than doing exercise! Now I exercise in front of the telly with a DVD. I move all the furniture, put my stuff on, sweat buckets, run around and look a complete idiot but I do it. I'd be mortified if anybody came to the door – but I do it four or five times a week, and that motivation has definitely grown. It's thinking like a person who isn't controlled by food. A slim person doesn't think 'oh I don't want to do any exercise.' It might not be something they particularly love doing, but it's something they know is a necessary part of being the way they want to be, it's something they've got to do. Like brushing your teeth. There are times I don't want to do it, but I bypass that now, put my stuff on and do it and feel great.

"There are times I think I could possibly push it and overeat if I wanted to, but I don't really want to. Because I'm a very controlling person, in my conscious mind after the G*m*B session I knew obviously I hadn't had the procedure. My conscious mind was saying 'no you haven't'. But because I'd started to lower my portion sizes before the 'band' was fitted, I was already eating a smaller amount so I didn't really test it to begin with. But then later I found I couldn't overeat. I have actually been sick.

"At Christmas I think I must have tried to overeat and I did actually get to the point I was feeling quite ill, the food wouldn't go down and yes I was sick. It was a very powerful demonstration, especially because I was very sceptical. Part of me was always a little bit unsure, but now it has made a big change which I can't explain which infuriates me because it's been so subtle.

"I think I'd reached a point where I was desperate, or unhappy, with the way things were going and there's a part of the therapy – the CBT – which I found very helpful. The imagery of standing at the fork in the road. I could go down one way, the way you're used to, the way you eat, regret it, see how you look, feel unattractive, know this could go on for years, feel depressed.. all visualised with son and husband at your side. It was such a horrible image. (* *author's note…*

just to illustrate how powerful the subconscious imagery can be....... I hope Joh won't mind me saying she was in tears even re-living this for our taped conversation) Then you go back to the crossroads and you have the option to go the other way.

"It's harder – it's not a miracle, wand-waving kind of thing. A friend said she'd love to have that done and not have to do anything and I told her it's not like that. You have to be committed to it. Keep yourself focussed and motivated. I think if I were to get to the point of wanting to 'fall off the wagon', that imagery is so strong and the positive reaction I felt looking at the other side as well would make a difference. Very much so.

"I can remember Martin asking me if I'd considered the health risks of being overweight. I hadn't. In all my time of feeling fat and frumpy and not being able to feel socially acceptable, the health risks came really low down on the list of priorities and now I'm quite disgusted that they did because I owe it to my son to be healthy and have that kind of pride in myself and I need to show him. He's going to have learned behaviour. If he sees that not only Daddy goes out running but Mummy does exercise too and we don't eat crap at home......"

She sees that her weight issues affected other relationships too. "I'm aware that probably my relationships with women were affected by the way I felt about my weight and the way I saw myself and the way I saw them. I always felt a bit insignificant, a bit as if nobody would ever say anything complimentary about me in terms of my physical appearance. That was quite upsetting. But now I don't feel that. I met family I hadn't seen for donkey's years, and they were saying I looked well and this time I didn't take that as meaning big and fat!

"I'm finding that I'm much more open to social relationships. I think obviously my husband notices I don't have crises like I used to, however even though I'm three and a bit stone lighter than I was, I say to him 'Do you think I'm getting fatter, are you sure my tummy's not getting bigger?' And he says 'No don't be an idiot!'"

—

If you can feel a craving below your neck, that is actual hunger. From the neck up, chances are you're not hungry at all - it's a craving. It's not an emergency!

—

Joh's attitude to food and drink looks to have changed fundamentally in quite a short period. "My normal thing now," she says, "would be if I think I feel hungry, have a glass of water, wait a bit and see if I still am. But it's not an emergency. It's not something you have to act on immediately! As an overweight person, you tend to feel that you think I must have a cake, I must stop what I'm doing immediately, get one now........

—

I always thought I might lose weight but I'll never look slim because I've had a big chest but now I've lost it all over... It's made my husband less happy though!

—

Apart from the expense of a new wardrobe, Joh reckons there aren't any downsides. And even needing new clothes isn't a downside because it's fun! "For me I don't think there are any negatives", she says. "Positives – well too many to try to explain. Things come up on a daily basis. It's made me much more positive."

"I think everything you learn as part of the process although it may be painful to admit it because there have been things you've been deluding yourself about, home truths, they're all difficult to swallow at the beginning. But once you can deal with that and look at it from a positive viewpoint, which is very much where this process is different from diets I've done; I've reached the point of being very unhappy and disappointed, and feeling unworthy. And that's no place to start a positive change in your life. You shouldn't start anything because you hate the way you are."

"Pride comes into it. I think I have more pride in myself now. Being able to be proud not only of what I've achieved, but of not being insignificant."

So having seen the changes possible with the Gastric *mind* Band, just how close did Joh come to having weight loss surgery? "I hadn't got to the point of actually considering surgery, she says. "I'm a bit of a coward about anything like that so I probably wouldn't have gone that far. But I think I was running out of options. I'd done this diet and that, they hadn't worked. You name it I'd tried it. I thought 'I've either got to do this and it's going to work' or I have to face the possibility that I'm going to stay like this.

"Maybe that's why the crossroads visualisation worked so well for me. Seeing, feeling, where I'd be in a year if I hadn't made the change. I'd pretty much got to the point I thought if I don't do something now I don't think I'm going to be able to make the change. Which is crazy because you can always change....

"I can remember being on diets before and forcing myself to go the gym, and if it got to a month on the diet or at the gym and I considered I hadn't lost enough to be sufficient recompense for the work I'd put in, that'd be it. I'd think 'there's no point; obviously I'm going to be fat no matter what I do', and I'm going to give it all up and go and console myself with a packet of biscuits.' That was probably the biggest difference for me. There are 365 days in the year, three meals in the day."

Joh recognises so well the mindset of many overweight people: "I'm 3 stone overweight I want to lose it in 12 weeks..... But you didn't put it on in 12 weeks. You're so desperate you forget that. "You're willing to put yourself and your body through all these extreme things. Looking back now it seems so ridiculous. I'm quite cross with myself that I put up with that kind of ridiculous behaviour – my own stupid behaviour, of course - and endured it for so long.

"If you were told that sugar gave you an allergic reaction, you came out in massive hives on your skin, you wouldn't eat it. But knowing that we're putting on fat by eating too much isn't enough for us," Joh laughs.

"I've got a very strong visual image of my lovely sister in law a couple of years ago. Us on a beach. Me with my little boy, the classic of everyone saying let's have a photo. Me with lilos and small child in front of me, she comes bounding over the beach, running towards me in this yellow bikini looking fabulous, she was a member of my extended family, not some horrendous person – and there I was, thinking 'right you've completely ruined my day, I'm going to end up feeling rubbish and I didn't feel great before but now you've put the tin lid on it. Thank you very much'. It was almost laying the blame on her. But it's not her fault she looks after herself!

—

It's almost as if I didn't like to admit I needed help

—

So when it comes to the crunch, what part does Joh think the 'band' element has played? "I can remember one part of the operation under hypnosis….. I remember snatches but not the whole thing ….. I can remember something touched my hand at about the time I was 'having the pre-med' and I actually jumped.

"When I came out I didn't believe it, I almost feel like a bit of a traitor saying that. I understand that the gastric band element is the hook. It's the thing that catches people's imagination but for me it was by quite a long way NOT the most significant part of the process."

Joh says her eating habits changed almost immediately after the first session, and to begin with she was ultra-strict on herself, doing a lot of controlling in her conscious mind.

"For me it was never an issue about losing weight – I always felt I could lose it…" she says. "I remember Martin saying I didn't have to consider the fear about putting it back on again. I just had to think what I was doing. He would make sure I didn't put it back on again.

"Now I have the information and the knowledge; though of course I probably already had it. It's wrapped up in a way I can relate to. I can remember one time Martin said in answer to me bemoaning something in my life, 'Well boo hoo. What are you going to do about it, are you going to spend the rest of your life worrying about that or are you going to draw a line and move forward?' I'd felt I had a right to feel like that and in one fell swoop he said 'get over yourself'. Well to be honest that was what I needed!

Joh's problem, she says, was snacking, picking at food. "No matter what it was. Not particularly sweet or savoury, I used to just pick at anything. Boredom. Even though I was aware I shouldn't be doing it. I try now not to eat between meals. Sometimes I fancy something, but I'm capable of eating one biscuit now, if I want to. And for me that's **so** not normal. If there are crisps around, or my little boy's eating something I'd normally have fancied, I'm now able to resist eating any.

"If I go out with a friend and she has cheesecake for dessert, and says do you want some, I'm able to say no, I don't want any. Maybe because I'd eaten sufficient with the main course, maybe because the cheesecake is just a load of excess calories sitting on a plate. And it doesn't feel like a hardship to say no to it. Before I'd have thought I can't have it because I'm horrible and fat – or eaten it and felt immediately hideous because I shouldn't have. Whereas today I could have eaten it but chose not to and I don't feel bad. I've never felt bad at any part of losing this weight.

"And if I had had that cheesecake I wouldn't have felt bad either. If I'd thought 'well I've done my DVD I can afford to have some' or thought it looks nice I'll try it, I'd probably have had a couple of spoons just to try it. Whereas before I'd probably have had the whole portion."

—

Cheesecake is just a load of excess calories sitting on a plate

—

Joh's final words? "It was a revelation to me to eat the things I like first off a plate, and only eat the things I like less if I've still got room….. simple!"

Joh's observations are truly compulsive; no punches pulled thinking not a million miles from Martin's own. "I do think there are overweight people who say they are 100% happy in their skin", she says. "I think if that's true, bloody great. Fabulous. I know I wasn't. If you're not you can't just moan about it. If you've got something you don't like and want to change it, why don't you."

Summary

- **Be clear what your reasons are**
- **You can stop being scared of being around food once you learn to control it rather than it control you**
- **Don't be frustrated at losing weight slowly – every pound lost is a pound less than you were before**
- **Eat less, move more**
- **Try picturing fat- and sugar-filled foods as excess calories on a plate**

19

SESSION 4
THE GASTRIC *mind* BAND

The fourth of the main sessions is the one in which the Gastric *mind* Band itself is implanted into the subconscious mind using hypnosis.

Before getting to this stage, you should have developed a clear idea not only of how you became overweight in the first place, but also why you want to get rid of it and what tools you're going to use to achieve this. The imagery of 'implanting' a Gastric *mind* Band is there to back the whole process up, to give you another, final, tool in your toolbox.

This is the last main session, so a bit like with a surgical gastric band, the process is reaching the point where it becomes 'all up to you'.

Some of this session you'll have read elsewhere in the book, but it does no harm to repeat things if it helps you learn how to change your flawed relationship with food, now does it!

Reading this chapter will add the finishing touch to your journey towards shedding your excess weight. You will have your own way of imagining a tightening, or shrinking, of your stomach. As you read, keep reminding yourself the size of the smaller 'pouch' sized capacity you are aiming to achieve for your stomach..... think of a golf ball. Get one if you can. Hold it in your hand as you read this chapter.

Just before that, though, let's take another last look at the surgical gastric band.

A typical adult stomach measures about 12in long by 6in at its widest point, and holds around 4 cups (32 fl oz, or 1 litre) of food and liquid. The whole purpose of the gastric band is to restrict the amount of food a person can physically eat at one sitting, by reducing the capacity of their stomach. The band works on the same principle as a cable tie, with a one-way locking catch. It is wrapped around the outside of the top part of the stomach and clicked into place, and because the stomach is soft, this has the effect of pulling the tie tight, almost like a drawstring bag, creating a small pouch in the upper section of the stomach – this is literally about the size of a golf ball.

Once the gastric band is fitted, whatever food is eaten simply gathers in the pouch, and as soon as this is full, then the person experiences the feeling of fullness (though higher up in the abdomen than usual) and cannot physically cram any more food in. The size of a meal someone with a gastric band can eat is only around six tablespoons of food on the plate, compared with a meal size of around two clenched fists which it would take to fill a normal capacity stomach.

The food then very slowly 'drip feeds' through the narrow opening at the bottom of the stomach pouch, and passes into the lower part of the stomach, where the digestive enzymes in the stomach acid break it all down, so it can then pass through the intestines in the normal way. So basically, the person feels full after eating just a very small amount of food, and then they will stay feeling satisfied for a long time afterwards, because it takes so long for all the food to filter down through the narrow gap.

If you imagine eating such a small amount of food without having the band in place, firstly you wouldn't actually feel very satisfied, but also you would start to feel hungry again in a short time, because the food would be able to pass relatively quickly through the stomach and into the intestines. The band simply slows down the whole process and allows the person to feel very satisfied on a tiny amount of food. Just as it is designed to do.

An overweight person will be used to eating larger than necessary portions of food, and their stomach will be over-stretched – it can stretch up to three times normal size. And of course this means they have a big hole to fill every time they eat! Then after the surgery things change drastically.....

From eating vast quantities before the operation, the person then has to get used to a typical portion size of literally around six tablespoons; on top of that they have to take mouthfuls no bigger than the size of the rubber on the end of a pencil, or roughly like the nail on your little finger. Then each mouthful has to be chewed at least 10 times before it can be swallowed, otherwise the food particles will be too big to pass through the pouch opening, so the food will sit there causing a blockage until it ends up making a sudden reappearance, as the body rejects it! They even have a special name for this phenomenon – it's called suffering from 'productive burping'. How nice!

So the actual surgery is all pretty drastic really – what a difference going from gulping down massive portions of food, shovelling it in as fast as possible, chewing a couple of times and it's gone; to suddenly taking forever to eat tiny amounts of food in mousetrap sized pieces and chewing it to death!

With G*m*B therapy, it doesn't need to be anywhere near as drastic as with the surgical band. You're obviously going to be eating a lot less than you were before, but it doesn't need to be as little as six tablespoons of food per meal. You'll be eating sensible, normal quantities, rather than eating too much. That's the difference. Take smaller bites, chew it properly, eat more slowly and concentrate on what you're eating. Notice the taste of your food and appreciate it. You may even find your tastes will seem to change. Maybe you'll notice that you no longer like foods you really thought you were enjoying before.

If you don't enjoy something, what's the point in eating it? Tell yourself: 'It's full of empty calories, it's processed, it's not doing my body any good, and on top of that, I'm not even enjoying it anyway – why am I bothering?

Try allowing some different healthy foods, such as fresh fruit, to spend longer in your mouth than usual. Savour the flavour, chew properly, eat slowly, and the taste just gets better and better – especially if it's a fruit you really enjoy! It's almost as if you can feel it doing you good. Now do the same thing with a food that is full of 'empty calories'. Be honest with yourself: You don't really get that same feeling you get with the fruit; if you let a piece of cream cake linger in your mouth for example. What you might find is that it starts to taste a bit too sickly sweet, and then the grease starts to coat the roof of your mouth....Is that really such a pleasant experience for you? My guess is probably not!

Having the gastric band fitted does not teach you how to eat normally. It's what's going on in your head that controls everything, and if your head isn't sorted out properly, then you will find ways to cheat on the band.

Not only is the surgical procedure cheatable, but it also carries a certain risk of death – around 1 in 2000 people will die as a result of going for the operation. Now, if you imagine somebody selling you a lottery ticket with a 1 in 2000 chance of winning, you'd want to buy quite a few, wouldn't you – after all, those odds are pretty good. Suddenly, though, when it's your life you're talking about, maybe you should be thinking: 'No, hang on a minute. I don't know if I want to take that risk.'

We had a lady who'd gone to her doctor about having a gastric band fitted. They did all the medical checks and in the end the doctor turned round and said to her that she wasn't overweight enough to qualify for this operation on the NHS. "You would need to be about another stone (14lb) heavier than you are now and then you would qualify". She went home and thought "Well if I eat all the rubbishy things I can think of for the next few weeks I can go back and I'll have put a stone on. Then I'll qualify to have the operation." Luckily she came to her senses and thought, "My God, what am I doing?" and that's when she heard about us and came here instead. If you read the national press this situation is far from unique.

You see, you get this idea in your head and you think it's totally logical. It's only afterwards you say to yourself "What was I thinking of?" The idea of putting weight on to enable you to take part in a weight reduction procedure is ridiculous. Of course, when the person has the operation, the first three weeks before they have it they're going to be following a strict diet anyway. So they're just putting on weight to take it off again soon afterwards!

After gastric band surgery, you have to change your eating habits in more ways than one. You're advised to eat your food in a certain order – for example choosing the meat first, because you have to chew it thoroughly, which takes time – and also the meat will stay in the pouch for a long time. Then vegetables are next in line, as they will sit on top of the meat in the pouch; soft, mushy things like mashed potato have to be saved until last. If you ate the meal in reverse order, then the food would pass through the pouch easily and you'd be able to eat more, which of course defeats the whole object of having the band fitted in the first place!

Using your visualisation of a golf-ball sized pouch to help you, you'll find it relatively easy to cut back your portion sizes.

It's only healthy solid food that needs chewing that gets restricted by the gastric band. Things that can be reduced to liquid consistency very easily – things like chocolate, ice cream – typical comfort foods – will actually pass through the band very easily.

—

Having the gastric band fitted does not teach you how to eat normal food normally. It takes you away from normality; you haven't developed a relationship with normal food. It's what's going on in your head that controls everything.

—

Chocolate milk shake for example – no problem at all – suck that down as if the band wasn't there! You can get away with it! People can and do cheat on the band! In the end it's just another diet really – a pretty invasive way of doing a diet, but it is one. You've got a list of rules and regulations and things you're supposed to do and things you're not supposed to do and if you choose to follow the rules it will work for you. But if you choose to cheat on it and get round it and break the rules, you can. And it's not going to work!

If someone is a comfort eater, makes the wrong choices, eats food at the wrong time and has the operation, they will wake up afterwards and nothing will have actually changed. They are still going to be a comfort eater, they're still going to eat the wrong food at the wrong times and make the wrong choices. The band won't actually stop them from doing that. They still have to make that effort to be aware of what they are eating and why.

—

If the patient is pretty much at the stage where they're killing themselves anyway, you can just about see that this is something that could help them in conjunction with therapy. On its own it's far from guaranteed. A 70% success rate tells you that.
However, you need to be in control yourself.

—

The gastric band operation is not foolproof. It's not 100% guaranteed. A lot of people don't seem to realise that. They think that it's this magic wand, it's 100% guaranteed, it will solve everything, and they are not going to have to make any changes or put any effort in because the band will do it all for them. The reality of it is very different. It only has a success rate of about 70% in the end. About a third of people who have the operation will get round it and cheat on it. It is just like another diet. It doesn't sort out what is going on in your head.

Another thing that people will do – this is really gross – if they are into fast food, the burgers, the fries and everything else – of course you can't eat the solid food in vast quantities, but you can have the liquid form. So what do they do? They get the burger, fries, milk shake and put it all in the blender, liquidise it and drink it down. It just goes to prove how powerful your mind is. If your head is not in the right place, it can just sabotage what you want to do.

You're also advised not to eat and drink at the same time. Not drinking for anything up to an hour before and an hour after a meal is a rule which seems to vary from provider to provider, the reasons also seeming to vary:

- Liquids can help to flush food through the pouch faster, thereby making it possible to eat again sooner
- Liquids taken after food can 'settle' on top, making the contents of the pouch heavier and increasing the likelihood of stretching and band slippage
- Some patients experience vomiting if they drink during a meal

Obviously none of this applies with our Gastric *mind* Band therapy. We want eating to be an enjoyable experience, and for it to be perfectly normal to sit and have a meal and a drink at the same time. As we've said, the operation doesn't change the thinking of a comfort eater, or the way they make their choices.

In the end, if you just change your approach to food, you shouldn't actually need to have a surgical gastric band for the rest of your life. People tend to rely on the band to do everything for them, rather than relying on their own mind, so they often expect to have the band for life. And, of course, if they are not successful and don't lose weight, then it's very easy to blame it all on the band, rather than accept responsibility for their failure.

Having the operation doesn't actually help people to build up a normal, healthy relationship with food; it's just like a diet in which you end up being even more obsessed with food. You'll be forever thinking "Oh, is that mouthful too big? Did I chew that mouthful enough? Oh no, I didn't leave long enough between having a drink and eating my meal'. You're always going to be on edge.

In preparation for the operation patients are told that they have to follow quite a strict diet for about three weeks beforehand that is low in the fat, starch and sugar. The purpose of that is to get the person's liver to shrink back down to normal size, as the body reduces its glycogen stores. When somebody's seriously overeating the liver becomes really enlarged and fatty; you may have heard of people being diagnosed with having a "fatty liver" when they've been over-indulging. It's exactly like what is done to geese to make foie gras. They get hold of the goose, force-feed lots of food down its throat so that its liver swells right up, gets unnaturally large and fatty so they can make paté out of it, and people pay a fortune for it!

So that's what an overweight person's doing to their own body. The only difference is that the poor goose has no choice in the matter, whereas an overweight person is actually choosing to do it to themselves. A lot of people actually say "Oh no, I don't eat foie gras because I don't agree with the principle of what they do to the geese." But they're doing it to themselves without giving it a second thought!

OK. At this point our clients, and you, the reader, have all the tools in your toolbox. All but one.

Clench your fist. That's about the size of your stomach (or at least it would be if you hadn't stretched it through overeating). Look at it again. Not very big, is it. How on earth do you fit all that food in there when you overeat? Well the next step is to picture your stomach shrinking. Hold that golf ball in your dominant hand. Hold it and squeeze. Shut your eyes and feel the size of it. Now that's really not very big at all, is it….. but it's the size of the pouch created by a surgical gastric band and it's what you'll be visualising as your capacity for food. Squeeze it again.

Visualisation: Picturing a band being wrapped around the top of your stomach. Clenching the golf ball in your hand at the same time as you picture the band being put in place. Squeezing the ball tighter as you imagine the band finally being clicked in its final position. Feeling the golf ball as it signifies your new smaller stomach capacity; recognising the restriction on your stomach and being unable to eat as much as before. Being satisfied eating much smaller portions. Eating only in response to hunger rather than for any other reason. Making healthier eating choices. Eating more slowly and mindfully. Recognising that this is a whole new way of life.

And when you next eat, you notice the difference…………

Your stomach is located on the left side, quite high up in your abdominal cavity. So take hold of your golf ball in your dominant hand. Squeeze it. Picture your stomach shrinking in size at the same time.

In the clinic, our clients will, under hypnotherapy, go through the entire process of having a gastric band fitted in hospital; they will be 'taken' down hospital corridors, hear reassuring voices, receive all the imagery to suggest they've had sedation and anaesthetic….all under hypnosis.

If you are reading this, your motivation has carried you this far – if you want to shed your excess weight enough, you'll be working hard by now to retrain your conscious mind. And through self-hypnosis, visualising the golf ball should be enough of an image to convince your subconscious that your stomach has a smaller capacity now.

We also give clinic clients a G*m*B wristband to signify the control the *mind* Band will now be having on their everyday eating choices. You might like to get yourself a thick colourful rubber band, or a knitted/coiled string bracelet; it should fit your wrist snugly without being uncomfortable.

Now, every time you look at that band – your own *mind* Band - you'll have a tangible reminder of the changes taking place in your mind and stomach.

If you'd had surgery, your next few weeks would involve consuming soup, and nothing to get your teeth into. But without surgery there's obviously no actual band so no need.....though don't be surprised if, like some clinic clients, you experience significant restrictions in your eating following your experience of the Gastric *mind* Band procedure, as the mind is a very powerful tool. Take it gently to begin with, starting with very small portions of healthy nutritious food – which you'll almost certainly have been doing since the first session anyway, because you will have been questioning all your food choices.

But if there are times when you really do want a piece of chocolate, then just allow yourself – because this whole process is not about having forbidden foods. When you set up the idea of something forbidden, it's typical to want it more and more. Deprivation creates a stronger desire. You can eat whatever you want to eat, but always consider first whether what you choose to eat is going to help or hinder you. And above all, make sure you are definitely hungry before you eat anything – it doesn't matter whether it's a chocolate or a carrot – if you're not hungry you DON'T need it!

Everything you're doing now, all your actions, are supposed to be helping you achieve this ultimate goal, this thing that is the most important in your life, the reason why you've picked up and read this book.

If you've got this far, surely you wouldn't want to spoil it all and binge on bars of chocolate? In the end nobody is forcing you to put that food in your mouth. You are the one in control. Wouldn't you rather choose the healthy option that'll help you to slim down? You are the only one who can question why you are doing it.

Your *mind* Band Self Hypnosis is in the following section; first you might like to think about what happens once the initial G*m*B process is complete:

.....A FEW WEEKS LATER!

In the same way as you would if you'd had a surgical gastric band fitted, we suggest you have a 'post treatment' session to assess how you're progressing and if necessary adjust the 'grip' the band – in your case the *mind* Band - has on your eating habits.

You will probably have been checking your weight/measurements weekly, or possibly more often. As we've said before, beware weighing yourself too often because that can give a misleading view of what's happening in the bigger picture. Four to six weeks after you started this process is a good time to sit back and assess how much you've changed your thinking and how much this altered thinking has changed your eating. These new eating habits should in turn have had an effect on the scales; if it's not quite as fast as you'd like you could re-visit the earlier sessions and see what hit home for you the most and whether there's a way to 'tweak' your thinking still further.

What you should avoid is expecting miracles yesterday, it's been said before but it could do with repeating. Gastric *mind* Band is a life change – not a diet, not a quick cure but rather a weight management system that you design for your own way of living because everyone's different.

To help you remember.......how long did it take you to put the weight on? Getting rid of the excess weight won't be an overnight thing!

There's no point at all in doing this for a few weeks and then letting go and reverting to your old ways – although if you've read carefully from start to finish and really got the picture from your questionnaire, you'll have had the best chance of putting into practice our techniques for avoiding overeating from that point on.

If you're starting to doubt yourself and how much you've really changed, shut your eyes and take yourself back to the fork in the road. A year ahead being exactly the same as you are now, or maybe even heavier, or a year ahead having lost weight consistently and feeling good about yourself. Which makes you feel better? No question! Besides, if you've shed any of that excess weight, you should be in a better place mentally than you were a few weeks back, don't you think?

As you approach your target, you should allow yourself another period – maybe an hour, maybe a day – frankly, whatever time you need - for reflecting on how your life, your eating habits, your choices, have changed and what a difference it's made to your life. There's every chance you'll have altered all the patterns of your attitude to food in such a way that you realise you don't really need to think about it. You're there. Not necessarily at target – but then target is what you make it. But certainly you're a different eater. Probably a different shopper. Maybe even a different person. But you're the person you've always known you could be yet until now hadn't found the motivation to be.

At target and beyond

When they reach their target weight, Elite clients are invited to return for a final session of hypnotherapy to 'release' the grip of the Gastric *mind* Band in the same way that surgical gastric band patients would have some saline removed from the band. This enables the person to start eating the right amount of food to maintain their weight rather than to continue to reduce it.

You, having read the book and started on your journey to shed your excess weight, will be taking sole responsibility for your own follow-up, and you may very well be the best person to do so!

If you're shedding, or have finished shedding, your excess weight, you need only re-read the book from time to time (or those bits which caught your imagination most powerfully).

Allow yourself a self-hypnosis session every so often, choosing as your Positive Thoughts those elements of your journey which mean the most to you. Whether it's something you feel particularly proud to have achieved, or something you're aware is a weak point, it's up to you. But every time you reinforce what you've learned, your subconscious is a stronger ally in your journey to be and remain a healthy weight.

Summary

- **Your subconscious should begin to help you notice a restriction in your stomach capacity**
- **Eating smaller quantities will come naturally**
- **To maintain your loss, read re-read and keep re-reading. You know it makes sense!**

SESSION FOUR
SELF HYPNOSIS

In the first self-hypnosis session we explained how, with the motivation for change, you can yourself provide a boost to the subconscious by relaxing yourself deeply. If you want to remind yourself before proceeding, you will find the section near the end of Chapter 10.

Please note that self-hypnosis should never be practised when driving, operating machinery or carrying out any other activity that requires your full attention

For this session it will help if you can have a golf ball with you.

Read your Positive Thoughts and make sure you feel completely focussed on what you are trying to achieve before you set about relaxing, so you don't have to 'wake up' to refer to notes or remind yourself what you meant to concentrate on. It's the subconscious you want to target, and that is best addressed when deeply relaxed.

Choose up to 3 suggestions from the list that are relevant and appropriate and read and revise them. You need to be able to repeat them to yourself mentally at least 3 times. They are your 'mantra', the messages to your subconscious to change your behaviour for life, starting now.

If there are more than 3 appropriate suggestions, then you can alternate and choose a different set each time you do this session.

You now need to 'talk' yourself into a state of deep relaxation.

Pick a spot (real or imaginary) on the wall or ceiling in front of you so you have to raise your eyes slightly in order to fix your gaze on it. Keep staring at the spot and mentally repeat to yourself at least three times "As I count from 5 down to 1, my eyelids are feeling heavier and heavier and when I get to 1 my eyes will close and I will completely relax."

Then slowly, mentally count down from 5 to 1, taking a deep breath in between each number. As you reach the number 1, close your eyes and allow yourself to let go and relax.

Now starting either with the tips of your toes, or the top of your head, focus your attention on each part of your body in turn, and gradually release all the stress and tension and relax every muscle one by one, while mentally repeating to yourself, "Relax", "Let go", "Deeper and deeper relaxed".

Then imagine a beautiful staircase with 10 steps leading down to a special place where you will feel totally safe, comfortable and relaxed. (It can be anywhere you want it to be, whether its a country garden, a tropical, deserted beach, or just your own bedroom).

Now count down from 10 to 1 and when you get to 1 picture yourself in your special, private, safe place. Spend a few moments allowing yourself to experience all the sensations, familiarising yourself with any sights, sounds, smells, feelings and tastes. The more senses you bring in to the visualisation, the stronger the experience will be.

This is the start of a brand new life for you and you're so carried away with all those wonderful, positive feelings that you hardly notice yourself pick up the golf ball in your dominant hand… squeeze that golf ball in your hand, really focussing your attention on the size and dimensions of your stomach much, much smaller – the size of that ball. Squeeze again and become aware of a tightening feeling in your stomach now. Picture in your mind's eye a band being wrapped around the top of your stomach. The tightening feeling is much stronger now, and you can picture how your stomach's been reduced in size.

For session four, your key points will be:

- You know your brand new life starts now
- You're on your journey to becoming permanently slimmer and healthier
- Your excess weight, which you're going to get rid of, has been weighing you down and holding you back from being the person you really want to be.

- Your lifestyle now will include smaller portions of food, total control of your weight and size.
- Thinking about this is relaxing and not at all stressful – you are confident, positive, and full of excitement about how your life is changing for the better.
- Your golf ball in your hand is going to help you identify just how much smaller your stomach capacity is going to be.
- You are now more aware of your stomach as if you were having gastric band surgery – squeezing the golf ball helps you focus your attention on the size of your stomach in the past and now.
- You can picture how your stomach's been reduced in size.
- The more you squeeze the ball the tighter your stomach feels.
- You will find that just a small amount of food is all you want and need to eat at each meal, though you feel totally satisfied.
- If you try to eat more food than you need your stomach will feel very uncomfortable. If you stop eating, you'll feel more comfortable and completely satisfied.
- Food is no longer a comfort or an emotional crutch, it's a source of nourishment and nothing more
- You can adjust your 'golf ball' when you choose, shedding your excess weight at a rate to suit you
- This is a permanent way of life
- You're now ready to start your new healthy life

Now..... Count yourself up from 1-5 suggesting that you have enjoyed a wonderful relaxation and on 5 you will open your eyes, feeling refreshed and energised.

If you decide to do your self-hypnosis before going to sleep, you can suggest that on 5 you will move into a normal and natural sleep... until it is time for you to wake.

20

OR WOULD YOU RATHER HAVE A TAPEWORM?

Did you know one of the current fad weight loss systems involves eating a portion of a UV and antibiotic-treated beef tapeworm known as a cyst, and allowing it to grow for nearly three months in the intestinal tract? A modern fad? No, actually a very old practice dating back well over 100 years - some research suggests as far back as Elizabethan times. It causes weight loss because it secretes proteins that affect how efficiently the host human can digest their food – but it targets specific nutrients/calories that it needs to develop (some people report getting cravings for specific foods while hosting a tapeworm). After nearly three months you take a medicine to kill the worm and have to have a month's rest before considering a follow-up 'course'.

Possible side effects range from abdominal pain and nausea to constipation, diarrhoea and intestinal perforation. On top of all that, as with all 'diets' or fad weight loss techniques, there is no guarantee that any weight lost will remain lost unless there is a significant change in eating habits – and it costs around $1000, too!

The first gastric band was a tapeworm - Elizabethan times - it's not even a new concept!

Do you think giraffes eat tapeworms to stop themselves getting fat?
Of course not. They only eat what they need.

Why don't we all go to giraffe school....

And how about other ways people have dieted over the years?

A tapeworm cyst may be an extreme choice for some, but the list of diet alternatives which have been tried over the years – centuries in fact – is long and fascinating.

Among others, in no particular order, there have been:

The **Coconut Diet** – mainly substituting coconut oil for butter

The **Sugar Busters' Diet** – 14 days of 30% protein, 40% fat, and 30% carbohydrates

The **Beverly Hills Diet** – Mainly nuts and fruits. 10 days fruit only, one day carbs only, no protein until day 19.

The **Cabbage Soup Diet** – eat all you want; very few calories in cabbage soup, and notably flatulent side effects!

Lemonade Diet – 'Flushing out the system' by consuming only a special lemonade mixture, salt water flush and herbal laxative tea for 10 days.

Slimming Soap - According to manufacturers, the algae extract in this seaweed soap penetrates the skin breaking down fat, increasing metabolism, and reducing cellulite.

Vinegar & Water Diet – 19th Century, followed by Lord Byron. Diluted vinegar drunk, as it was in ancient Egypt.

Cigarette Diet – almost inconceivable today, but in 1925 before restrictions on tobacco ads, some cigarette manufacturers tried to sell the appetite-suppressing qualities of their brands.

Eat Right for Your Type – meaning eat as if a vegetarian if you're blood group A, balanced plant/animal for group B, meat and high protein fruit and veg for carnivorous Type Os.

Grapefruit Diet – High protein diet including a lot of bacon with half a grapefruit a day.

Maple Syrup Diet – a detox system involving drinking a mix of water, maple syrup, lemon juice and cayenne pepper for 10 days.

The Great Masticator – devised by San Francisco art dealer Horace Fletcher, this suggested constant chewing but absolutely no swallowing.

Ear Stapling – a metal staple pierced into the cartilage of your ear intended to suppress your appetite.

Diet Sunglasses - Blue-tinted sunglasses are supposed to make your food look less appealing so you will eat less of it.

Then there's the Caveman, Cheater's, Scarsdale, Atkins, Zen, Hay, Graham's...........

And of course when a diet ends, what happens? You go back to your old way of eating, and put all the weight back on again, that's what happens!

21

SO....DO YOU REALLY NEED TO BE TOLD ANY MORE OF THE EFFECTS OF OBESITY?

Having given you a brief glimpse of some of the better known obesity-related illnesses earlier, it's definitely worth labouring the point: The list was by no means complete. Even what you're about to read is not the full story. Just do some research for yourself. In the meantime, here's something to think about:

TYPE 2 DIABETES

Diabetes is reckoned to be the fourth or fifth largest killer in most developed countries. Statistically, overweight people are twice as likely to develop Type 2 diabetes as people who are not overweight. Research has indicated that in the western world, over 90% of cases of Type 2 diabetes are attributable to weight gain. Women with a BMI greater than 35.0 are over 93 times more at risk of developing the disease than women with a normal BMI. The connection between obesity and diabetes is as strong as that between smoking and lung cancer, but it just doesn't seem to get the media attention.

Complications mean you can end up losing your sight, having kidney trouble, and more. Diabetes UK says research shows losing weight can reduce the risk of developing Type 2 diabetes by 58%. With the more severe cases, sufferers have to keep a very tight watch on what they eat and drink, test their blood or urine daily or several times a day, maybe inject themselves with insulin.

Type 2 diabetes is often referred to as adult onset diabetes, as it was rare for it to develop during childhood, but in recent years an increase in the number of overweight and obese children has resulted in an alarming pattern of premature type 2 diabetes.

Being overweight makes a person resistant to the hormone insulin, which carries sugar from the blood to the cells, where it's used for energy. When you are insulin resistant, the sugar can't pass into the cells and so it stays in the blood, making the blood sugar levels higher than normal. This puts extra strain on the cells that make insulin as they try to bring the blood sugar levels back to normal and eventually these cells could fail. Prolonged exposure to high blood glucose increases the risk of heart disease, stroke, high blood pressure, nerve damage, blindness, kidney failure and poor circulation in the extremities, which can lead to amputation.

GALLBLADDER/GALLSTONES

Overweight people are seven times more likely to have gallstones, than people who are normal weight. Women are often sufferers, and also people who've recently followed an unhealthy weight-loss regime. Over 80% of cases develop when the liver produces high-cholesterol content bile – possibly due to a high cholesterol diet or an excess of refined carbohydrates like those found in white bread and cakes.

In women, the risk of developing gallstones or having the gallbladder removed completely (cholecystectomy) is about 20 per 1,000 women per year for those with a BMI greater than 40 compared with three per 1,000 in normal weight women. And also, unlike other weight related conditions, weight reduction in the morbidly obese patient actually increases the risk of gallstone formation, especially if the weight loss is rapid.

OSTEOARTHRITIS

—

Being just 10lb overweight increases the force on the knee by 30 - 60lb with each step you take

—

Osteoarthritis is the most common cause of pain in older people and the knees are the most affected area. When you walk, every step exerts a force on your knees of one and a half times your whole body weight, and when you run, this force is increased to up to 6 times your body weight. The force exerted on the hips is estimated to be around 3 times body weight.

Carrying extra weight puts a lot of pressure on all your joints, and especially the knees. The extra pressure eventually wears away the cartilage, which normally forms a cushion between the bones, so the bones then grind together, making movement difficult and painful.

Research has shown that obese women are 4 times more likely to develop arthritis in the knee joint compared with women who are normal weight. For obese men, the risk is nearly 5 times greater. Even just a small amount of weight loss reduces the risk of developing osteoarthritis of the knee, and can also help to reduce the pain experienced by people who already have it.

Joint replacement operations on obese patients have a higher rate of complications than on people who are normal weight. Obese patients spend more time on the operating table, they need to stay in hospital for longer to recover after the operation, and often require more nursing / rehabilitation during their prolonged recovery period.

CORONARY HEART DISEASE AND STROKE

Heart disease and stroke are the leading causes of death and disability for both men and women in the Western World. Overweight people are more likely to have high blood pressure, and are 3 times more likely to be at risk from heart disease and stroke, than people who are not overweight. Very high blood levels of cholesterol and triglycerides (blood fats) can also lead to heart disease and are often are linked to obesity. Being overweight also contributes to angina (chest pain caused by decreased oxygen to the heart) and sudden death from heart disease or stroke without any signs or symptoms. Reducing your weight by even 10 percent can decrease your risk of developing heart disease.

As you know, risk of heart disease and strokes are dramatically increased in overweight people, and neither is a condition reserved for the elderly. We once had a client at the clinic who wanted help with depression. He told us it was caused by the pressure he was under having to look after his 43 year old wife following her stroke, which resulted in her losing virtually all use of her left arm and leg. Visiting the toilet and cleaning herself were virtually impossible.
He said she had been overweight prior to the stroke.

Stroke

Obesity and poor diet are high risk factors for stroke, which the NHS says is the third largest killer in the UK. Conditions such as diabetes and hypertension – both also linked with overweight – can cause strokes too.

HEART ATTACK

Twenty per cent of heart disease in the UK can be attributed to obesity, which increases the risk of cardiovascular disease, namely all diseases of the heart and circulatory system including angina and heart attack.

GOUT

Gout is a joint disease caused by high levels of uric acid in the blood. Uric acid sometimes forms into solid stone or crystal masses that become deposited in the joints. Gout is more common in overweight people than people of normal weight, and the risk of developing the disorder increases in parallel with an increase in weight.

BACK PROBLEMS

People who are overweight are more likely to have, or to have worse, back problems. In the UK, 1 in 6 working days lost is due to back pain, and osteoporosis, osteoarthritis, rheumatoid arthritis and lower back pain are all exacerbated by the extra strain that obesity exerts on the spine.

CANCERS

Cancer Research UK say major studies confirm that obesity increases the risk of developing various cancers, and the WHO says it is the most important known avoidable cause of cancer after tobacco. Some 13,000 people a year in the UK could avoid getting cancer if they were a healthy weight.

The NHS website says that combined with a lack of exercise, obesity contributes to one third of cancers of the colon, breast, kidney and stomach. In women, cancers associated with obesity include cancer of the uterus, gallbladder, cervix, ovary, breast, and colon. Overweight men are at greater risk of developing cancer of the colon, rectum, and prostate.

The doctor of the future will give no medication, but will interest his patients in the care of the human frame, diet and in the cause and prevention of disease.
Thomas A Edison

COLON CANCER

Research has revealed that people who are obese are two to three times more likely to develop colon cancer than people who are normal weight. The five-year survival rate from colon cancer is just 50%.

BREAST CANCER

Cancer Research UK say scientists estimate some 7%-15% of cases of breast cancer in the developed world are linked to obesity, and although obesity doesn't increase the risk of breast cancer before menopause, obese women have a 30% higher risk of post-menopausal breast cancer. If the average lifetime risk of breast cancer is 1 in 9, an obese woman's is 1 in 7.

Young women too need to be aware: after the age of 18, putting on about 4st increases the risk of breast cancer by 45% and putting on 7st 12lb doubles the risk.

Recent studies show obesity not only increases the risk of getting breast cancer but also shortens the time between return of the disease and lowers survival rates.

OESOPHAGEAL CANCER (cancer of the gullet)

Being overweight doubles the risk of developing this, being obese can triple it. According to Cancer Research UK, it is estimated that about 37% of this type of cancer is linked to being overweight.

> **When diet is wrong medicine is of no use.**
> **When diet is correct medicine is of no need.**
> *Ancient Ayurvedic Proverb*

CANCER OF THE UTERUS

Up to half of all cases in the UK are calculated to be linked to overweight or obesity.

PANCREATIC, KIDNEY and GALLBLADDER CANCERS

– studies suggest clear links with overweight/obesity.

BRAIN CANCER, LEUKAEMIA, HEPATIC (LIVER) CANCER, MULTIPLE MYELOMA (cancer of plasma cells in bone marrow), NON-HODGKIN LYMPHOMA, OVARIAN, AGGRESSIVE PROSTATE, THYROID CANCERS ……

Cancer Research UK says there is evidence of increased risk of all these with overweight/obesity.

ASTHMA

A Harvard Medical School research study, published in the *Archives of Internal Medicine* in November 1999, showed that the risk of developing asthma increased with increasing BMI, and so obese people can be almost 3 times more likely to develop asthma than non-obese people. The study, led by Dr Carlos A. Camargo Jr, involved 85,911 female American registered nurses.

SNORING/SLEEP APNOEA

Sleep apnoea – short (usually no more than a few seconds) periods without breathing during sleep followed by rousing when breathing re-starts again – may sound a relatively minor side-effect of obesity, but for people who suffer from it, stopping breathing up to 300-500 times a night has a major impact on daytime performance.

Obesity is the main risk factor for sleep apnoea, with neck diameters of over 17in being the critical dimension. Not only are sufferers depleted of vital oxygen but their night time rest is so disturbed that they can have severe problems of sleepiness during the day – whether at work, driving, or whatever they are doing. Overweight people are more likely to snore and have general sleep disorders resulting from disturbed sleep.

ARTHRITIS

Obesity/overweight gives an increased risk of developing arthritis or of it being a greater problem you have it already.

One UK health authority has decided not to refer obese patients for NHS hip or knee replacements, 'to ensure that taxpayers' money is used for maximum clinical effect' because anaesthesia for the obese patient is more difficult and they do less well after the operation.

HIP REPLACEMENTS

The obese are more likely than normal weight people to get osteoarthritis of the hip and end up needing a hip replacement – but are then at higher risk for surgical complications, and more likely to need follow-up surgery later.

Let nothing which can be treated
by diet be treated by other means.
Maimonides

KNEE REPLACEMENTS

Obesity puts greater strain on lower body joints and causes more wear and tear – and fat produces chemicals which attack cartilage. The connection with increased waist measurement means you are up to four times more likely to need a joint replacement.

FATTY LIVER DISEASE

Fatty deposits in the liver can ultimately lead to fibrosis and in the worst cases cirrhosis and liver failure.

DEPRESSION

So often you'll have heard (or said) the cliché about being fat but happy – however the statistics suggest otherwise. According to research published in the Archives of General Psychiatry, there are links between obesity and depression. They found people with a BMI of 30 or more had a 25% increased likelihood of major depression, bipolar disorder and panic disorder. The suicide rate among morbidly obese people is higher than that of people of normal weight.

INFERTILITY

The effects of obesity on the hormones in women of childbearing age can lead to irregular cycles, less success in IVF treatment and also to increased risk of miscarriage.

When fat is concentrated around the abdomen and in the upper part of the body (the apple shape), this poses a higher health risk than fat that settles around the hips (the pear shape). Fat cells in the upper part of the body appear to have different qualities from those found in the lower parts. In fact, studies suggest a higher risk for diabetes in people with the "apple shape" and lower risk in those who are "pear shaped."

Some researchers are now questioning whether the lymphatic system – the body's first defence against disease, including cancer – struggles to such an extent under the sheer volume of products taken into the body in an overweight person's unhealthy diet that it is unable to provide that defence efficiently.

Summary:

- **So DID you really need to be told more of the effects on your health?**

22

WEDDING DRESSES, WEIGHT MAINTENANCE and TEENAGERS

If you've got this far in the book you should have already started your own weight loss and healthy eating process. Maybe you've already lost a few pounds: well done! Enjoy! And here's the rub – you've possibly, even probably, been here before, having lost weight. This time, though, that sinking feeling that you're on the verge of putting it all back on within the next few weeks, months, you'll be lucky if it lasts a year, will not affect you. Because you know you've changed, right?

You took all those long hard looks at yourself and your previous bad eating habits, and you've got Martin and Marion's words ringing in your ears about why would you eat if you're not hungry, and don't be a prisoner if you go out to dinner, don't fool yourself about how much you need to eat, a lapse isn't a disaster, etc., etc., – so this time you've got all the tools you need to deal with each and every time you need to make food choices. Whether it's in the supermarket or your own kitchen, a 3 star Michelin restaurant or a friend's dinner party, you need never make the same mistakes again.

You've learned how to relax yourself so deeply you can re-visit all your affirmations any time you choose, knowing they'll keep you on that high road to success.

So if you're expecting a chapter about what to do to maintain your new weight, that was it. Just keep doing what you've been doing.

Eat mindfully, enjoy your food because you're eating because you're hungry and above all be happy! The toolkit worked!

G*m*B for Successful Dieters

Of course you may be one of the many people who manage to shed excess weight easily enough on your own, but find the problems start just when you should be beginning your new, happier, slimmer, healthier life. What problems? Keeping that weight off, we hear you say. And why? Because you revert to your old, bad, eating habits, it's as simple as that.

You might not even have returned to your bad relationship with food, you might have just shed that weight for the first time and have heard so much about the vicious circle of yo-yo dieting that you want to avoid it at all costs. Then again you could be one of those unfortunate yo-yo dieters whose lives have been caught up in a repeated battle to shed weight, only to seem incapable of keeping it off.

So how G*m*B can help is pretty straightforward. You've done what many would see as the hard bit, you're all set to feel and be positive. Now having read the book and, at the same time beginning to enjoy your life as the new, slimmer, you, you've begun to learn how and why you got fat in the first place and how to change your approach to food

Reading this book, doing the self-hypnosis sessions, (or of course visiting one of our clinics), is probably the best way you can be sure of not slipping back and undoing all the good you've done.

Shifting your excess fat, as you'll know if you've read the book this far, starts with two things: understanding how you became overweight in the first place and identifying your motivation for wanting to change. Anyone who's already reached their goal weight should be able to identify their motivation very easily. They may even be able to identify their previous poor eating choices because they will presumably have overcome them – maybe only on a temporary basis – in order to achieve their current weight loss.

If you've done both of these things and have now read the sessions through from start to finish and reinforced all the Positive Thoughts in self-hypnosis, you should have put the toolkit and manual in place on a subconscious level, ensuring you have the means to avoid all those previously poor food choices in the future.

So far we've been looking at how to deal with long-term weight issues, making sure you know how to shed weight safely while learning how never to gain it back again.

Of course some of you will be, or know, people who don't have a long-term weight problem but may have a short-term reason for being sure they're going to lose that little bit of extra weight. Weddings being a classic example, or an upcoming exotic beach holiday, or a school or college prom....

Well never fear! This approach is equally applicable, because although it's not a 'crash diet', if followed accurately, it will guarantee weight loss at the widely accepted safe rate of 1-2lb a week. So a bride-to-be sized 14 who wants to be in a 12 or 10 in a few months' time can be sure she'll reach target. If she needs, or chooses to, remain following the system afterwards, it's entirely up to her. The ideal is to eat healthily, of course, so if any changes made for a short-term loss lead to a better level of nutrition, less fat, more fibre, more water .... only good can come of it.

From Session One you can start the change – and although you're likely to alter your relationship with food and food choices generally every bit as much as someone coming to the book with a high BMI and considerable amount of weight to shift, you'll have a relatively shorter journey reaching your target.

There are other groups of people who could benefit, those with chronic illnesses or debilitating conditions either caused by, or made worse by, excess weight. Diabetics are perhaps the most obvious group – if you are diabetic, changing your eating habits is one of the first things your doctor will advise, and in the case of Type 2 diabetes there are indications that you can improve, or arguably completely eradicate, the condition, by losing weight through a healthier diet coupled with more exercise. Kay's experience (re-visit Chapter 16) supports this.

Teenagers Too.....

The numbers of obese children and teenagers is soaring; not far short of a million youngsters – some 10% of six year olds and 17% of 15 year olds, according to the NHS website, are classed as obese, so overweight that their health is in danger. In fact there are researchers now predicting that in the near future a generation of parents will start to outlive their children because of the obesity-related problems their children will begin to suffer. Leading nutritionist Professor Andrew Prentice, from the London School of Hygiene and Tropical medicine, estimates being clinically obese shortens lifespan by some nine years. He describes the mix of obesity and a more sedentary lifestyle – with 25% of British youngsters watching four hours TV a day – as an explosive mix.

The WHO says at least 20 million children under the age of 5 were overweight globally in 2005. The International Obesity Task Force calculates that up to 155 million school age children worldwide are overweight/obese. Rather than the cliché puppy fat, obesity as a child is a strong indicator that they will be obese adults.... And we've already looked at what that can mean.

Health problems which can affect overweight teenagers **include** the following: (This is not an exhaustive list!)

- **Blount's disease.** Excess weight on growing bones can lead to this bone deformity of the lower legs.
- **Arthritis.** Wear and tear on the joints from carrying extra weight can cause this painful joint problem at a young age.

- **Slipped capital femoral epiphyses (SCFE).** Obese children and teens are at greater risk for this painful hip problem. SCFE requires immediate attention and surgery to prevent further damage to the joint.
- **Asthma.** Obesity is associated with breathing problems that can make it harder to keep up with friends, play sports, or just walk from class to class.
- **Sleep apnoea.** This condition (in which a person temporarily stops breathing during sleep) is a serious problem for many overweight kids and adults. Not only does it interrupt sleep, sleep apnoea can leave people feeling tired and affect their ability to concentrate and learn. It also may lead to heart problems.
- **High blood pressure.** When blood pressure is high, the heart must pump harder and the arteries must carry blood that's moving under greater pressure. If the problem continues for a long time, the heart and arteries may no longer work as well as they should. Although rare in most teens, high blood pressure, or hypertension, is more common in overweight or obese teens.
- **High cholesterol.** Long before getting sick, obese teens may have abnormal blood lipid levels, including high cholesterol, low HDL ("good") cholesterol, and high triglyceride levels. These increase the risk of heart attack and stroke when a person gets older.
- **Pseudotumor cerebri.** This is a rare cause of severe headaches in obese teens and adults. There is no tumour, but pressure builds in the brain. In addition to headaches, symptoms may include vomiting, an unsteady way of walking, and vision problems that may become permanent if not treated.
- **Polycystic ovary syndrome (PCOS).** Girls who are overweight may miss periods — or not get their periods at all — and may have elevated testosterone (the male hormone) levels in the blood. Although it is normal for girls to have some testosterone in their blood, too much can interfere with normal ovulation and may cause excess hair growth, worsening acne, and male-

type baldness. PCOS is associated with insulin resistance, a precursor to developing type 2 diabetes. Women who are overweight also might have fertility problems.

- **Insulin resistance and diabetes.** When there is excess body fat, insulin is less effective at getting glucose, the body's main source of energy, into cells. More insulin becomes needed to maintain a normal blood sugar. For some overweight teens, insulin resistance may progress to diabetes (high blood sugar).

Information taken from:

http://kidshealth.org/teen/food_fitness/dieting/obesity.html

With some experts now saying gastric banding should be considered on people as young as 15, perhaps it's time to educate these youngsters about only eating when they're hungry. Given that the UK Government's Change4Life programme suggests that 90% of today's youngsters will be overweight or obese by 2050 unless there is a radical change in eating habits and activity level, (and in these crunch times let's not forget that obesity is reckoned to cost the British economy more than £2 billion annually) the change needs to start, and start now.

In today's high speed high tech society, often households don't share mealtimes, don't sit at a table together – and you can find all sorts of psychological implications from that apart from dietary. But fast food, if that's the choice of the teenager, or schoolchild in a rush, is as we've identified back in Chapter 7, generally high-fat, low nutrient, high sugar, quick fix food, the classic 'beige food' which anyone conscious of their weight and health should avoid, favouring fresh fruit and vegetables and other unprocessed foods.

Gastric *mind* Band is equally relevant for young people as anyone else – there is no dangerous fad, no nutritional food groups to cut out, no coding, points, bans - just a way of recognising how to alter your view of food, what and when to eat.

Just because you're young doesn't mean you can't understand the blindingly obvious; if you eat more than your body needs you'll get fat. And if you're fat you won't be as healthy as if you're slim and if you're fat you won't be able to buy clothes as easily, and buying size 16 or 18 or 20 clothes won't be nearly as much fun as grabbing a standard 12 from the rail..... and so on and so forth. The youngsters themselves may not be thinking long term, or even thinking health at all, but parents be aware: Type 2 diabetes, which is closely related to obesity, could knock 20 years off your kids' lives. It's usually diagnosed in the over-40s but rates in children are rising with about 2 youngsters a week being identified with the condition.

Experts from various countries have been saying for a number of years that it's increasingly likely parents will start to outlive their children due to the high incidence of obesity in young people.

Ironically, maybe the first step to ensuring young people eat a healthier diet and address any weight problems they may be developing, would be to learn to cook. If you can make yourself a tasty nutritious meal, and enjoy the process as well as eating it, you've less need of junk food!

You must learn it's not too late, in fact it's never too late, to make the changes that help you get a grip on your weight and prevent the health problems you could be heading for. It's no different from the rest of this book. Not big changes.

In your teens you have bodily changes that are hard to live with even if weight isn't an issue. Girls' hips broaden, breasts develop. You may not match up to your ideal of how the girls on TV and in magazines look. Especially if you haven't taken on board the significance of airbrushing to the impression given by those images. Guys develop at different rates, and washboard abs are usually found only on models in their 20s.

If you find it hard to control how much you eat, you may decide to follow an extreme diet – but often that's followed by eating huge quantities of food and because you then feel guilty about your binge, you might make yourself vomit or take laxatives. Eating too little to remain at a healthy weight (anorexia) and eating followed by throwing up all the food (calories) you've eaten (bulimia) are both harmful eating disorders and if you recognise these symptoms in yourself or anyone you know, you should contact the doctor.

If you want to lose weight, the best way is:

- Cut back on sugary drinks.
- Don't have seconds.
- Do more exercise, as much as you can – start with five minutes a day if that's what you have time for.
- Ask anyone for help if that's what you need
- Eat a wide variety of food, choosing more fruit and vegetables
- Drink more water
- Use your bike more
- Don't kid yourself chips count as potatoes!
- Swap some of your usual 'plastic' bread for whole wheat bread
- Eating a healthy breakfast is good for weight loss as well as school results!
- Do not consider pills or fad diets
- Plus, of course, many of the other ideas mentioned throughout the book.
- Particularly……. Eat When You're Hungry, and only when you're hungry!

So - what if you come off the rails?

Everyone will have a plateau, maybe more than one, when shedding excess weight; these are of course nothing more than temporary blips, which you pick yourself up from and move on. There might come a time, though, when some crisis occurs – perhaps a loved one dies, emotional trauma, financial meltdown – lots of possibilities which would understandably knock your focus totally away from the time and effort you'd put in dealing with your food issues.

At the time you will almost certainly think there's no getting back on track, or no interest in getting back on track; you won't feel remotely inclined to even think of turning a corner, never mind doing it.

In fact although traumatic and upsetting, with regard to weight loss these are actually no different from a plateau. They may feel worse and be emotionally worse, but all you need do is start afresh. Read the book from scratch. You haven't relapsed, you've had a lapse – and you <u>can</u> get over it.

Summary

- **So you've shed excess weight already? Be sure to keep it off.....**
- **The Gastric *mind* Band can be used for shorter term weight loss**
- **Teenagers will be quite safe using our methods too**
- **It doesn't matter how many times you start**

23

POST SCRIPT

We originated the seeds of the Gastric *mind* Band therapy back in 2007 and have been treating clients since early 2008. However, it was following major UK media attention and the visits of US and Japanese TV crews in 2009, that our waiting list grew beyond our wildest dreams as we welcomed a massive influx of new clients to our clinic. Soon after our amazing worldwide press coverage, not surprisingly a number of clinics started offering mental gastric band type treatments. You might choose to call it coincidence, or imitation being the sincerest form of flattery……..

In the last year we've often found ourselves working seven days a week and hardly stopping to take breath; we were even talked into travelling to the Greek Islands to undertake a final session for a G*m*B client living there. Not really something that needed much persuasion, if we're honest!

Our base in Fuengirola, southern Spain, has had to grow to cater for our growing client register, and we are now in a spacious top-floor suite almost (but not quite) overlooking the Mediterranean. Not a bad place to meet clients!

The G*m*B treatment - which may be the best known, but is of course only one of many therapies we offer - has kept us busy with continual research, development and functional improvements. During 2010 we plan to launch the Post-Diet Gastric *mind* Band©. This further process caters for those who find it relatively easy to lose excess weight but almost impossible to keep it off. The early building blocks of this new Post-Diet G*m*B© therapy are contained in this book.

G*m*Band therapy is now available in clinics in the USA; London should be open by the time this book reaches the reader. We hope that with the expansion of our treatment into other continents, that we will also be training other therapists in the intricacies of the one-to-one therapy within the G*m*B process.

The WHO recently stated that obesity has reached epidemic proportions with more than one billion adults being overweight - 300 million of them clinically obese - creating a global burden of chronic disease and disability. As the battle against obesity and obesity-related illnesses continues to cause financial headaches on a global level, we trust that some time soon we will be able to offer our treatment to a greater audience by obtaining recognition from the appropriate government departments, especially in the UK and the US.

Whatever happens with the expansion of the G*m*B brand, our own immediate plans are to continue offering the G*m*B treatment personally at the Fuengirola clinic. We know that through meeting clients, providing therapy face to face, and working with their feedback, we are guaranteed to stay at the 'sharp end' of the treatment process and are in the best position to improve and develop the G*m*B treatment. We believe that Gastric *mind* Band has a significant part to play in the lives of the people we treat and in the global battle against obesity.

Fuengirola
Spain
Summer 2010
www.gmband.com

—

We are proud, and often surprised, that we see so many new clients each week from across Europe and beyond. We hope that the trust and confidence placed in us as therapists is based on our dedication to always strive to exceed our clients' levels of expectation in every aspect of the treatment provided. If you should have any questions regarding the book, us, the clinic, or indeed the therapy, we would be genuinely pleased to hear from you.

—

YOUR G*m*B JOURNEY DOESN'T STOP HERE

You reached this point with our help, maybe with support from your family and friends. From here on, though, you will most probably be relying on your own resources and what you read in and learned from this book.

Whenever you need our help we'll still be here – all those little stories, reminders, anecdotes, examples, proverbs... all the ammunition you'll need against the diet terrorists and the sting merchants will still be right here within these pages.

Before you consign us to the bookshelf, though, (only to be dusted down when you next have a bad day or a stressful week!) here is a reminder of the key points to keep at the back (front?) of your mind for when you face food choices – which after all is likely to be at least twice a day.

When you are eating something, be sure:

- Why you are eating it. If you are not hungry you don't need to eat.
- Might you be thirsty? Don't forget some of the sensations of thirst are the same as for hunger. If you think you're hungry, drink some water & don't eat unless you still feel hungry 10 minutes later.
- Are you eating slowly enough for your brain to have time to let you know when you're no longer hungry?
- Are you tasting the food and truly enjoying the flavour of it?
- You remember your reasons for wanting to become a healthy weight. What is more important, the quick fix or the longer term goal & a healthier future life?
- You can always picture your fork in the road – where will you be and what will you feel like next month, or next year?
- You remember your pause button. It can make all the difference if you just use it to put your thoughts on hold & give you time to reconsider the choice you're about to make.

As we said at the beginning, this book can never truly replicate the personalised Gastric mind Band treatment as provided at our clinics; should you require more information, details of locations or availability, please visit www.gmband.com

READER OFFER

If you've read this far, well done…. As a thank you, if you're interested in visiting one of our clinics we've got a special reader offer, details at the front of the book

Biographies

Martin, born in London, and Marion, born in Newcastle, undertook a diploma course in Clinical Hypnotherapy together before moving to Spain where they established the Elite Clinic in central Fuengirola, in Southern Spain, in 2004 putting into practice their shared love of helping people – overcoming addictions, helping with panic attacks, raising their self esteem or in many other ways – including losing weight and feeling better about themselves!

Martin, a former PR and marketing director who's worked in places as diverse as London, Los Angeles and India, met Marion whilst they were both on a training course in the UK. It was time when she was a disenchanted language teacher looking to change career having become frustrated at having to deal with disinterested, unmotivated youngsters.

Intrigued by psychology since taking a course on the psychology of sales and marketing many years earlier, Martin added to his skills over time and undertook a primer CBT course at the school of Psychology at Birmingham University along with many courses in NLP. He's a member of the International Hypnosis Research Institute. Both Martin and Marion hold Diplomas in Clinical Hypnosis and are certified and registered with the American Board and British Institutes of Hypnotherapy. Marion is also a member of the UK IBS Register, and during 2010 is planning to undertake additional training, specialising in diet and nutrition.

Martin and Marion have become prolific article writers on the subject of their therapy and hypnosis in general in recent years, and in true plain-speaking style, however, Martin defines the knowledge gained in colleges as less significant than the life experiences of being married, divorced, burying close family members and time spent travelling the world. He and Marion also have an extensive library, buying and reading five or six books on psychology each month.... they say they are possibly Amazon's best customers!

Most of Marion's family was involved in matters medical – her mother a trained nurse, brother a doctor, sister a midwife. However being 'far too squeamish' to consider doing anything that involves 'blood and guts' etc., the idea of being able to help people in a therapy situation seemed perfect. Always slim, fit and active, she clearly loves being able to help people achieve something they've maybe wanted most of their lives. Marion gained an Honours degree at Durham University.

In the book, the couple talks about variations and new approaches to the concept. They see it as an ongoing project that they embrace 24/7, with every client providing new insights and solutions to different aspects of weight management.

Martin's hobbies include flying and sailing. He holds a UK private pilot's licence and a RYA Offshore Yacht Master's Licence. Marion's number one pastime is cooking; she enjoys cooking Thai, Chinese and Indian food alongside contemporary classics.

'We are not doctors, but as far as obesity and weight management is concerned, between us we have built up literally thousands of hours of one to one experience, working with individuals who are often desperate to take charge, to make a change in their life, with regard to their weight. Through them we have heard first hand what worked and what failed, and what contributed to both outcomes. This detailed information formed the foundation of the G*m*B therapy and continues to contribute to its ongoing development.

'We are grateful for the sometimes painful stories that many of our past clients have shared with us.'

I once met a child suffering with what I believe to be called 'selective mutism' – she was about 10 years of age, had never spoken a word in her life to anyone other than to whisper to her mother.

Not to make too long or big a deal out of it, she had seen the best of the best in Europe as far as specialist doctors were concerned and attended the leading children's hospitals. I met her one morning with her parents. They explained her condition to me, I spent the whole day talking with her, sitting on the floor, at her level; she always looked uncomfortable looking up at people. I wanted her to start looking down. That night I sat on the grass with her and she started talking, and to my knowledge has never stopped to this day. Her dad went and got a camcorder in case it was a one off, he wanted to show the doctors in London. It was probably no more than a fluke, that I'm sure, but the feeling it gave me will go with me to my grave, and that's the truth.

Martin Shirran, 2010

At the time of writing, we are in the process of opening clinics in the United States and in London. Who knows where may be next! For details of the locations of the clinics, or to contact them, or for more information about us or the therapy, go to www.gmband.com

About the Authors

Martin Shirran and his wife Marion, trained clinical hypnotherapists, pull no punches. Their belief in their Gastric *mind* Band therapy is absolute and absolutely passionate, and this extends to their belief in their first book.

Martin, an ex marketing and PR man, is a gregarious, persuasive individual whose written style reflects this. His natural ability to 'sell' his beliefs about obesity and the G*m*B therapy shines through in person and on the page. Marion, a former teacher, has done much of the backroom development and fine-tuning of the various techniques involved, and her thoughts on the subject are equally clear and articulate.

They both prefer to talk straight to the reader just as if you were in the therapy suite with them. It's a bit like tough love.

Tough love that they've put to the test first hand....when they started developing the therapy Martin was a hefty 264 lb and Marion a seemingly effortlessly slim 124lb. They worked sometimes 24/7 much of the time for two years testing, tweaking and developing their therapy.... Martin now weighs in 57lb lighter and Marion's understanding of her relationship with food has played a key part in how they approach 'The Hunger Question'. She, naturally, has remained within a few pounds, the same weight throughout. Now Martin understands why!

Fiona Graham is a former London journalist working as a freelance writer from her home in Spain.

1676458R0021

Printed in Great Britain
by Amazon.co.uk, Ltd.,
Marston Gate.

A Golden Mist

John Wheatley

Visit us online at www.authorsonline.co.uk

A Bright Pen Book

British Library Cataloguing Publication Data.
A catalogue record for this book is available from the British Library

ISBN 978 0 7552 1214 9

Authors OnLine Ltd
19 The Cinques
Gamlingay, Sandy
Bedfordshire SG19 3NU
England

This book is also available in e-book format, details of which are available at www.authorsonline.co.uk

for Alma

The Author

John Wheatley is a Lecturer at Stockport College. He first visited Anglesey, as a child, in the 1950s, and his interest in the story of 'The Royal Charter' began with walks along the coastal path from Moelfre and Lligwy, and exploring the stretch of coast by boat. He is married with two sons and two step-daughters and lives in Cheadle Hulme, Cheshire.

Acknowledgments:

I would like to pay tribute to Alexander McKee, whose work **The Golden Wreck** has been, for generations of enthusiasts, the definitive account of the Royal Charter tragedy; also, Chris and Lesley Holden, whose beautifully presented book **Life and Death on The Royal Charter**, with its wealth of illustration and primary evidence, has provided a new source of inspiration in the year which commemorates the 150th anniversary of the shipwreck.

- Alexander McKee (1986). *The Golden Wreck: the tragedy of the `Royal Charter`: Middleview, an imprint of Avid Publications.*
  ISBN 978-1-902964-02-7

- Chris and Lesley Holden (2009). *Life and Death on the Royal Charter: Calgo Publications 2009.* Calgo Publications. ISBN 978-0-9545066-2-9.

'A Golden Mist' is a work of historical fiction. Some of the incidents and names are taken from fact; the characterisation, however, is fictional, and except in cases where there is a well documented historical record – as, for example, with Stephen Roose Hughes – no actual resemblance is claimed to the people who once played their part in the tragedy of `The Royal Charter`.

Part 1

Chapter 1

Text Message, from Saffy Williams to Charlie Robson [Jo`berg] 21st May, 2009, 6.25pm
Tchd dwn 1800 mchstr. Gd flite. Wll cntct u wen on-lne.
Sff xxx

Text Message, from Saffy Williams to Elizabeth Williams [Jo`berg] 21st May, 2009, 6.28pm
Arivd safe manchstr. Ant Liz at airprt. Wll ring u 2nite.
Lv Saffy.

Text Message, from Saffy Williams to Sally Whitelock [Cape Town] 21st May, 2009, 6.35pm
Hi Sal. How r u? Am in Englnd, vstng lng lst rels! Wll b in tuch.
Saff.

***

"Hi mom!"

"Is that you, Saffy?"

"Yes. Why, does it sound like someone else?"

"Is that you, Saffy? It is?"

"YES!"

"Good. Did you get there safely?"

"No, we nose-dived into the Atlantic just off the coast of Spain."

"Try to be serious, Saffy."

"Didn`t you get my text?"

"Your what?"

"My text."

"Oh. No. I haven`t had my phone switched on."

"Mom, what`s the point of having a mobile phone if you

don`t switch it on?"

"Well, I so rarely use it. I don`t like to waste the battery."

"Anyway, yes, I`m fine."

"Did Aunt Liz meet you?"

"Yes, she was there at the airport. I recognised her straight away. She looks just like Aunt Mags."

"Goodness! After so long!"

"Well they are the same family."

"Yes, but they`ve never even met each other. Isn`t that strange?"

"If they did, they`d think they were looking in a mirror."

"I can`t believe that."

"No. It`s just the hair, really."

"Oh, that! The Williams` hair! Now you`re telling me something that doesn`t surprise me. Don`t forget to write to her, will you?"

"Aunt Mags?"

"Yes. She`ll be keen to hear how you`re getting on."

"OK. Is dad there?"

"No. He went over to see Janie and Mike."

"OK, well, tell them all hi from me, and don`t worry, I`m fine."

"Have you called Charlie?"

"No. I texted him from the airport."

"Do call him, Saffy. He`ll be calling here, if you don`t."

"Tell him I`ll e-mail him soon as I can get on-line."

"I`m sure he`d much rather have a phone-call. It`s so much more personal."

"He`ll be fine with e-mail, mom."

"Have you thought any more about what he said?"

"About getting married?"

"Yes."

"No."

"Well, I think you should."

"He only said it because I was going away. He didn`t really mean it."

"What a terrible thing to say!"

"Why?"

"When he`s gone to the trouble of asking you."

"It wasn`t any trouble. It was completely off the top of his head. Even he was surprised by it."

"Well, you know what I think."

"Yes, mom. I know what you think. Better go now. Phone you later in the week. Love you. Bye."

"Take care Saffy. Bye."

***

"Thanks, Aunt Liz, that was lovely."

"It was nothing special."

"After two days of aeroplane food, that was very, very special!"

"Would you like a drop more wine?"

"Mmm, yes, please, why not!"

"There we are. I thought we might take the dogs for a little walk afterwards. If you`re not too tired."

"No, I`m fine. It probably won`t catch up with me until tomorrow, and then I`ll be out like a light for two days!"

"Well, there`s no rush to do anything. You can rest as much as you like."

"Do you mind me calling you Aunt Liz? I don`t suppose `aunt` is very accurate really, is it?"

"Well, as far as I can work it out, my great grandfather and your great great grandfather were brothers."

"Wait a minute! Just let me try and work out how many *greats* that is!"

"It was in the 1880s, I think. Your side of the family moved to South Africa."

"Yes. There was a row about something dad said. But he doesn`t know anything more about it than that."

"Nor do I really."

"So you and I are the first people from the two sides of the family to meet for over a hundred years?"

"Yes."

"Well, I`ll drink to that. Cheers."

***

"Have you always lived here?"

"At New House?"

"Yes."

"Not always. When I was a girl, of course, but when I got married, we went to Exeter, and Cambridge, all over the place, really. Then when my husband died, that was eight years ago, I came back here to look after my brother."

"Who was living on his own by then."

"Yes. His wife was killed in a motorway accident in the eighties. Very sad, really, only in her forties. Then he died two years ago, and left me here on my own."

"It must seem like a big place for one person."

"Well, it`s always been too big, really, even when we were kids, my mother used to complain. It was obviously built with a Victorian size family in mind, and servants to boot."

"You`ve never been tempted to sell it, then?"

"Tempted, yes. When my brother died an awful lot of work needed to be done on it, and I nearly sold up then, but my son, that`s Stephen, said we couldn`t let it go out of the family, and he agreed to pay for the work."

"And will he come and live here?"

"Well, at the moment, he lives in California, so I don`t think it`s very likely."

"But your other children still live in England?"

"Oh yes. And their children. You`ll meet Lucy on Friday. She`s nineteen. Robert`s still at school, doing GCSEs, and Stephen`s pretty much the same age as you, he`s a teacher in Sheffield."

"Another Stephen!"

"Yes, I`m afraid so."

"Like my dad and his dad."

"Really?"
"Yes."

***

From: Saffy Williams
To: Sally Whitelock
Tuesday 26th May, 2009

Hi Sal, thanks for yours. Congrats on the new job, hope it goes well. Let me know. I`m here in England for two months. Staying with the ancient line of the Williams family in Cheshire. Charlie`s fine, thanks. Actually, he proposed to me before I set out but we were both quite pissed at the time so it probably doesn`t count! Suzy Randall told me to look her up in London, but will need to see how the time pans out. Keep in touch. Saff.

Wed 27/5/09
From: Saffy Williams
To: Charlie Robson
Hi Charlie, did you get my texts? If so, reply! Settled in here at `New House` with Aunt Liz. We eat, talk, walk the dogs and drink wine. Her grand-daughter, Lucy, is coming here for the weekend tomorrow. Hope you`re OK. E-mail me when you get this. Have fun. Be good! Sff xxx.

Wed 27/5/09

Dear Aunt Mags,

Hope you`re all well. I expect mom told you I arrived safely. I`m having a really nice time and thought you`d like to know how I`m getting on.

New House is quite an imposing place. I`m going to upload some photos, and will get dad to print them off for you to see. Apparently it was built in the 1860s, in the parkland of a much larger estate, going back centuries, but the old hall was demolished early last century, and most of the land now has housing developments, and the like. New House still has about four acres, with a stream crossing one corner and some woodland, which the dogs – three Labradors – love!

Aunt Liz is going to dig out the family snaps, so I`ll let you know if anything interesting turns up.

Give my love to Uncle Ben and Phyllis.

Saffy

Chapter 2

"So, when was this one taken?"

"It`s on the back."

"New House. 1894."

"That`s it."

"It`s much more open isn`t it? Before all the trees were planted."

"Yes. I think it was more or less open parkland when they bought the land. You can just make out the chimneys of the old hall over the hill. There, look."

"Oh, yes. And the bridge over the stream."

"Yes."

"There`s something else that`s different, though."

"Yes, that`s right. If you look on this side, here, that`s where the kitchen garden is now. There was a fire, sometime in the early 1900s, and this part was destroyed."

"And they never rebuilt it."

"No."

"What was it?"

"The bottom floor was the nursery, and above that was a library, well, the study – the first Richard Williams, collected books, and paintings."

"So nothing remained then, after the fire?"

"Nothing to speak of. It was all they could do to save the rest of the house. Mainly charred remains, though there were a few bits collected. Nothing of any value."

"Paintings, too, what a pity! But you still have some nice paintings in the house."

"All recent, I`m afraid. Apart from the one in the hall. The churchyard scene. That was one of the original collection."

"Oh yes, I saw that one. `The Churchyard at Eastry`."

"Yes."

"By Robert Wheeler. Is he famous?"

"No, I don`t think so."

"Even so, you should get it valued. Might be worth something if it`s Victorian."

"Well, I doubt if we`d sell it, anyway. It`s a bit like a family friend, really."

"I`ll look him up for you, anyway."

"On the internet?"

"Yes."

"It`s a marvellous thing, isn`t it?"

"Is this one the family?"

"Yes. There you are. Taken on the terrace at New House, in 1873. The oldest photo there is. That`s Richard Williams himself. "

"The one who had this place built?"

"Yes. And that`s his wife, Elizabeth, and the three sons, Isaac, the eldest, Stephen and Simon, the youngest. Stephen of course is your great great grandfather, the one who went to South Africa."

"They look quite young, about thirty? And the photo is taken here at New House, so they must have made their money very quickly, or inherited it."

"She looks very determined, doesn`t she?"

"Stubborn. Family trait like the hair!"

"And she was Elizabeth, too."

"Yes. She was still alive when my mother was a child. She died in 1932. My mum remembered her quite well. All her marbles and a wicked sense of humour, apparently."

"You wouldn`t think so to look at the photograph, would you?"

"Well, it was all very formal wasn`t it? Everyone had to look dour and respectable for photographs in those days. She gave my grandmother this necklace, look. It came down to me eventually."

"That`s pretty. What does the inscription say?"

"`RW:EW`."

"I suppose that`s Richard and Elizabeth."

"Yes."

"I wonder what the argument was about."

"Well, you know what families are like. Sometimes the least thing!"

***

From: Saffy Williams
To: Steve Williams
Mon 1st June 2009

Hi Dad , I`ve uploaded some photos for you to print out and pass on to Aunt Mags. It includes one of Liz and Lucy together. See any resemblances? Getting quite into the family history. Will you ask Aunt Mags if she knows anything else about things? Tell mom I`m eating properly and looking after myself. I do tell her myself but she doesn`t believe me! Take care. Saffy.

From: Saffy Williams
To: Sally Whitelock
Tue 2nd June 2009

Hi Sal, how`s it at your end? The new boss sounds dishy. Don`t do anything outrageous! Met my `cousin`, Lucy on Thursday – took me out for a girlie night in Manchester at the weekend, with some of her friends from uni. Reminded me of us five years ago at Wits! Ended up in a taxi at four o`clock in the morning, spent most of next day recovering! Getting too old for this kind of thing! Not heard from Charlie yet, apart from a sarky five word text. I guess he thinks he`s punishing me for taking this trip. Getting quite caught up in the family saga. Trying to discover my roots! Keep me posted re. you know what! Saff.

Chapter 3

"Aunt Mags gave me this to show you, by the way. I`d forgotten about it until you showed me the necklace."

"Tiny shells."

"Yes. She said it was part of a necklace once, and that it had some green beads with it at one time. Not worth anything, but she said her mom told her it went back a long time. Anyway, Dad spoke to Aunt Mags, she says she thinks the family came from Ireland originally."

"Yes. That`s what we`ve always thought. Some time in the 1860s."

"Williams doesn`t sound particularly Irish."

"Well, no. Welsh, really, but there must be thousands of families called Williams."

"Millions. Like John Smith."

"Who?"

"Most common name."

"Oh, yes, I see."

"I suppose lots of people moved around during the nineteenth century."

"There was a story that he worked as a sign-painter for a time."

"Richard?"

"Yes."

"Wouldn`t have thought there was much money in that."

"Then they came over here, and he started the business."

"And built New House."

"Yes."

"Which was completed in..?"

"1870. It`s on the keystone over the front door."

"1870. Quite impressive. And what exactly was the company?"

"It was called `Bridgecastle Munitions` to begin with apparently. Then it became `Williams Iron and Steel` sometime in the 1890s. We don`t really know whether he bought out a company that already existed or whether he started the company from scratch. In any case he changed the name later on."

"Munitions. They made weapons, then?"

"Yes, apparently, to begin with anyway. It was quite a business – the Crimean War, then The Boer War, later – apparently the Empire had an endless appetite for new and better weapons."

"And the first world war, too, I suppose."

"Yes. Of course, Simon – my grandfather`s brother – was killed in the trenches. At Ypres."

"Really, how sad."

"But the company had already become part of a larger conglomerate by then. After that the family were just shareholders rather than managers."

"Right. I see. And there aren`t any other records?"

"Well, I suppose there would be public records, to do with the company and everything. But apart from the photographs and a few books and bits and pieces that survived the fire, nothing really."

***

From: Saffy Williams
To: Steve Williams
Tue 9th June

Hi Dad, Thanks for downloading the photos, I`m glad Aunt Mags liked them. Tell her I think I may have found some evidence that our origins are Welsh after all. Aunt Liz showed me some books and papers that survived the fire here in 1907. Nothing of great interest really apart from a couple of poetry books that were kept in a different part of the house. One is a copy of some Byron poems, and the other is an edition of `Lyrical Ballads` by Wordsworth and Coleridge [which I had to study in my first year at Wits]. It`s pretty old, though not a first edition, unfortunately [or it would be worth something!] but in the flyleaf is an inscription, *S.R.H.*,

Moelfre, 1853 - for R.W., September, 1858. Nobody has any idea who S.R.H. is, but presumably R.W. is Richard Williams, our venerable ancestor. So somebody in *Moelfre* gave him a copy of Wordsworth in 1858, and *Moelfre*, I have checked, is a place on the coast of Anglesey, which is separated from North Wales by a thin strip of water called the Menai Strait. So, it looks as if he may have been there in the 1850s, wherever he went afterwards. So, how`s that for detective work! I`m going to London for a few days next week, but may pay Moelfre a visit when I get back. Lucy says she`ll go with me, so we`ll make a weekend of it. I`ll let you know how it goes. Love to everyone. Tell mom I`ll call her before I go to London. Take it easy! Saffy.

Part 2

Chapter 4

I was born in Porthaethwy, on the island of Anglesey, in the year 1839. My father, Richard Williams, was Master of the Customs House in that busy maritime thoroughfare, and it was with his name that I was christened in the Church of St Tysilio, close by the Afon Menai, on November 27th, some five weeks after my birth.

My mother, Elizabeth, was native to the town, and as soon as I was of an age to understand, the bed-time tales I favoured were of the times when the great iron bridge spanning the water to the mainland was built, times she had witnessed in her youth. No man, she would say, certainly no man in Porthaethwy, believed such an enterprise possible, and it was, as my father insisted, with the enthusiasm of a practical man, a marvel of science of which the age could stand proud.

My mother recalled the tumult and excitement as the populace of the town swelled with an incoming workforce of engineers and surveyors and labouring men; the din of industry by day, the rowdiness of the streets by night: a sense of danger and adventure from which she elaborated tales, largely fanciful I fear, of deeds and misdeeds, romance and mischief which thrilled my childish imagination.

Taking me on walks, on warm summer evenings, or on Sundays after the church service, my father would point, from various viewpoints, to sections of the giant structure and instruct me on the principles of physics by which the great forces and strains were held in counter-balance; when she joined us on these excursions, my mother could describe, from her own recollection, the day when the chains of the central span were hoisted, foot by foot, by a hundred men and more with their pulleys and scaffolds and tackle, to the sound of the fife and drum, whilst the whole town watched in awe, and applauded to the heavens when the seemingly superhuman task was complete.

My early education was at home, in the hands of a Miss Swithens who had once been a Governess to the Bulkeley family of Baron Hill, but who now, approaching advanced years and largely in retirement, was able to supplement a modest annuity by taking charge of my instruction. My lessons were in Arithmetic, Grammar, and what Miss Swithens termed French, though the latter consisted mainly in the repetition of certain polite phrases with the emphasis on refinement of enunciation which she took to be a virtue of the highest order. The reading over which she presided was Shakespeare, Milton and, of course, the Bible. All my instruction was in the English language. My mother spoke to me a little in Welsh but my father did not encourage it. "You`ll turn the boy into a `gwerin`!" was his warning, meaning, I think, that he feared I would be swallowed up into the undifferentiated masses of the common people and make nothing of myself.

It was very clear that my father had ambitions for me, even at that early age. A great believer in the inventions of mechanical science, he had visited the shipyards of the Mersey, the Dee and the Clyde; he had seen the furnaces of industry, as he called them, of the cities of northern England, and his dearest wish, I believe, was to see his son taking a part in that onward surge of human progress.

One day, a short time after my seventh birthday, he took me to the central point of the great bridge, and pointing to the south west, beyond the swirling waters below, and beyond the treacherous rocks by which the pilots steered, he explained to me that soon another, even greater bridge would cross the strait, and this one, he added, would carry steam locomotives, all the way from London, to the port at Holyhead.

He seemed, as I recall, on that day, to be in a strange fever, almost a turmoil of excitement. The world, he said, was being transformed every day by new inventions in transport, new industrial processes and discoveries in medicine. He said that I would be sent to school, not, as I had always imagined, to the Grammar School in Beaumaris, but to a college in England where I would be in the hands of teachers of truer and wider learning, and then to University in Edinburgh or even Caen in France, where I would study architecture and physics.

Whether it was the weight of expectation being placed upon me, or whether by some odd intuition or premonition I sensed the illness which was to overtake my father early in the following year, I do not know, but a dark foreboding troubled my sleep that night and for many nights to come.

What neither of us could know that day was that by the time that second bridge was built, carrying, as my father predicted, the railway to Anglesey, my fortunes were to be very much changed indeed, and not for the better.

Chapter 5

Nature, in her wisdom, has so composed the infant mind as to protect it from full consciousness of the worst that fate may inflict; how else would we survive those shocks and blows which, truly known, divide us forever from all that is most trusted, and most sure?

That my father had fallen ill, I knew; that he was growing weaker I could perceive from the short visits to his bedside, which, until the final days, I was permitted. I was aware of the soft tread of strange people coming and going about the house, of hushed whisperings, of doors closing with respectful quietness, and I played all the more intently at my game of tin soldiers and imaginary castles to allay the anxieties they caused me. As if in a cocoon, I had no real notion of there being a harmful circumstance to which there was no remedy, or a sorrow to which there was no immediate and loving solace.

At the funeral, I was aware, more than anything else, of my mother`s tears behind her veil, and was distressed for her sake, that her vulnerability should be shown in so public a way. I looked, when instructed, into the grave and cast down the handful of rose petals I had been given, but I had no sense, even then, of the finality of death. Afterwards, men shook me by the hand, which I found odd, having only known that gesture before as a sign of greeting or congratulation.

In the days and weeks that followed, I experienced a strange sense of freedom. The usual routines of the house were suspended, including my lessons; my mother, as I was often told, was resting, a state which, as I deemed it conducive to feeling well, I was happy to respect. In short, I went unmonitored, and the novelty of that was its own gratification.

I let myself out of the house, and let myself back in more or less as I pleased. I wandered along by the quay, and watched the mariners and the shoremen about their business, loading and unloading their cargoes, sometimes marble from the island`s quarries, sometimes livestock, sacks of grain, bales of wool. I talked to the old sea-dogs who frequented the quay, chewing their plugs of tobacco, their sea days over, and learned from them the meaning of the tides and the winds; and all the time, I partly believed that I would see my father coming out of the Customs House, or turning a corner from the quayside to meet me and take me home.

He had made for me, a special present for my seventh birthday, a model schooner, its hull carefully moulded from strips of seasoned timber, perfect in miniature detail as to the masts, the sails and the rigging, and many an hour I had spent, lying with my face flat against the soft pile of the nursery carpet, watching as it ploughed through imaginary seas. It was in such an occupation, about a month after his death, one Sunday when the constant rain prevented me from my usual outdoor pursuits, that I suddenly realised the enormity of what had happened. There would be no more father`s hands to craft such loving gifts, no more ships like this, not ever.

I cried inconsolably until at last, though I had been exhorted to desist for her sake, my mother was called. She took me in her arms and cradled me until I fell silent. It was then, looking up, that I saw her smile, the first smile I had seen for many weeks, and almost immediately my sudden fit of black and boundless mourning was over.

Chapter 6

We were, for the next six months or so, inseparable. In place of Miss Swithens, my mother now became my tutor, and though she adhered to my father`s prescription that I must be well schooled in grammar and the branches of mathematics, she also read to me in Welsh, stories from the Mabinogi, and told me of the Welsh poets, including the great poet of Anglesey, Goronwy Ddu o Fon.

In the October of 1847, just after the Fair, we visited my mother`s cousin, Agnes, in the village of Cheadle, in the county of Cheshire, a journey of two days. From a vantage point close to Aunt Agnes` house, the city of Manchester was visible as a smudge of hazy smoke in the distance and my Uncle Harold told lurid tales of the grim misery and poverty which was to be found in quarters of that city. We visited Lyme - Uncle Harold, a supplier of coal, having business there - and saw the great hall, set out with its lake and formal gardens, and, imagining the fine lives of those who lived within, it seemed to me to be a perfect haven of peace and tranquillity. The mild Cheshire countryside with its rolling panorama of open field, hedgerow and wide horizon equally pleased my youthful gaze, but though there seemed to be an endless feast of new things to see and learn, it was not long before I was homesick for Porthaethwy, and particularly for that homely sense of nearness to the sea.

That my mother should re-marry was an idea I had never entertained. It was not that I felt her to be under some debt of eternal loyalty to my father, though one part of me may have struggled with that concept; quite simply, I could not grasp that she should wish to seek anything beyond the complete [as it seemed to me] sufficiency of the life we had together.

There were some hard realities, however, which I was about to learn. I had always supposed that the disappearance of Miss Swithens from the nursery school-room had been a matter of choice; that in replacing her, my mother had sought to cushion my loss and surround me with all that was most soothing and familiar.

It did not occur to me, not until it was pointed out, much about the time that Dilwyn Jones began to pay court to my mother, that Miss Swithens had been allowed to go because she represented an expense which could no longer wisely be met.

My father had not left us to fall on the parish; indeed, there were some trusts set aside by which he had attempted to provide for my education, and, presumably, for his own and my mother`s welfare in later years; but to some extent, the suddenness and rapidity of his final illness had made it impossible, it now transpired, for him to provide for our comfort and subsistence for any length of time without the need for a significant reduction in our circumstances.

That we might otherwise be poor, however genteelly so, somewhat softened the blow dealt me when my mother told me of her intention to accept Mr Jones` proposal of marriage. It allowed me to see him as something in the nature of a benefactor; it removed, almost entirely, however blindly, any need to regard him as someone my mother loved.

Dilwyn Jones was a farmer, a cattle-man, as he liked to style himself, and his presence in Porthaethwy, and other places about the island, corresponded with the times of the markets and fairs. He was a man of thirty five, then, as I guess, clean-shaven, though with dark shoulder length hair, and, with the wide hat and high boots of the horse-riding drover, which made him cut something of an imposing figure, he was a man who, you might say, stood out from the crowd.

He had been, in earlier years, on the great cattle runs, which, in the old days, started with the herds crossing the shallowest part of the strait at low water, progressing thence through the passes of Wales and onwards to the Marches, sometimes to Shrewsbury, even as far, sometimes, as London itself. In this respect, in my early acquaintance with him, I was somewhat in awe, for it had to me then an air of high adventure; though when I learned that we were to be transported, with all that we possessed, to the lands in the parish of Llanallgo where he held his tenancy, the image of the cattle farmer took on a different and less heroic aspect.

Chapter 7

My mother and Dilwyn Jones were married in the Methodist Chapel in Porthaethwy on the 8th February, 1849, just over two years after my father`s death. There was no great ceremony either before or after. Immediately afterwards, Mr Jones set out on horseback for Llanallgo, and a day later, in an open coach which he sent for us, and with trunks behind carrying our possessions, we followed.

It was a wearying journey. The way was muddy from three days of rain, and on the steeper climbs the horses fretted and struggled, so that several times we had to alight and walk beside so that they did not tire. The upland tract was as bleak and forlorn a piece of country as I had ever seen, rough pastureland, with black stunted trees, and with the wind blowing constantly from the north-east. In clear weather, as I was later to learn, the mountains of the Welsh mainland are visible from this route, in all their changing glory, but on that day the air had closed around so that in no direction was the view any greater than half a mile.

In the late afternoon, we came down into the village of Pentraeth, and stopped for a while at the inn to warm ourselves and take some refreshment; then we began to climb again, past the wide expanse of Traeth Coch to our right, and just before dusk, I saw for the first time that stretch of rugged coast which was to become my new home.

It was too dark, when we finally arrived, to make out more of the farmstead than its outward appearance, a long building of hewn stone, with small windows, and returning a little at one end to make the shape of a letter L. My new step-father met us at the door, embracing my mother and offering his hand-shake to me, and though his welcome was affable enough, I detected in his smile the self satisfaction of a man who feels he has made a cunning bargain.

A blazing fire within lit the gloom and gave out an ample warmth so that despite my low spirits from the journey and other apprehensions, I could not help but be somewhat cheered. My step-father barked an order in Welsh, and some minutes later a white haired lady, of perhaps fifty, appeared with plates of meat, cheese and bread. We ate, not in silence but without conviviality, my mother responding to Mr Jones` enquiries and remarks with polite brevity so that I found myself glancing at her and wondering if her misgivings were not as great as my own.

After our supper, the white haired lady reappeared, and on Mr Jones` instructions lit me the way to my own chamber. A staircase at the corner of the scullery led to an attic room secluded from the rest of the house. A small fire had been burning in the grate though now only the embers remained.

The woman said something in Welsh which sounded kindly but because of her strange accent I could barely make out the words. When she had gone, I stooped to look out of the room`s single window, and could make out a strip of pale moonlight across the sea, giving the scene, in accordance with my mood, a ghostly aspect.

My sleep that night was fitful, troubled by strange noises, imaginary, no doubt, or the figment of dreams, distant sobs and murmurings that left me momentarily in terror that the place was haunted indeed. I was shocked out of my sleep the next morning by a dull boom that made me jump up in bed as if someone had fired a cannon through my dreams. The repetition of the sound some minutes later confirmed that it came from the world outside and not from the darker regions of my mind. I discovered later that it was the sound of dynamite being set off in the quarry at Bychan, a short way down the coast.

Daylight revealed a fuller picture of my new surroundings. The farmstead stood on the slope of a hill, half a mile above the line of the sea; a small harbour was visible to the left – which I soon discovered to belong to the herring village of Moelfre – and beyond that, on the skirt of the bay, perhaps a hundred yards off-shore at the high tide, a small rocky island where the sea birds flocked. To the side of the farmhouse itself, rough stone walls formed an enclosure with outbuildings surrounding an open yard where fowl and pigs roamed loose: a barn, a stable for the horses, a sheering house and other sheds with tackle and equipment.

As for the dwelling itself, nothing could have been a greater contrast to our house in Porthaethwy. Where there had been the quietness of ticking clocks with their silver chime on each quarter, the smell of polished wood, and small tapestries and prints to adorn the walls, there were now bare whitewashed walls and solid stone floors; where once neat fireplaces with pretty tiles and scrolled ironwork, now the great open hearth with logs piled high on each side. My father`s study had instruments of brass and silver for mathematical calculation, leather-bound books, and an ivory chess-set; Dilwyn Jones kept the ledgers of his business in a side-room adjacent to the scullery, and in a cabinet to the side was an assortment of fowling pieces, hunting knives and pistols.

When I came down at six o`clock on that first morning, my stepfather was sitting by the ashes of last night`s now extinguished fire, smoking a pipe and taking a mug of ale, his usual practice before going out on his business; he told me my mother would lie in for a while to recover from the rigours of the journey and instructed me to go along to the scullery to get myself fed. The old woman was in the yard outside hanging clothes to dry, and though there was no doubt it was the same woman I had seen the night before, her fleecy white hair was now loose, hanging, like a young girl`s, almost to the line of her waist. Seeing me, she came in, greeted me in a similar kindly mumble to the night before, and then brought me some hanks of bread, some ham and a jug of milk.

I had little appetite, but I drank the milk, which was warm and sweet, and took some bread and a little ham so as not to appear ungrateful, and began to wonder how I should now spend the time until my mother appeared; by now, the old woman, I noticed, had contrived to take her hair up, drawing it tightly up from her forehead and temples and fastening it closely behind. It was as if I had discovered her in a realm of unguarded privacy which she now sought to conceal.

Chapter 8

Not wishing to return by the main room and risk further converse with Dilwyn before I had spoken to my mother – I was still hopeful that she might be persuaded to see the folly of the venture and return with me to Porthaethwy – I let myself out by the scullery door and yard gate onto a cobbled lane which ran alongside the farmhouse.

This I followed for some two hundred yards down the hill until it joined a rough track which led in the direction of the village. Stopping for a moment at this point, and wondering whether to return or explore further, I became aware that I was not the only person present in the scene. Some creature, a child to judge from what I glimpsed in the fleeting moment before it stepped into the concealment of a rocky wall by the side of the lane, was following me.

I waited to see if it would reappear. When it did not, I carried on, a further twenty yards, and then turned back suddenly. Again, the creature – this time I could see that it was a girl of six or seven – hurriedly stepped off the lane and hid. I repeated this process once more, and again there was the same attempt at concealment. A little further on, where the track turned suddenly, I pressed myself against a bush, and waited. When, a few moments later, she appeared, I stepped forward.

"Why are you following me?" I asked.

The girl stood as if frozen, like an animal that thinks that by absolute stillness it will be camouflaged from its foe. She was wearing a rough woollen jacket and fustian skirt, and broken leather shoes, but the most striking thing about her was her hair which was the strangest colour of red I had ever seen, darker than chestnut, almost as dark as the copper beech.

"Why are you following me?" I repeated, this time in Welsh.

At this, the girl`s eyes grew darker, and then began to fill slowly with tears, filling to the brim as if they could hold many tears` worth before letting them spill onto her cheeks.

"You don`t need to cry," I said. "I`m not going to eat you."

At this provocation, the gathering flood at last broke forth in large droplets, and she turned, without making a sound, and fled.

I watched as she ran back up the lane, and then, fifty yards distant, she again darted into the concealment of a bush, and after a moment I saw her peeping out in my direction again. Not wanting to perpetuate this childish game further, I set forth in the direction of the village at a pace which I judged would make it difficult for her to follow me further.

The path joined a wider lane, wide enough, to judge from the wheel ruts and imprint of horse hoofs, for two carts to pass each other, and then descended directly into the village. The harbour which I had seen from the house was little more than a tapering shingle beach, bound on each side by low cliffs, and crowded with some thirty or forty fishing skiffs, with their baskets, nets, oars and sails. At the head of the beach were several small stone cottages, and a public house with the sign of the *Talyfron* above the door.

Some men were standing there, smoking pipes and drinking ale, talking, pointing and nodding seawards, as if weighing up wind and tide and weather. A handful of boats, which must have been out at dawn or before, were landing baskets of small fish which leapt and flipped, flashing silver, as they were carried off, whilst overhead the sea-birds mewed and wailed, hovering as if to pounce and steal their share.

There was sufficient business going on for the presence of a stranger not to be a matter for undue attention, I thought, and wishing to view the small island I had seen from closer quarters, I began, albeit a little self-consciously, to make my way across. There were some mutterings as I passed, and hearing Dilwyn`s name in their quiet phrases, I realised that they had already surmised my identity. There were also, when I looked up, some half nods of greeting or acknowledgement, and on the whole I felt that there was some warmth rather than otherwise in the interest I awakened.

On the other side of the bay, the main thoroughfare turned away from the cliff to follow a hill with houses on either side, and the sea path followed the line of the shore, along the cliff top. The prospect from here, and all along the coast, differs greatly depending on the position of the tide; blackened rock shelves, falling away amidst a wilderness of boulders, visible, as they now were at the low tide, are submerged and hidden when the tide is full. The channel between the mainland and the island – Ynys Moelfre as I later discovered it to be named – varies accordingly, and the higher the tide, the smaller and more distant appears the island itself.

On its rocky margins now, I could see clearly the black cormorants drying themselves with their wings held aloft, like witches or griffins, terns and gulls of various sizes and coloration. My father had once said to me, there are as many types of gull as there are religious denominations, and like religious denominations, you can be sure that they will all be fighting one another. I was reminded of that now, with the island seeming to be a screeching colony of competing sects.

I made my mind up then, that on my return, I would seek out from our travelling chest, the brass spyglass, which, along with some of my father`s other instruments, my mother had said I might keep, and on my next visit use it to inspect more closely the island`s inhabitants. At the same moment, I recalled the conflicting resolution I had made, not an hour before, to persuade my mother of the wisdom of returning, as hastily as might be arranged, to Porthaethwy, and it was to this purpose, now, as I retraced my steps through the village, and up the hill, that I set my mind.

Chapter 9

It was some time before I was able to speak to my mother alone. Dilwyn Jones, in order, as he put it, to celebrate the honourable estate into which he had entered, declared that the farm work could go hang itself for a few days, and during that time he scarcely left my mother`s side. I suspected that his motives were to do with keeping me from a mission in which he knew that I would succeed, but sensing that further familiarity with her new circumstances and surroundings could only possibly serve to alienate her from them, I thought it no bad thing to play a waiting game.

I used the immediate opportunity to discover, as I have said, the cause of the explosion which had wakened me at dawn, and which I had heard repeated several times since, and also to determine the identity of the creature who had followed me down the lane.

"There was a little girl, just near here," I said, "with red hair. I think she was following me."

"She`s a witch child," said Dilwyn, with a mirthful smirk. "Have nothing to do with her."

"That`s Izzy," my mother said. "She`s the daughter of Mrs Parry. Mrs Parry," she added, at the sign of my bemusement, "is the lady who keeps house."

"The lady with the white hair?" I asked. "She seems more likely to be her grandmother."

Dilwyn cackled with hearty approval at this my honest, but unintentionally cruel, assertion.

"Hard work and much care make us all appear old," said my mother, with a sigh.

"Then you must have neither," said Dilwyn, now in high spirits, "for I`ll not have my bride a day less beautiful than she is now!"

I did not care to see how my mother responded to this flattery, but momentarily turned my eyes to the dog which, teased by Dilwyn`s prodding, was trying, much to his master`s amusement, to worry the sole of his boot.

"Izzy," I said, going back in the conversation. "Is that a name from these parts? I`ve never heard it before."

"Richie!" said my mother, with a laugh. "It's the same name as my own. Just shortened a little to suit a girl."

"Did they call you Izzy when you were a girl?"

"No," said my mother. "But I was sometimes called Beth."

"And Beth," said Dilwyn Jones, "is what I shall call you from now. No more of Elizabeth. Too much of an English name, too much of a Tudor name! My sweet Beth, that`s what we`ll have you as now. My own sweet Beth!"

Having tired somewhat of this conversation, I asked if I might find the travelling chests in order to unpack some things to take to my chamber. One of the things I had in mind was my father`s spyglass.

Chapter 10

The conversation with my mother, when it took place, some four or five days later, did not follow the simple form, or reach the simple decisive outcome I had earlier hoped for. Nor, by that time, to be perfectly honest, did I expect it to.

"You will soon settle down," said my mother. "Look how busy you`ve been already. I`ve hardly seen you."

I tried to explain that my having been busy was a matter partly of dealing as best I could with time that would otherwise be irksome, and partly a means of avoiding the house when Dilwyn was there with his overbearing attempts at gallantry, but my mother`s look was far away, as if she barely heeded the words I said. I noticed that she had stopped wearing the silver necklace which my father had given her many years before, on which both their initials were engraved in tiny scrolled writing, and I supposed that this was at Dilwyn`s behest.

Dilwyn himself, by this time, was back to the work of the farm, and was away from the house most of the day, but when he returned, it was still with the overtures of amorous turtle-doving which he made no attempt to disguise in my presence, and to which, it pained me to observe, my mother responded with winning looks and smiles.

"We`ll let things settle down for a time," she went on, in the same even, distant tone. "And then we`ll start to think about school."

"School?" I said. "Is there a school here?"

"I mean sending you away to school," she said. "As your father wished. You`ve mentioned it often enough yourself."

This invocation of my father`s wishes, at this particular time, seemed to be the clearest indication of all that there was no going back; and with it, my sense of having been replaced in the affections of my mother was now complete.

After this, and for the several months which followed, as those times present themselves to my memory now, day merges into day, and week into week, so that I can't say precisely when this happened, or that happened, though certain events in themselves remain as clear to me now as when they occurred.

Since the time when my mother had ended her solitary grieving for my father, my comings and goings had been monitored at almost every turn; I never ventured from the house alone without her knowing where I was going and when I would return: now, instead, I was once more allowed to roam at will, and by choice I was more from the house than in it.

Sometimes, waking with the first light, I would make my way down to the village to watch the boats setting out in search of the herring, and often enough I would be there to greet them on their return; if the catch was good there was always great business in the little harbour, with the womenfolk gutting and salting the fish before they were sent off to market. Sometimes the shoals stayed away and the mood in the village was more sombre. When the herring season finished, in the spring, some of the men set out to be hired as labourers on the land – Dilwyn Jones himself often hired half a dozen men, or so - some went to work in the quarries of Bychan and Traeth Coch, even as far as the mainland, and the slate quarries of Dinorwic. Some went to Amlwch, though they said that the copper extraction there was not what it had once been, and joked that soon the place would only be fit for painters and poets.

There were always, however, a few boats putting out, some with lobster pots, some for the mackerel shoals which returned in the summer months, and as I grew to be a familiar figure about the harbour the men would joke with me about how rich my step-father was - *moneybags*, they called him - and asked if my mother bathed in milk. I got to know their names: Mesech Williams, Owen Roberts, Israel Hughes, and so on, many of them with the same surname, and the same surname as my own, and many of them with sons who bore the same Christian name as their fathers and grandfathers before them; and though they would never accede to my request to be taken out to sea with them, they were, apart from one or two of the naturally sullen ones, amicable enough and patient as I plied them with questions about their trade.

With the boys of the village, my relations were not, to begin with at least, so amicable. Not long after our arrival, I put into practice my plan to unpack my father`s spyglass and take it to the cliff top on the far side of the village to examine more closely Ynys Moelfre and its teeming bird life. There I found myself beset by a group of three or four boys, one of whom promised to knock me down if I did not make a gift of the spyglass to him forthwith. This I refused, and though he did not knock me down, he made a bid to wrest the spyglass from my hand. I held it so close to my body, for its own protection, that he could not prise it from me, though when he invoked the other boys to pull my arms from behind, a greater struggle ensued, one that common sense told me that I could not ultimately win.

Before I could capitulate, however, a voice from above, six feet away on the cliff top, bade them desist. It was a boy, much the same age as myself, though obviously with some authority, for the other boys obeyed him immediately.

"What is this?" he asked, jumping down to level where we stood. "Here we have a stranger, a noble youth who should be honoured amongst us, not trampled as a slave!"

At first I thought this somewhat poetic vein was in mockery and possibly the prelude to a renewed siege on the spyglass, but it soon became clear that his intention to defend me was pure.

"Have you heard the way he speaks?" said one of the other boys.

So far our rough exchanges had been in Welsh, and though I could hold my own, much as with the spyglass, I was at a considerable disadvantage in the present hostile company.

"He speaks like a Sais," said another, *Sais* being a term which I knew to be associated with the contempt some of my fellow countrymen felt towards the English.

"You shall not know a man by his tongue," said the newcomer, in a manner which again I thought might provoke laughter, "but by the thoughts of his heart."

The other boys, however, perhaps despite themselves,

seemed to be impressed by this high-minded sentiment. Turning to me directly, and now speaking in English, the newcomer said, "welcome to our humble but beautiful island of Mon, friend, pray tell us your name."

"Richard Williams," I said.

"See," he said, turning to the others, "a Welshman. Now may I introduce myself. My name is Isaac Lewis."

We shook hands and then he introduced me to each of the other boys in turn and we all shook hands.

"Now," said Isaac, finally, "if you will be so kind as to let each man look through your glass for a few moments, we can all be friends, and turn our attentions once more to the defence of our island from the marauder."

The bargain was sealed, and together we trotted along the coastal path, as if on horseback, searching the coves and the horizon for the appearance of enemy ships.

And so began my friendship with Isaac Lewis. With the other boys we were alternately Men of Mon or the marauders themselves, depending largely on Isaac`s mood, but whatever the guise my spyglass gave me the authority of a lieutenant, and my largesse in letting others look through it was always extolled by Isaac as a mark of nobility.

Sometimes, when he was not in the heroic vein, Isaac, whose father owned a fishing skiff, and who, unlike myself, had been out several times with the catch, would tell me of the hardships of those who earned their living from the sea, and confided in me that he believed the day would come when he would be forced to leave the island, and seek for bread elsewhere. On other occasions, we would walk along the cliff path in the direction of Bychan to get as close to the dynamiting as we could before the quarrymen shouted us off. And it was Isaac, too, who taught me, in his own meticulous way, the names of each twist and turn of the coastline around Moelfre. "That is Porth y Ross," he said, pointing away to the right, "and then Porth Aber, and this is Porth Moelfre, here at the village. Then, Porth Nigwyl and Porth Lydan, and then the Swnt, that`s the shingle beach opposite Ynys Moelfre, and then

Porth Helaeth which goes away to the big beach at Lligwy and Dulas Bay. Porth Helaeth, though," he repeated, "that`s the place to go and watch when there`s a big storm blowing!"

Chapter 11

Dilwyn Jones` farm, one of several tenancies on the land of Lord Boston, covered an area of forty acres, partly on the seaward side of the road, and partly on the rising slopes towards Marionglas. It had been in the family for three generations, going back to the Napoleonic Wars, and during that time much of the land had been turned over to grazing, though some fields were kept for barley and other crops needed for winter food for the animals, and for the kitchen. At the busy times of the year, up to a dozen men were hired as labourers, but apart from Mrs Parry, the only permanent hand was Ivor Reece, who acted as a kind of under-manager, and his wife Margaret who sometimes helped in the kitchen; they occupied a cottage adjacent to the main farm buildings.

Along the coast, farmland came as close to the cliff-top paths as it could reach; on the coast itself, from Traeth Bychan to Benllech, and the from Traeth Coch across the wide sandy bay to Llandona, quarrying was, besides fishing, the main occupation, and often the air was thick with the dust and smoke of explosions. This was all part of the world which, during my first few months in Moelfre, I began to explore.

It was not an infrequent occurrence, as I set out on my each day`s roaming, for the little girl, Izzy, to repeat her curious game of following me at a distance, and hiding from view whenever she thought me about to turn and look. Sometimes I humoured her and pretended not to notice her pursuit; sometimes I deliberately doubled back and took a different route to confuse her, but I rarely spoke to her, mainly, I suppose, because I was loath to provoke another demonstration of the strange capacity of her large eyes to carry volumes of tears without spilling them.

That she was the daughter of Mrs Parry, whom my mother had described as the housekeeper mainly, I think, to dignify her own sense of our new establishment, I already knew; in addition, I found out that they inhabited a small room behind the kitchen, which backed onto the walled enclosure, but more than this, neither my mother nor Dilwyn Jones told me anything, and I was not curious to find out.

It was Izzy`s normal custom, when she followed me, to persevere as far as the bottom of the lane, to the point where convenient camouflage grew scarce, and then to retrace her steps, or, as I occasionally discovered, to await my return so that the game could be played in reverse. On one occasion, however, unbeknown to me, she extended her pursuit through the village, and as far as the Swnt, where my fellows and I were initiating an imaginary raid on the life boat house.

"Look," said Dafydd, the boy who had once tried to take my spy-glass, "look, there`s one of the *gwragged causa*!". I knew the phrase to mean "cheese-gatherer", the same as saying someone was a vagabond who went round the village begging.

This set the other boys laughing, and Izzy spat something back, in the nature of a curse, though with language no child I ever knew would dare to use in the house. She was obviously used to the taunting of these boys.

"Go and tell your mother she`s a copper lady!" shouted John Owens.

This, at first, I did not understand, but mistakenly thought it might be an obscure reference to Izzy`s hair, or to her mother`s, which was possibly once the same colour. Later, Isaac explained to me that a copper lady was one who had had lowly employment in the mining trade at Amlwch, and again it was meant as an insult.

"Leave her," I said. "Let`s get back to what we were doing."

"Ask her where she`s from," said Dafydd.

"I know where she`s from."

"No, go on, ask her. Come on, Izzy, we don`t mean you any harm. Come down here and tell Richard where you come from."

Cajoled by the treacherous gentleness of his tone, Izzy picked her way down.

"Tell us again where you`re from."

"My dadda," said Izzy, proudly, "is the King of Tara in Erin."

"And tell us how you got here."

"A wicked sorcerer cast a spell, and my mam and dadda, and myself a weaning one, were transported by magic and cast in the darkness of night into a dungeon on Ynys Moelfre."

The boys, who up to now, for their better sport, had preserved a respectful silence, now began to give signs that the pent breath of snorting laughter could not be held in much longer.

"My mam and I escaped," Izzy went on, still in the sad illusion that her specialness was being acknowledged, "but my dadda lies there still, chained in a hall of marble, and guarded by a unicorn."

This was too much for the boys who, one by one, set each other off with the kind of laughter which contorts the body, and which, even at the point of exhaustion, sets itself off again until the very ribs ache.

Long before this had run its course, however, Izzy, her eyes filling to the brim just as on that first morning, had turned and fled. I was glad that I had managed to suppress my laughter until then, but as soon as she was gone I, too, joined in the mirth.

"God forgive us," said Isaac, solemnly, when it had at last subsided and even though he himself had laughed as uproariously as anyone else. "Wickedness is not the preserve of the English after all."

We all thought about this for a moment, as if there were some genuine moral to be drawn, and then, almost as loudly as before, we began to laugh again.

Chapter 12

Though Dilwyn Jones never gained my affection, I cannot say that I ever found him to be a bad man, certainly not in those early years. If he expressed little interest in me, it was perhaps because I expressed no desire to be of interest to him, and apart from the common factor of my mother, we lived, on the whole, in separate worlds.

He took me once, however, at my mother`s behest, to the market in Llanerch-y-medd. Whether she thought it would cement a greater bond between us, or whether she simply wanted to have two days of peace and quiet without us, I do not know, but the experience was one that left a vivid impression on my mind.

We set out just after dawn in a wagon which was also carrying the sheep, a dozen of them, which Dilwyn was to sell, together with two dozen pullets in cane boxes, so that if our own conversation was lacking, there was no shortage of ill-sorted noise and chatter to accompany us on our way and fill any awkwardness of silence there might have been.

We took the road to Marionglas and then began the climb inland with the dark ridge of Mynydd Bodafon away to our right, passing tidy cottages with white linen stretched out on the hedges, and folk who greeted us and wished us luck, and men who looked up from the field to wipe their brows and watch us as we passed.

I was preoccupied on the journey with what my mother had said just before we left. "Take care the boy isn`t shown any lewdness, mind!" Dilwyn grunted, his characteristic shorthand for laughter, and pulled on the reins to set the horses on. "You mind, now!" said my mother, more loudly, though she, too, seemed to have a flicker of laughter in her eye.

"What did my mother mean?" I ventured to ask, at last.

"What did she mean?" he replied, as if to indicate some fundamental lack of clarity in my question.

"About lewdness," I said, directly. "She said I shouldn`t be allowed to see any lewdness."

"Why, would you like to be allowed to see such a thing?"

"I`m not sure that I`d know it if I did."

"Well, then, that`s the best protection of all."

"I know it`s something bad," I said, hoping to get more from him than this.

"She meant I musn`t let you see men drunk."

"I`ve seen men drunk before."

"And she meant I musn`t let you see women drunk."

"Is there any great difference?"

"Indeed, for when men are drunk and women are drunk together, then it`s a good sign that there`s whoring going on. Do you know what whoring is?"

I admitted that I didn`t.

"Well, then, so long as you keep your eyes judiciously closed through life`s long journey, you shall see no such thing."

Deciding that any further questioning would be likely to prompt only more in the way of evasive half-riddles such as this, I allowed the conversation to be complete; at the same time, however, I resolved that I had no intention of keeping my eyes closed, judiciously or otherwise, when we reached our destination.

"Do you have any money in your pocket?" he asked, as we drew near.

"Yes," I replied, for my mother had given me three pennies in case I wished to buy any gewgaw.

"Then, keep your hand firmly over your pocket, and mind anyone who calls you dearie, and you`ll be all right."

I have been on streets in many busy places since, but until then I`d never seen anything to match the merry pandaemonium that greeted us when we reached the high street of Llanerch-y-medd that day.

The street was athrong with people and animals so that at first it seemed that there was hardly a way through. Notwithstanding, Dilwen edged the wagon forward, and howsoever they grumbled and gesticulated, men stood aside, and at last we reached an inn yard, where an ostler was given charge of the horses, and the stableboy helped Dilwyn to unload his cargo.

The sheep were penned on the street outside, and Dilwyn spoke to a man he seemed to know well, who took some money from him, smoked a cheroot with him, and then went off to find another man who, he said, would pay a good price for the sheep. The method of buying and selling animals seemed to me at first to be entirely chaotic, but as I watched, over the period of an hour or so, I began to see that there was a system, with runners carrying messages up and down the street, and with men who appeared to be acting as stewards, keeping an eye open for those of dubious intent.

On each side of the street were hawkers and pedlars of every description, calling and haggling, and shouting remarks which now and then caused a burst of loud merriment around their stall. Behind them were shops, general stores that sold everything from sacks of meal to copper pans, lanterns and chinaware, haberdashers, and, more numerous than any other, bootmakers.

Some stalls that I came across at the lower end of the street boasted curiosities from across the oceans, conch-shells and strange coloured birds, spices from the east, snake-skins and animal paws which, some of them claimed, had magical properties. I looked closely at the paw of some creature, which still had fur and talons, and the fellow there said I might hold it and stroke it for luck, and then made a joke which had the crowd about laughing, and I guessed that this was probably the closest thing to lewdness which I had witnessed yet. Just after that, an old woman took me by the elbow and said she would show me where the mother of our Lord lay buried, and this I would have taken as profaneness, if not lewdness, had it not been obvious that the poor old woman was mad. I shrugged her off and hurried on my way.

Fifty times or more I was on the point of buying something, and the same number of times exactly I refrained. It was not, I hasten to add, a parsimonious nature which thus prompted me, but more the pleasure of anticipation, denying myself now only in the hope of finding something better, something more exciting at the next turn.

And so, as Dilwyn had advised, I kept my hand firmly over

my pocket, though as to his other admonition, I could only judge from the many terms of endearment that passed quite naturally from the women to friends and strangers alike, that it was a private joke of his.

I met him later, as agreed, at the yard where we had alighted, and where he had arranged with the innkeeper for us to have supper and a bed. There was stew of mutton and potatoes, and an apple pie, and Dilwyn, flushed with good humour at the success of his transactions, improved his spirits all the more with a bottle of claret from the innkeeper`s cellar.

I stayed there as late as I might, but yawning at last, and drowsy from the mug of ale which I had been given to drink, I acceded to Dilwen`s assertion that it was time for me to be abed. A tall girl with a hare-lip lit me with a candle to the top of the house and warned me to take off my boots before getting into bed, and then left. It had been my intention to open the shutter and see, from the remaining activity on the street outside, if there was any lewd behaviour to behold; but, instead, having dutifully removed my boots, I lay on the bare mattress, and hearing the sounds of merriment from below, fell almost immediately into a deep and dreamless sleep.

When I awoke, the next morning, I found myself covered by a thick rug which I supposed Dilwyn to have put there though whether he had stayed, or slept elsewhere, or not at all, I had no way of knowing.

The business of the second day of our visit was to do with the acquiring of provisions. The farm was self-sufficient in milk, eggs, butter and cheese, and, of course, meat, and Dilwyn kept a field of oats and a field of barley, so there was no shortage of these cereals unless the harvest was especially bad, as some years, due to the weather, it was; there was also a kitchen garden which provided us with potatoes, peas and herbs; but other goods had to be brought from the market.

So it was, that day, that we loaded the wagon with sacks of flour from the mill, with bags of coffee and tea, salt and sugar, jars of oil, soap and candles; also some things my mother had requested for herself, some lengths of woven cotton, some lace material, some wool, some coarse calico, thread and needles and so on. For my own part, I decided at last to buy a little trinket to give to her, a necklace of beads, all in different shades of green, with three tiny whorled shells threaded at the middle. The woman selling it wanted four pence, but allowed me to haggle her down to three, which pleased me, though I doubt if it was worth half of that, if the truth were known.

Chapter 13

My mother had set about the business of adding some civilised and more feminine detail to the internal décor of the farmhouse. Trips to Beaumaris and Bangor, and one, on which I accompanied her, to Amlwch – my first view of the sulphurous air and blackened terrain surrounding Parys Mountain - furnished a walnut dining table and chairs, a satinwood wardrobe and a rosewood chiffonier with a mirror, for her own room.

Lace patterned silk brocade curtains added a touch of lightness to the rooms, and embroidered cushions and antimacassars softened the aspect of dark leather armchairs that were probably half a century old. Mirrors, vases and decorative ornaments, with picturesque designs all contributed to the transformation she attempted. Dilwyn, though he affected to mock the expense on such fripperies, looked on with a kind of proprietary indulgence as her work progressed.

I had brought with me some favourite volumes from my father's study, books on astronomy and the natural sciences together with some works by Daniel Defoe, Thomas Payne and Walter Scott. These had stayed on a cabinet in my chamber since being unpacked, but I now asked if I might set them up, in a small alcove next to what Dilwyn called his counting room, as a kind of library and study for my own personal use. Dilwyn at first seemed less than enamoured of this proposal, but when he saw that it would please my mother to have my whim humoured, he agreed.

It was a quiet corner, which caught the light of the sun on days when the sky was not overcast, and it was pleasant enough to sit there for an hour or two when the mood took me. The visits to Beaumaris and Bangor enabled me to add one or two new volumes, an illustrated book of flora and fauna written by an English Vicar, and a novel by Thomas Love Peacock, which was a parody of novels in the melodramatic romantic vein, though I did not realise this at the time.

I began, I suppose, though I did not fully acknowledge it at the time, to form an attachment to Moelfre even in those early months. My acquaintance with Isaac, more than with any of the other lads of the village, soon turned into a lasting friendship, and, with Izzy sometimes shadowing us, or appearing from some unexpected hidden vantage point, we explored the various pathways that led to and from the village; but it was the place itself, with its seascapes of changing mood that began to impress on me the wild beauty of the spot.

Sometimes it would rain for days, even weeks, on end; sometimes the sudden shifting of the wind to the north easterly quarter would bring high seas and bitter cold; sometimes the clear weather would reveal amazing expanses of sea and land and mountain; sometimes, a thin mist would hover all about the sea, so that the sun`s rays penetrated like a haze of shivering gold.

It was not something which I would have sought to put into words then, for in the youthful imagination, those things which are simply there from day to day require no formal utterance, but when I left Moelfre, in the autumn of the following year, when I was sent away to school, those impressions and memories were the subject of a good deal of melancholy reminiscence.

Chapter 14

Since leaving Porthaethwy I had had no formal schooling. There was a parish school which the other boys of the village attended – unless their fathers` work required their assistance, which happened quite frequently – but the level of tuition was very rudimentary. The Rector, the Reverend John Griffiths, encouraged girls to join the school too but with mixed success, most families finding better occupation for them, as they saw it, than learning to read and write. Izzy, so far as I could tell, had never been to school at all. My own case was different, as I had received instruction at home for several years, and my mother did not press me to join the class.

With my eleventh birthday now approaching, however, my mother informed me that the time was now come for my education to continue. Having been uprooted once, I put up some resistance, but my mother was insistent, and, from motives which I believed had little to do with my better interests, Dilwyn lent support to the wisdom of the plan.

I had a period of some five weeks to reconcile myself and prepare. Meantime, letters were exchanged with the Rev. P. W. Levison, the High Master, as he styled himself, of the Eastry School in Shropshire, and arrangements were made with the bank for funds from the trust to be set against the fees due for my tuition and accommodation.

And so it was that on the fifteenth of September, 1850, I set out for Eastry. My mother`s farewell was as tearful as could be wished for, so that you might easily have thought her the one whose wishes had been over-ruled, but that was little consolation to me. Izzy stood by the gate and waved as I left, and Isaac was at the top of the lane, near the school-house, with Dafydd and Ivor to shout their farewells as I passed.

During the seven years I was at Eastry it became common for the main stages of the journey to be undertaken by train, a minor excitement which thrilled many boys like myself at that time when such travel was a novelty, but my first journey was the slow progress of horse and coach. The first leg was to Bangor, then by public coach to Chester, and thence to Eastry, some twenty miles from Shrewsbury.

I arrived in the sombre hall at Eastry School at seven o`clock in the evening, some two days ahead, I was told, and not without a sense of reprimand by Mrs Hodge, who we called matron, of my fellow pupils. My immediate instinct was to call back the coachman and bid him take me home, but this not being possible, I was directed to the kitchen, given some broth and corn bread, and after that to a dormitory with twelve empty beds and told to say my prayers and go to sleep.

Chapter 15

There must be many thousands of boys, sent away from home to school, who have experienced the same acute loneliness that I felt that night. If it did not quite rank with the moment, some two and a half years before, when I had truly realised that my father had died, it was the more prolonged for there being, on this occasion, no loving arms to console me, or comforting words to beguile my despondency.

Had my fellows been present, there might possibly have been some camaraderie to lift the spirits. As it was, the emptiness of the dormitory, when it grew dark, compounded my misery with terror, as I was not beyond the age of believing that ghosts walked the earth and visited dark spots such as this with malevolent intentions.

The morning brought little relief. If I had wished for some company the night before, now I began to dread the arrival of the other boys, fearing that I would appear to them ignorant and weak and become the victim of their scorn.

Not all my fears were ill-founded. Whereas the boys in Moelfre had mocked my English manner of speech, now I was mocked for my Welsh accent which earned me various nicknames which I had to outface and endure before I became inured to the intended scoff, or indeed until, by familiarity, it became a kind of affection.

During the early weeks and months at Eastry my despondency was somewhat offset by the belief that my father`s design with regard to my education was now to be realised. He would have had me trained so that I might become an engineer, a designer of buildings, a doctor. How long exactly it took me to realise that Eastry was not the kind of academy he had envisaged, I do not know, but in truth, as one can see retrospectively, it was a school of mediocre ambitions and an uninspiring curriculum.

The Rev. P. W. Levison was a small rotund man of sixty, with a ruff of grizzled hair at the back of his head, and plump white fingers, who took little interest in the classroom, but who could sermonise endlessly in the school chapel mainly on the subject of the moral benefits of hardship and deprivation, though to judge from his household he deprived himself of little and suffered few hardships beyond the inconvenience of turning himself out to walk the fifty or so yards to the chapel each morning at nine o`clock, and the fifty or so yards back.

The masters, twelve in number, were a mixture of all sorts. One master, Mr Roper, who professed Mathematics, was of a dark, melancholy disposition; there were two or three for whom life`s disappointments had transformed into a rigid educational philosophy, though only one, who, during my time there at least, practised outright cruelty; but in the main the masters were benignly complacent to the point of laziness.

At the very beginning, when I was most isolated – the boys of my form having for the most part been together for two years already so that their friendships and alliances were already established – I counted the days as a means of giving some purpose to my existence, but time is too long, especially to a child, to live by such abstract goals, and I found myself, before too long, adapting, like the chameleon, to my surroundings, and making the most of what was there to be had.

Chapter 16

I returned home for the first time on Christmas Eve, and stayed just over a week, until the New Year of 1851 had been welcomed in. The herring fleet was frequently busy during this season so I saw little of Isaac or the other boys. Izzy, by now, was employed with her mother in the kitchen and about the house each day, and so, I guessed, her perambulations and her espionage had been curtailed. On one occasion I found her sitting in my library alcove pouring over a book of verse; rather doubting her ability to make sense of the letters she traced with her finger, I maintained a tactful silence, and sat down to read my own book. I was somewhat amused to notice that, for my benefit, her eyes began to travel quickly from side to side, and to note the rapidity with which she turned the pages.

"You`re doing very well with your learning, Izzy," I said.

She demurred, shrugging her shoulders slightly, as if to signify the remark to be quite superfluous.

I happened to notice, at this point, that she was wearing the shell necklace that I had bought for my mother at Llanerch-y-medd over a year before.

"I like your necklace, Izzy," I said.

A high colour came into her face. "Your mother gave it to me," she said, taking hold of it protectively.

"It suits you well," I said.

I wondered whether to take the matter up with my mother, but Izzy was clearly so proud of her piece of `jewellery` that I decided not to make any fuss.

At Easter, I was told by the Reverend Levison that I must stay at school instead of returning home; a letter from my stepfather, he informed me, said that my mother was unwell and must have tranquillity. My mother did not write to me during this period and so I had no idea if she received my own letters. I blamed Dilwyn for this and saw him as the chief instigator of my exile, though it later transpired that my mother had miscarried during this time, and that her illness was, indeed, severe.

I spent the two weeks with Simon Wheeler, a boy a year older than me, though from his frail frame and blanched complexion, you might have taken him to be three years my junior. Simon, `wheezer` as he was known, not just because of its similarity to his name, but because of his frequent attacks of asthmatic wheezing, was left at the school because his father was an artist, travelling in Italy, because his mother was dead, and because he had no other living relatives.

He was, without doubt, the most sickly child I have ever met; he could not walk above a certain pace without the fear of something flaring up, and he could not go outdoors in the sun without the fear of something else flaring up: "one of these days," he used to say, "I have no doubt that I shall flare up altogether, and that will be the end of me!"

Consequently, our companionship that Easter, consisted largely of sitting in the `Crib`, the room designated for holiday boarders such as ourselves, playing backgammon and talking, a skill in which, as if to compensate for everything else, he excelled.

In all my time at Eastry, and perhaps even since, I can honestly say that I never made a friend to compare with the friendship I had with Isaac; but poor Simon, with all his ailments, came to seem almost like a brother, the kind of brother you want to protect because his frailness and vulnerability break your heart.

At the beginning of June I finally received a letter from my mother telling me that her health had much improved and saying how much she was looking forward to seeing me in July when the school term finished. I wrote back, and included a note for Isaac which I suggested Izzy might be able to pass on.

Though Simon and I were in different forms, we maintained our friendship over the occasional game of backgammon after prep., and, curiously perhaps, it was a friendship which the other boys respected without any of the usual schoolboy jibes at anything slightly odd or out of the ordinary.

Three weeks before the end of the term, I came across Simon, one day, in a state of great nervous excitement: he had received a letter from his father.

"He`s in London," Simon explained. "He wants me to stay with him for five weeks during the vacation. And he wants you to come too."

"Me?"

"Yes. I wrote to him to say what a good friend you`d been to me when just the two of us were here at Easter, and he says he would like to meet you."

"The trouble is," I said, "I`m supposed to be going home, too."

I saw his face drop.

"I couldn`t go for five weeks, or anything like it."

"No, just few days. A week at the most."

My strongest inclination was to refuse, for I was, intermittently, very homesick for Moelfre, but at the same time, I truly believe that apart from me he had never had a friend at all, and I could not bring myself to disappoint him.

"I`ll write to my mother, and ask," I said, half hoping that she would forbid the excursion.

My mother, however, seemed to think that it was a delightful prospect, and urged me to profit from the opportunity to see the capital. I returned her letter, with details of the journey, and enclosed another letter for Izzy to deliver to Isaac, if the time could be spared from her duties at the house.

I found myself wondering, as the day approached for our journey, what sort of man I might expect to meet in Simon`s father. I had been, to some extent, pre-disposed to think ill of a father who could leave so poorly a child alone, but now, as the time approached for me to meet him and be in his company, I thought I should try to find out a little more about him.

"You said your father was a painter?" I asked as the coach took us from Eastry to Gobowen.

"Yes," Simon replied, furrowing his brow thoughtfully. "He doesn`t earn much money from his painting yet, that`s the trouble, he hasn`t quite made his name yet."

"Enough to send you to school, though."

"Well, not exactly. He inherited a little money from his father, and that just about keeps us going. He`s been plagued by bad luck. He made a rather unfortunate marriage in his youth, doubly unfortunate in that it landed him with me."

"Surely that`s not his opinion!"

"Oh, no, not at all."

"What does he paint?"

"Well, being an Irishman he has a natural love of horses, so that is the subject he likes most, but all manner of things, hounds, cats, birds."

"Mainly animals, then."

"Well, yes, though set in landscapes, and gardens."

I tried to take this in and formed the impression that he must be an odd sort of artist.

"He`s been travelling around France and Italy, meeting people, you know, other artists, it`s very important to do that, you know. Oh, he is fairly sure to make money, soon," Simon continued, "and then I shall leave Eastry and we will set up house. That`s my ambition, to set up house and sit in a comfortable chair and watch him painting."

"Like a cat?"

"Yes, I should like to be a cat. You don`t see cats flaring up all the time."

I mused at Simon`s apparent trust, his philosophic acceptance of things; for all his ailments and weaknesses, he seemed much more at one with the world than I felt myself. My musings, however, were short-lived, for soon we were approaching the station at Gobowen, and the imminence of my first ever journey by locomotive drawn train began to fill me with excitement.

Simon, who had completed the journey three or four times already, was my guide, and he exuded an air of familiarity which was reassuring. To me, everything was new, not least the sense of danger that came at every turn: the approach of the engine with its thunderous noise, the hissing of pistons and the screech of wheels as it drew to a halt; then the motion, sometimes high above the surrounding fields, flying across bridge and viaduct, at a speed of forty miles an hour and more.

When I had overcome the terror that I might, at any moment, be hurtled to my death, I began to experience the true exhilaration of railway travel. Farms and villages sped by; here and there the rail tracks ran alongside a canal, and we passed barges making their slow progress; sometimes the billows of smoke and steam swept across the fields, and, then, with a change of the train`s direction, swept back across the window, filling the carriage with the fumes of smoke.

This, at one point, caused Simon to have a flaring up of the eyes, and again, a little later, a flaring up of the lungs, but these were both of a minor nature, and, for the most part, he was as vigorous and spirited as I had known him.

The only remaining fear lay in my being far from convinced that the locomotive would be able to stop when we reached our destination, where, as I understood it, the track ended abruptly at a stop rather than running on beyond. However, several stops to take on fresh water and coal, and others to allow passengers to alight or join the train, finally persuaded me that some reasonable level of control could be exercised by the engineer, and when we finally arrived at the station at Euston Square, I was only sad that the journey was over.

If I had any doubts as to how I would like or approve of Simon`s father, they were soon dispelled. Bob Wheeler was an open-faced man, with large features and a shock of ungovernable black hair, and a warmer or more loving greeting than he made to Simon, I have never seen.

He shook my hand, thanked me, with tears in his eyes, for being Simon`s friend, then laughed heartily, and hugged me in much the same way as he had Simon. Then he summoned a hansom cab and took us to his lodging which was in the vicinity of Pimlico and just above a chop house, so we did not go without a cheerful repast that night.

The following morning, Simon, evidently the worse for the rigours of the journey, was kept in bed by a bad attack of the wheezing, and whilst Bob tended him – and not wanting to roam out on the streets of the capital alone lest I should lose my way – I went up to the attic room which Bob called his studio, and looked at his paintings. My experience of art was very limited indeed; at an exhibition in Bangor, once, my father had shown me paintings of heroic action at the Field of Waterloo, and I recall some rather grand biblical scenes, portraits of aristocratic people, and pastoral landscapes. Whether Bob`s paintings had any true merit, I could not judge, but they seemed to me to have a curious appeal. As Simon had told me, his main theme was animals – horses, greyhounds, badgers, cats, foxes, all painted to look very real, though with something quite whimsical, too, it seemed to me, quite in contrast to the bleak and mountainous landscapes in which they were set.

When I returned, Bob was holding Simon`s hand and talking. "Never mind, old chap. It won`t be too long now. I`m very hopeful of one or two commissions in the autumn, and maybe I`ll take on some portraits."

"It`s a pity Miriam isn`t a bit older," said Simon.

"Yes, well, that`s a long time off yet, and who knows but that she might change her mind."

"I don`t think she`ll ever change her mind, dad."

"Anyway, one more year should do it, and then we shall have you out of Eastry, and we`ll set up that house of ours, that`s for sure."

"In Dublin?"

"In Dublin, where else?"

I felt so sorry for them both, father and son, at that moment, that I only wished I had enough money to purchase some of Bob`s paintings and set them on the way.

We had a meat pie with pickled onions for our lunch and then, with Simon now fully refreshed, Bob told us that we were going to set out to see the `Great Exhibition`.

At first I misunderstood this, thinking that Bob merely meant an exhibition of art. I could not have been more mistaken.

A short carriage journey brought us to Hyde Park, and there

we came upon a building of great splendour, all of glass and ironwork, which was called the `Crystal Palace`. The exhibition, Bob explained, was the brain-child of Prince Albert, and its aim was to bring together, for the people of London, all that the genius of science and art had produced, across the world, to enhance and modernise our lives.

It is almost impossible to describe the magnificence of the exhibition or the effect it had on me. Many hundreds of people were there, moving quietly, as if in awe, from one hall to another, inspecting the exhibits. My only sadness was that my own father wasn`t there beside me, for he more than any other man would have been delighted at what there was to see.

"Perhaps he will be watching you," said Simon.

"Here in spirit?"

"Yes. I`m a great believer in spirits. Do you think they roam the earth?"

"Possibly," I said, though the question seemed quite at odds with the place we were in, with its vast assemblage of mechanical invention.

"I hope so," said Simon, "for I`m sure mine will be glad to be free to roam when it`s let loose from this wheezing old carcass."

"You don`t feel a flaring up coming on?" I asked, concerned that a repeat of the morning`s indisposition might be at hand.

"Not at all," he said. "Lead on!"

We were, at that moment, entering a compartment filled with engines and boilers, great and small, some designed to power the machinery of mills, some for the new locomotives, much bigger and much faster, it seemed, than the one which had pulled our train: rows of gleaming pistons, and polished brass, and metal plate studded with iron rivets.

"They do say," said Bob, catching up with us, "that engines such as these will drive the new iron ships and motor carriages that will run without tracks, so that by the next century there won`t be a sail on the ocean or a horse on the streets."

"Does that make you sad?" I asked.

"I regard the horse, young Richard, as a friend. Now why

should I be saddened if I see an old friend gain some remission from his labours?"

We came presently to a chamber which demonstrated agricultural equipment.

"Your step-father`s a farmer, is he not?" said Bob.

I nodded, as we both looked at the mechanical reaping machine on display, and, picturing the barley fields at home, with four men working abreast with scythes, I wondered what Dilwyn would think of this.

Not all the exhibits were of great size. Handicrafts and ornaments of great beauty, the intricate work of the silversmith and the goldsmith, stood side by side with baskets of pearl and precious stones to create a dappled blaze of colour. "Come and look at this, boys," said Bob. "The Kohinoor diamond, the biggest in the world! Now, if we had some shares in that, we would no longer need to fret over the earning of our bread."

There were implements for the household, too, machines and devices to carry out many menial chores, and equipment for the creation of daguerreotypes which much interested Simon, musing that an image could be produced in few moments which might take an artist many hours of patient application to achieve. He was much amused, too, at the discovery, in the Retiring Rooms, of Public Conveniences, the first it seemed, anywhere in the world, a service which could be purchased for the sum of one penny.

To complete the day, Bob later took us to a musical soiree at the Hanover Rooms. I had heard my mother playing on the pianoforte and singing at our old home in Porthaethwy, and I had heard two or three musicians together, in Moelfre playing working songs and fishing songs, but a full orchestra, and the sound it made, filling the room with pulsating music was an experience which overwhelmed me. My favourite piece was one called `The Egmont Overture`, by Mr Beethoven, a German composer; it seemed to have a heroic purpose, as if to challenge tyranny across the earth, and make it forever a wiser and more just place.

I was also intrigued by the other members of the audience, the gentlemen in their frock coats and cravats, the ladies in their fine gowns and hats, and, in particular, a group of three young ladies sitting close to us, with pale powdered faces and necks, and tumbling ringlets of hair, so elegant and so lovely that you could almost fancy them made from the finest porcelain.

On the way home, by contrast, on the shadowy streets, we saw beggars, and men and women drunk, and the girls they called streetwalkers. "God preserve us," said Bob, "for all the richness and beauty we`ve seen and heard today, there`s an awful lot of misery in the world still."

The following day, we rested until noon, then took a dog-cart to the river – wider than the Afon Menai, and with great buildings along each bank, - though when we went by boat to Richmond Park we were all somewhat troubled by the bad smell which came off the water.

"Who is Miriam?" I asked Simon, suddenly recollecting the conversation I had overheard the previous day.

"Miriam. Oh, she`s an American. She mixes with all the artistic people, you know, poets, painters. She`s what they call an heiress, and she says she wants to buy all my father`s work. Trouble is, she doesn`t inherit until she`s thirty – it`s written in someone`s will."

"How old is she now?"

"Nineteen."

"Quite a wait, then."

"Yes. You`ll probably meet her. You might find her a little strange."

It is perhaps true to say that when I met her, a day or two later, I found Miriam to be a little strange, but it was only one strangeness amongst many that I discovered that day, and I cannot really say whether oddness or wonderment was uppermost in my thoughts.

"I`m going to take you to meet some friends of mine," Bob said, on the evening in question. We summoned a carriage which took us to an inn in the area Bob called Soho. "They call themselves `the Brotherhood`, said Bob, affectionately, "I`m sure you`ll like them."

"What does `the Brotherhood` mean?" I asked Simon, summoning images of an order of monks or something of that description.

"Oh, it`s nothing really. They`re just artists. Artists are always calling themselves something or other."

The inn was crowded and noisy, full of colour and mirth, and Simon and I sat in a corner, unnoticed, we hoped, and took it all in.

"Which is `the Brotherhood`?" I asked Simon, wondering if it was everyone who frequented the inn.

"That`s Will," he pointed out, "and over there, talking to a woman, is John, and the woman is Ruskin`s wife, Effie, though she also models for paintings, and then there`s Gabriel, the one talking to Bob, and next to him is Lizzy, she`s a model, too, and that`s Edward, on the far side of the table, and he`s sitting next to Christina who`s Gabriel`s sister – she`s a poet – and the other one is Miriam."

I paid particular attention to Miriam, and thought her rather beautiful, though extremely pale, and also with a very faraway look in her eyes, which Simon said might be laudanum, or marijuana, though you couldn`t really tell, as it was actually quite fashionable to have that sort of look if you mixed with the Brotherhood.

I gazed at her, and at Christina, and the other women who were present, and they all seemed to have some magical luminous quality as if they had been taken out of paintings and brought to life, rather than being ordinary beings who belonged, like myself, to the ordinary world outside.

We stayed there for an hour, and then it was announced that the party was moving on to Gabriel`s house. "16, Chatham Place, Blackfriar`s Bridge," said Bob. "Remember it boys, for I`m tight as a tick and like to forget it if left to my own devices."

"16, Chatham Place, Blackfriars Bridge," we repeated to the coachman. It was nearly ten o`clock when we arrived; some of the others seemed to have disappeared altogether; others seemed to have been picked up on the way, but the party continued, albeit in a quieter vein, as people spread about the house.

There were paintings in every room I went to, some hanging on the walls, others stacked as if the whole house served as an extended studio, and I recognised some of the girls from the public house, in various costumes and poses.

One in particular, which was hanging in the hall, caught my attention and aroused my curiosity. It showed a man lying on the ground who looked, at first, as though he had been murdered, though it seemed from the rest of the painting that he was, in fact, merely unconscious with drink, and what had seemed like spilt blood was in fact mead or wine. On the left of the picture, behind another drunken man in a chair and some sleeping hounds, through slotted windows, some kind of dancing or revelry was visible, and on the right side, a young man and a young woman dressed in gowns of the medieval times, had emerged from a curtained doorway and seemed to be picking their way through the scene. The painting had a label attached as if it had been at an exhibition, which said: The Eve of St Agnes, by William Holman Hunt.

I studied it for some time, trying to work out its precise significance, and then took the opportunity to broach the matter with Gabriel, who was sitting alone by the fire, looking lazy and relaxed.

"Excuse me, sir, but may I ask a question?"

"So long as it`s not a request for cash, old chap."

"Could you explain the painting to me?"

"Which painting?"

"The one in the hall."

"The flight of Madeline and Porphyro? It`s one of Will`s."

"Yes," I said, though it had not occurred to me that the William Holman Hunt of the painting was actually Will.

He closed his eyes, as though he might go to sleep, and I sensed that he was a little tipsy.

"It`s from a poem," he said, at last. " `The Eve of St Agnes`. Chap named Keats. Dead now, poor fellow. Never got the recognition he deserved. Probably be discovered one day. That`s the trouble with art. Chap does the work, some other beggar gets the benefit when he`s dead."

He closed his eyes again, and I thought that that was the end of that, but, presently, he resumed, "Porphyro and Madeline. Complicated really. Eve of St Agnes, middle of winter, feast going on. Old tradition – virgin goes to bed, naked, says prayers and charms, and other such rituals, has dream vision of the man she will marry. Well, here`s the crux of it – chap`s hidden in girl`s room, you see, having bribed old crone to let him in, you see, something like that. Anyway, chap`s hidden, watches girl disrobing, very sumptuous, too…"

He closed his eyes once more, as though picturing the scene to himself, for there was the ghost of a smile on his face.

"Anyway," he resumed, once more, "girl`s in bed, chap comes out of hiding, leans over her, looks down at beauteous visage, girl opens eyes, thinks she`s seeing dream vision of husband to be, chap slips into bed beside her, and, well, virgin no more! When girl realises she`s not dreaming - which to my way of thinking must have been pretty damned soon - much lamentation from her and much expiation from him. Anyway, turns out they were pretty much in love beforehand, else why was she dreaming of him in the first place, and so they make it up, pledge eternal fidelity, and run away together whilst the revellers are all lying about drunk. That`s the painting. Make sense to you, does it?"

"Yes, sir, I think so."

He closed his eyes again and this time went soundly to sleep, leaving me to ponder my own thoughts alone.

The following day, I went with Bob to meet `the Brotherhood` again, this time in a tavern close to Charing Cross. Simon, feeling tired after the day`s activities, had decided to stay at the lodgings to rest, but I went because I wanted to ask Will to elucidate more of his painting of `The Eve of St Agnes`. Will, however, was in the middle of a heated debate about religion, arguing that all his paintings from now on would strive to express a new spirituality, far from the dross of lust, as he termed it, so the opportunity did not arise.

We had been there for about an hour when John arrived,

announcing rather breathlessly, "the old man`s sick. Not long to live by all accounts. I suppose we`d better pay him our respects."

"Who`s the old man?" I asked.

"Turner, " Bob replied.

"Turner who?"

"J. M. W. Turner," said John. "Joe to his friends. Not that he has many of those these days. More or less a recluse."

"Where is he?" asked Gabriel.

"Sophia`s."

"In Chelsea. Where else!"

"Come on then, boys. Drink up."

The references still meant nothing to me and so, on the way, I asked Bob to enlighten me.

"Turner?" said Bob, with some reverence. "Why, he`s the foremost landscape artist of his generation."

"Not that that`s our generation, mind you!" said Edward.

"According to Ruskin," said Gabriel [Ruskin, I had discovered, was not a painter himself but a critic] "it is Turner who most stirringly and truthfully measures the moods of Nature."

"Poor fellow," said John, "all he`ll be measuring soon is a length of earth."

We eventually found our way to Chelsea and were let into the house by a bemused servant at the door. "Just look," said Gabriel, "he doesn`t even need to sell his paintings, the house is an art gallery."

"But it isn`t his house, is it?"

"Even worse, his mistress` house is an Art Gallery."

In the hallway were several magnificent canvases, seascapes and riverscapes all of which seemed ablaze with golden light and steam and smoky clouds.

We made our way upstairs

"What do you want? " said a dignified and rather stern lady appearing from a door at the top of the stairs.

"Someone said Joe was dying. We came to pay our respects."

"Who says I`m dying?" said a gruff and irascible voice from inside the room.

Through the gap in the door, I could make out a figure sitting in a chair by the fire, with a rug over his knees.

"Who is it?" he called again.

"It`s the members of the Brotherhood," said the lady.

There was a long, impatient growl in Turner`s voice.

"Is Bob Wheeler there?"

"Yes, he`s here."

"Send him into me. Is his boy with him? Send him in too."

Everyone looked at each other, and then at me.

"Go on. Go in. He`ll not know the difference."

I followed Bob into the room.

"Bob," said the old man, reaching out a hand warmly, "old friend. It`s true, I`m dying."

"But you look well," said Bob. "I`ll wager there`s more to come from you yet."

"No. It`s done. What`s done is done. But you. You must settle down, now, and attend to your work. No more of your wandering."

"I intend to do as you say."

"Good. You never know when it might end. And the boy, well?" he said, turning to me.

"Yes," said Bob, "Quite well."

They continued to talk and I studied the face of Turner. It was gaunt and deeply lined though the eyes were sharp and lively; I did not think him upon the verge of death, but at the same time, with childish logic, I could not really imagine him living a great deal longer, any more than any other very old man.

My attention was drawn by a painting in the room which was framed with the title, `Dogano and Santa Maria della Salute, Venice`. In the hazy distance, the towers of a ghostly city arose above a waterway with indistinct wharfs and boats in the foreground, and as with the paintings I had glimpsed briefly in the hall, the sky seemed infused with golden hazy light, like the sun shining through a mist, very similar to that which I had sometimes observed at Porth Helaeth in certain weather.

"Well," said Bob, at last, "we must leave you to rest."

"Oh, plenty of that coming my way soon, I don`t doubt. Take the rest of them with you if they haven`t already gone."

"Goodbye, Joe."

"Goodbye Bob. Goodbye, young man."

"Goodbye, sir."

"He was my teacher once, twenty years ago," said Bob, as we made our way downstairs to find, indeed, that the others had already gone.

"He seems to like you."

"Yes. He always did. Can`t think why."

"Probably because you`re a thoroughly likeable chap, Bob"

"Nice of you to say so, Richie." He drew a long sigh. "It`ll be a sad day for me, though, when old Joe Turner goes. Ah, well, it`s the way of nature. Now, let`s get you back to something a little more cheerful, shall we?"

Chapter 17

Two days later, bidding Simon and Bob farewell at Euston Square, I began my return journey, travelling by train to Chester, then to Bangor, and thence, via the new Brittania Bridge, to Llanfairpwll. There, Ivor Reece was waiting with a dog-cart to take me home.

As soon as I was fed and decently rested from the journey, my mother insisted on my telling her the whole story of my stay in London. How coherent I was, I do not know, since there was much to tell, and some parts of my narrative developed a habit of interrupting other parts, helter-skelter fashion, so that more then once she was obliged to stop me and to encourage me to go a little more slowly; there were, too, certain parts of the story which I did not tell her fully, parts which had become more a matter for private consideration than for outward disclosure.

In turn, my mother told me that her health continued to improve, though in truth, she looked tired and slightly drawn about the face, as if she had been aprey to some illness that had had a wasting effect. Dilwyn had become morose and taciturn, and there were few glimpses now of the affable suitor and bridegroom of two years before. Sometimes, in the evening, he would sit by the fireplace, and if he spoke at all it was to bemoan his rents, or the poor state of the markets, or the cursed bad luck that had taken off a dozen lambs with sickness; sometimes, he would take himself off to the Talyfron, in the village, intending, no doubt, to drink himself into a better humour.

It was Izzy who told me the truth of my mother`s illness. "She miscarried a child," she said. "It was a terrible night. We feared for her life, and the doctor, when he came the next morning, he said that she might not last the day, but my mother nursed her, and if you think she looks ill now, you would not say so if you had seen her then."

If she had meant to reassure me, her account had quite the opposite effect, but I thanked her, nevertheless, for the earnestness of her intentions was clear.

"And I delivered your letters to Isaac," she added, as if to add a little more to the sum of my debt.

"Thank you," I said again. "And how is your reading progressing?"

"Very well," she replied, colouring slightly, recalling, I suspected, the afternoon in my study alcove at Christmas.

Meeting Isaac, the next day, and walking out to the Swnt, our usual haunt, it did not surprise me to find Izzy hovering by. Though I had not seen her following me, it was evident that her old habits had not deserted her entirely.

"She`s all right," said Isaac. "She found me to give me the letters you sent."

"Yes, I know."

She sat on a rock a few feet away from us, like a cat at the edge of a campfire, part of the company and yet apart from it.

Isaac listened with great curiosity to my account of London and the Great Exhibition, asking questions and nodding his head as I answered, and then he questioned me about every part of my journey by train. When I told him about Gabriel and `the Brotherhood`, he furrowed his brow thoughtfully, and when – exaggerating slightly – I told him about seeing the great artist, Turner, on his deathbed, his eyes widened like saucers. The only thing I did not go into fully was `The Eve of St Agnes`, which I felt I couldn`t properly explain, certainly not with Izzy listening in close by.

"Can you meet tomorrow?" said Isaac, as we made our way back towards the village.

"Yes," I replied. "At the Swnt?"

"No, here. I`ve got something in mind."

"Can you tell?"

"Make sure you don`t let anyone know," he said, "especially you," he added, nodding towards Izzy. "We`re going to go out round Ynys Moelfre. Meet me here an hour before the full tide."

I lay in bed that night in as great a state of anticipation as with any of my recent excursions. The prospect of rowing around

Ynys Moelfre was something we had talked of many times, but I had never thought we would do it. Now, in order, I think, to counterbalance my exploits with something of his own, Isaac had decided that the time was right. I only wished he had not told Izzy, partly because I feared she might blurt it out, and have the expedition banned, and partly, I admit, because I did not want the secret to have another sharer.

When I reached Porth Moelfre the next morning, with Izzy hard at my heels, the fishing boats had already left. Isaac was at the far side of the beach, with the tender his father sometimes used for sculling the shallow waters of the bay.

"The wind is just about right," said Isaac, importantly, as if any undesired variation would cause his superior judgement to cancel the exploit.

We pulled the boat down the shingle until she was perched on the edge of the water.

"Let me come too?" called Izzy.

"No," said Isaac, decisively. "Too dangerous for a girl. Jump in Richie."

I could see Izzy`s mouth set in a twist of spite and disappointment, as Isaac took the oars and pulled us away, leaving her behind.

We pulled out along past Porth Lydan, where, out of the shelter of the bay, a crosswind ruffled the surface of the sea.

"Let me row for a while?" I said.

We changed places, and in my new position, looking back towards the Swnt, I could see the forlorn figure of Izzy in the distance, her skirts, her shawl and her hair - blowing slightly in the wind - all shades of red or brown against the grey rocks of the shore.

As we approached the island, its rocky shelves and ledges became clear, and with the swell of the sea and the wind now stiffening, I began to wonder about the wisdom of making a landfall. I sensed that Isaac felt the same way too. "We`ll carry on," he said. "The important thing is the circumnavigation."

With this grand word to support our decision, we pulled away to the eastward side of the island, and soon the Moelfre shore was hidden.

"Look," said Isaac, pointing out to sea. Some fifty yards away there was visible a disturbance at the surface of the sea, with gannets circling round.

"Is it a shoal of fish?" I asked.

"It`s more than that. Watch."

I looked hard at the waves, and with my eyes focused, began to notice, every so often, a dark shape breaking the surface.

"Porpoises," said Isaac. "Now, watch the gannets."

Just then, from twenty or thirty feet above the surface, a gannet plummeted, as straight as an arrow, and plunged into the sea. Then it seemed that the whole flock was doing the same thing, and we watched, spellbound, for a good twenty minutes, seeing every now and then the amazing sight of a porpoise leaping clear of the water altogether.

When we finally rounded the island and the Swnt appeared again, there was no sign of Izzy. Secretly I wished now that we had taken her with us, so that she too could have enjoyed the spectacle we`d seen, and regretted the pettiness of motive which had made us exclude her.

During my remaining time in Moelfre that summer, I began to sketch. It was an exercise in which I had no great skill, certainly to begin with. If I attempted to represent people, either the face or the form, the results were poor indeed, little better than the attempts of a child, worse, in fact, since they lacked a child`s naturalness. I found, however, that the lines and shapes of the coast, the curves of the bay and the strong ridges of the cliffs and headlands, were a more manageable subject for my immature efforts, and so I was able to depict, in a simple way, some of the familiar scenes, and, through some basic shading and smudging, to convey some of their moods.

Imperfect as they were, I showed them to Simon on my return to Eastry, and he was delighted with them, making me talk through each one in every detail, until he could take up the tale himself. "This is Porth Helaeth," he would say, "and here`s the

Swnt, and that is the island you rowed round with Isaac," and so it went on. He lived out the drawings as if he were there, or as if they created a world into which he could enter; often, as I came into the room, I found him looking at them alone.

He was, after the summer spent with his father, in the best of spirits to begin with that term. He was full of his own stories of what Hunt had said to Christina, and what Gabriel had done, and what John had said about Miriam, and a hundred other things. He had been, too, to the seaside at Southend, the first time, he told me, that he had ever seen the sea, and it had done his health, he averred, a power of good.

His seeming good health persisted through the warm dry days of September, but as soon as the damper autumn weather began to draw in and cling around Eastry, the colour of his cheeks faded to the old pallor, and, as he called it himself, the flaring-up season had begun.

A chill which started one Sunday morning, had become, by the middle of the week, a settled fever; a week later, the matron pronounced that it was the rheumatics, and said that a doctor must be called and the bill sent to his father. The doctor said that he feared contusions of the lung, and prescribed a resinous mixture that looked like tar-water and smelled like sulphur. Amongst the boys, the whisper going round was that Simon had consumption.

The last time I saw him was in the sick-room at Eastry one gloomy Sunday afternoon in November. His breathing was hoarse, and his now pitifully thin frame was shaking, but still he asked me to tell him about the occasion when Isaac and I rowed around Ynys Moelfre, and though I had no spirit for it, I managed to push out the words from the dryness of my mouth.

By the time I finished, he had slipped into a sleep and spoke no more. The matron came in presently and sent me brusquely away. The following day, in the school chapel, the Rev. P.W. Levison informed us that Simon Wheeler had passed away during the night.

The funeral took place in the churchyard at Eastry that Thursday. A few of us, myself and the older boys were allowed to attend so that the school would be represented. I hoped that Bob would be there, but when we arrived there was no sign of him. The brief service in the church came to an end, and still he was not there. Then, just at the moment when the coffin was about to be lowered, I saw him, coming in through the lych-gate and taking off his hat. He stood at a distance watching, as if some terrible apprehension had frozen him to the spot. And then, as the rest of the party moved away, I turned to him, and saw that his whole body was racked with heaving sobs. I threw my arms around him and he threw his around me, and at last his sobs, and my own, grew less. "God bless, you," he said. "Don`t speak now, too painful, old chap. Write to me. Whenever you can. Write to me and tell me how it was." And with that, and one last, squeeze of my hand, he turned to go.

That I had something to occupy my mind, some purpose to be achieved, was, perhaps, however difficult the task itself, no bad thing. My letter to Bob went through several drafts, as I tried to strike a note that would give him some consolation without deviating too far from the sad facts of the truth. It was three or four days before I was happy that I had something which was worthy of the undertaking, and then I began to wonder where I should send it. I knew that the lodgings where we visited Bob in July were only temporary, but where he had moved to, though I knew it was still in London, I had no idea.

My only recourse was to ask the Rev. P.W.Levison. I knew he must have had a contact address in order to write and tell Bob of Simon`s death and of the arrangements for his funeral, and so I had no hesitation in going to his study to ask for the information I needed.

"Please, sir," I said, having been admitted to the room, and standing in front of the table where the Reverend Levison was writing, "I should like to write to Mr Wheeler."

"To whom?" he asked, not looking up from his writing, and as if the name meant nothing to him.

"To Mr Wheeler. Simon`s father."

"And why," he said, after a considerate pause, "should you

wish to do that?"

"I should like to try to console him."

"And what power do you think you have in yourself to achieve that end?"

I thought about this but I could find no way of expressing the care I had taken, in composing my letter, to say the right things.

"Please, sir," I said, instead, "he asked me to write to him."

"Did he, indeed?"

He looked up at me finally, and taking off his spectacles, pressing his eyes the finger and thumb of one hand, he stood up and moved to the window.

"Had it been known," he said at last. "Had it been known at the time when the party concerned was enrolled at this establishment, that his father was a wandering artist of here, there and everywhere, then that party would never have been enrolled at this establishment. As it is, I have an unpaid doctor`s bill which, I have no doubt, will remain unpaid until I pay it, and which, I also have no doubt, is the explanation for the late arrival and hurried departure of the person in question at the churchyard last week."

"I do believe him to be an honourable man, sir," I volunteered.

"Do you indeed!"

"If you would let me write to him, I would ask him to pay the doctor`s bill."

To this there was no reply. I thought, for a moment, that he was considering my proposal, and felt spurred to continue.

"If you have an address where I might write to him, I should be very grateful, if you have no objection."

"Ah," he said, returning to his desk, "but I do have an objection."

"May I ask what it is?"

"Do you question my judgement?"

"No, sir, but…"

"Then let that be the end of the matter."

He resumed his writing, paying me no further attention, and

I knew the interview was over.

I went away to consider my options. The most attractive option, and certainly the one to which my injured sense of justice turned most readily, was to run away to London and deliver the letter myself. This, however, when a few hours had tempered my better judgement, I realised would not be wise. I wondered if I might send the letter to his old lodgings and hope that someone might know where it might properly be forwarded. This, however, the more I considered it, seemed fraught with uncertainty.

Finally, I decided to send my letter to the only other address in London of which I was certain. I enclosed a covering note:

Dear Mr Rossetti, you probably don`t remember me, but I am the boy who enquired after The Eve of St Agnes. I would be much obliged if you would forward the enclosed letter to Bob Wheeler, the father of my friend Simon who passed away recently, as he expressly asked me to write to him. I am your obliging servant, Richard Williams.

It was some three months later, after I had almost given up hope of ever hearing from him, that I received Bob`s reply.

Dear Richard, thank you for your letter which has finally reached me in Dublin, where I am now set up, and will now stay here as I promised Simon though it grieves me sorely that he is not here to see it. Your letter gave me great solace, and my abiding sorrow is much lightened by the knowledge that a kind and loving friend was at his bedside to the last. If I can ever be of any service to you, you can be sure that I will give you my most devoted attention, the same as, were he here now, God bless him, I would give my own son. I remain your most grateful friend, Bob Wheeler.

Part 3

Chapter 18

From: Saffy Williams
To : Charlie Robson
Tue 9th June 09

Hi Babes, sorry things have been so madcrazy at work, thought you`d gone off me! A week in the Kruger sounds good though! Don`t get eaten by lions. Going to London for a few days to stay with Suzy Randall so may be off-line for a bit. Keep texting, so will I. Love you. S xxx

From: Saffy Williams
To: Sally Whitelock
Wed 10th June 09

Hi Sal, spending a week with Suzy, she sends her love. She has two kids now and is completely domesticated, you wouldn`t believe it! They live in Falconwood which is just inside Kent, twenty minutes from London by train. Joe, her partner, works for Stanley Gibbons, the stamp people, near Charing Cross. We went up to meet him yesterday, went to see `Jersey Boys` which had us all singing along. London is amazing but too much to take in at one go. Back tomorrow, then going to Wales for the weekend with Lucy. How was your dinner date? Do tell all! Saff.

Text Message, from Saffy Williams to Charlie Robson [Jo`berg]
Tuesday 16th June
Hi babes, hpe u gt ths. On trn bck 2 mnchstr frm lndn.Gd fw dys, hpe ur havn gd tme. Goin wales @ wkend. Wen u bck? Lv u, sfy,xxx

Wed 17th June, 2009

Dear Aunt Mags,
Thanks for your letter which has just arrived. I`ve just got back from a trip to London to see one of my friends from university who moved here. She`s now married with kids, but don`t tell mom that or I`ll never hear the last of it! Anyway, had a great time and am now back at New House.
Glad you like the photographs. I`ll try to get some copies of Aunt Liz` photos to send on to you, but they`re *very* old, so I don`t want to do anything that might damage them. Yes, it`s quite intriguing about the possible Wales link. I`ve downloaded some information about Moelfre which I`ll include with this. I`ll send it all by e-mail and get Dad to print it off for you.
I`m going to Anglesey this weekend to have a look, so I`ll tell you what I find when I get back next week.

Love Saffy

Attachment:

MOELFRE

Moelfre is a village on the Isle of Anglesey in Wales, and is on the Anglesey Coastal Path. It has a population of just over a thousand..

It was the site of the wreck in 1859 of the steam clipper The Royal Charter near the end of its voyage from Australia to Liverpool. The village today has just over 500 households and there is a post office, a bakery, a fish and chip shop, one restaurant, Ann`s Pantry, and a pub The Kinmel Arms Hotel which also serves food. There were no street lights in the village until well after the Second World War.

Moelfre RNLI Lifeboat Station is open to the public, and has a famous history, including the Hindlea rescue in 1959, when all the crew were rescued.

This area is popular as it is close to the large sandy beach Traeth Lligwy, which is an excellent spot for water and beach sports, and the early British homestead of Din Lligwy. It is also close to Traeth Bychan [sailing] Benllech [beach] and Red Wharf Bay. Close by, the small rocky island, Ynys Moelfre, is also a haven for birds, and seals and porpoises may be seen. The village is easily accessible being only 5 minutes from the main road from Menai Bridge to Amlwch, the A5025. The nearest mainline railway stations are in Bangor and Llanfairpwllgwyngyl. These can be reached in under half an hour by bus.

The Welsh language word Moelfre translated in English is 'bald or barren hill', which describes the land behind the village, as seen from the sea.

Part 4

Chapter 19

The years passed at Eastry and I reached the age of sixteen without having developed any clear purpose as to what career I was to pursue. After Simon`s death, my flirtation with sketching and drawing lost its newness of appeal, and with neither encouragement nor advice, the habit dwindled, and my sketch-pads and pencils stayed in the drawer.

The impression left on me by the paintings of Turner remained, as did my curiosity about the painting of John Holman Hunt, Madelina and Porphyro from `the Eve of St Agnes`, but in my isolation at Eastry there were few new influences to stir the embers into an active flame.

It was generally assumed, I think, that when I completed my education at Eastry I would find some clerical position in banking or commerce. It was a prospect that did not excite me, but I had no more stirring ambition to put in its place.

By this time, the Rev. John Griffith had been laid to rest, and he was replaced by the Rev. Stephen Roose Hughes, much younger, and a man who was ambitious to make his ministry effective.

During my vacation, I helped a little in the school, and on two or three occasions, the Rector accompanied me on walks about the lanes surrounding Moelfre, to his brother`s church at Penrhos Lligwy, or as far as the Mynydd Bodafon, giving me the opportunity to talk about my frustrations and disappointments. He it was who began to promote the idea that when I left Eastry I might progress to university to study for the ministry myself.

The idea of becoming a clergyman was one I had not, until that point, ever considered.

"I`m not sure that I have a true calling," I said.

The Rector leaned forward, put his clasped fingers to his lips in a characteristic gesture, and then, after a thoughtful pause, said, "a true calling is one which perhaps no-one knows he has until it is truly tested. And remember, even our Lord said at one point, `take this cup from my lips`. But think, Richard, first, of what you mean by a calling. It is not necessarily something like Saul on the road to Damascus, you know, a flash of blinding light, a magical revelation - a calling is seldom like that. If, however, you feel you could derive some contentment from serving ordinary folk, in helping them to find peace of heart through the word of God, and through understanding the nature and the beauty of Christ`s sacrifice, being there for them in their time of need, and, of course, too, in their times of happiness, then it is no bad thing. It is a very ordinary thing, but a very worthy thing to be a shepherd to a flock."

I turned all this over in my mind over a period of several weeks, and found myself inclining more and more towards it. The appeal was linked, perhaps inevitably, with Stephen Roose Hughes himself. The Rectory was next to the church at Llanallgo, and there he lived with his wife, Annie, and her two sisters, and about the house, with its air of patient and busy devotion to Parish affairs, which all four shared, there was nothing sombre; quite the opposite, there was often a mood of cheerful lightness: the conversation was lively and whimsical, and I was there more than once when some playful misunderstanding or double meaning of a word set off all present in a bout of spontaneous mirth.

It was possible for me to imagine a version of myself in such a mode; respected, trusted, admired - a life of tranquillity and contemplation mixed with purposeful activity. Perhaps it was only the outward trappings I saw, but nevertheless, it held something for me that was very attractive.

When I returned to Eastry for the Michaelmas term of 1855, I carried with me a letter from Stephen Roose Hughes to the Rev. P.W. Levison, requesting on my behalf some guidance from him in directing my studies and giving me advice. Somewhat begrudgingly, the Rev P,. as he was known to the boys, gave me access to his library and outlined some of the steps I would need to take to gain admission to the college at Lampeter when I reached the age of eighteen.

I set myself targets for reading: the Book of Common Prayer, commentaries on the gospels, the writings of Keble and Newman, the Anglican poets such as John Donne and George Herbert, and tried to be systematic in the notes I kept.

There came, however, another influence on me at this time, which began to exert an equal, though to some extent, opposite effect on my thinking. James Thurbrand was a graduate of Oxford who came to Eastry that term as a junior master. He was a colourful personality who entertained us with his satirical imitations of the Rev. P, and exuded at times an air of profound languor, which contrasted so strongly with the otherwise hectic and lively manner, that his character took on an interesting and unpredictable aspect.

When I told him that I had once met Dante Gabriel Rossetti and his sister, Christina, he showed a particular interest in me, since poetry was, he confided, the great love of his life, and an area where he had some aspirations himself.

On one occasion, he had a somewhat public row with the Rev P, over some petty matter of procedure, and this endeared him further with the older boys, myself amongst them.

"The man`s a sham," he declared to us openly in class, "A charlatan and a hypocrite!"

It was James Thurbrand who introduced me to the works of Lord Byron, and if, after reading a dozen or so cantos of `Childe Harold`s Pilgrimage` I saw certain similarities of attitude and temperament between the famous author and my school master, it in no way lessened my admiration for him, quite the opposite.

The poetry itself fired my imagination in a way which none of my more sober texts could do; my mind was filled with the splendour of the remote places of that poem: Spain, Albania, Greece – the endless quest for the wild and the exotic, the restless search for new and redeeming experience. If I had a strict timetable for my official reading, I needed no imposed discipline for my new found material, and it filled all my leisure time.

I ventured one day, after the class, to ask James Thurbrand if he had heard of a poet named Keats.

"Of course," he replied. "John Keats. Of course I have."

The following day he brought a volume of Keats` verse into the class.

"Do you mind if I borrow it?" I asked.

"Take it, take it!" he exclaimed, with a dismissive gesture of his hand.

As soon as the day`s lessons were over, I took the volume to the privacy of the `Crib`, the room where I had shared an Easter of backgammon with Simon nearly five years earlier, and was delighted and excited to find that it did contain the poem which had been lurking in my imagination since that same year, `The Eve of St Agnes`. I read through each stanza with rapt curiosity, using Gabriel`s commentary for assistance when the sense at first eluded me, but recognising at last every detail of the story as he had outlined it.

Chapter 20

I returned home as usual at Christmas, and again at Easter, and it was then I discovered that Izzy and her mother were no longer living at the farmhouse, but had moved to a dwelling on the edge of the farm, half a mile away, at the corner of the lane. At first, though I thought it rather odd, I had other matters to occupy me, and was not particularly curious about the reason, and as they were still working at the house during the day, it seemed no great change.

I went with my mother to the Easter service at St Galgo`s church, and afterwards we were invited to tea with the Rector and his family. Mr Roose Hughes asked me how I progressed under the instruction and guidance of the Reverend Levison; I said I had made good progress, though I didn`t make any comment on the rather passive nature of the Rev. P`s part in my education. We talked a little of poetry, but neither on this or on any other occasion during that Easter holiday did I mention Byron or Keats, though I sometimes wondered if he had heard of them, or read them, and if so, what his opinion of them might be.

I also met Isaac two or three times. Our usual meeting place was the Swnt, but gone were the games and adventures of our earlier friendship. A change had come over Isaac; he had lost some of his ebullience and confidence, and as we talked, sometimes late into the evening, a furrowed brow was his characteristic expression.

"I see you going away, Richie," he said, "making your way in the world, meeting people, making plans, and I look around here and see only… I must have some purpose, too, something to achieve…"

I tried to explain to him my own lack of certainty, the conviction that the education I was receiving was not the one my father had intended, and that I was deeply divided in myself about many things. It brought us closer together, but he still had the fierce longing to shape some ambition for himself away from Moelfre and its old customs and ways.

It was coming home from one such meeting, passing the Talyfron, that I glimpsed Dilwyn inside, playing cards at a table and laughing with the company; I took my leave of Isaac and made my way home. My mother was sitting by the fireside in a thoughtful mood.

"Are you happy at school?" she asked, when I sat down.
I affirmed that I was, though I did not elaborate.

"Why have Mrs Parry and Izzy moved away to the cottage now?" I asked, for want of another topic of conversation.

"Mrs Parry asked to move."

"It doesn`t seem a very comfortable place to live."

"I thought…" she hesitated, "I thought it best they should move."

"Why?"

"There were some things that were difficult. Izzy…"

"Has she done something wrong?"

"No, nothing like that."

"What, then?"

She took a deep breath. "I Dilwyn. You know, sometimes, when he comes home the worse for drink…"

"I`ll speak to him," I said, cutting in angrily.

"No," she said, emphatically. "No, Richie. Don`t make it worse. He`s not a bad man. He just…I think he is disappointed that there is no child. I thought it better for her, and for him."

"Are they provided for?"

"Yes."

I learned later that, besides the occasion which had kept me at Eastry, there had been several further miscarriages, and it became clear, over the next year that my mother`s health was failing. She would sit by the hearth most of the day, staring into the fire or the embers, and I often wondered if she was thinking of the old days in Porthaethwy, though I never asked her directly of what she was thinking.

Dilwyn continued to drink at the Talyfron as many nights as not, but she maintained a strange, persistent loyalty to him, feeling, I sensed, that she had let him down by not giving him a child. She would always sit up to wait until he came in, however late. Sometimes, when the hour drew late, she would ask me to go and bring him home. "Go on, Richie," she would say, "for my sake," and though I resented it, I went, knowing that she would fret otherwise, and it was not unpleasant, on a warm summer night, to take the horse and trap down the lane to the Talyfron. Once he was back, she would be at peace to go to bed. Often, he would stay up and sleep in the chair, but always, by the time I rose in the morning, he would be out and about his business.

Would it have pleased me if once she had said to me that she regretted ever leaving Porthaethwy, if she had admitted making a mistake? Would I have felt in some way vindicated? Perhaps so. The thought did cross my mind. But she never made such an admission, and for myself, I could not, in truth, conjecture what my life would have been like there by now anyway, and so it was not a question that had any purpose.

Returning to Eastry once more when the summer was over, I was somewhat surprised to find that James Thurbrand had married during the vacation, the daughter of a milliner of the town, a plump girl with pink cheeks and a commodious bosom, who wore a mop cap, and baked rather splendid apple pies which she occasionally sent, so the rumour went, to the Rev. P, as if to appease that gentleman in the way most likely to secure her husband`s preferment.

If this diminished his status as a hero in the mode of Lord Byron a little in my eyes, it did not prevent me from reading the poems he could supply. By now I had my own copy of `Childe Harold`s Pilgrimage`, and I continued to retrace the steps of that flawed and melancholic youth around the mountains and palaces of Europe; in Keats` `Endymion` I explored the realms of idyllic pastoral beauty, and in `Hyperion`, I was fascinated by the evocation of the very depths of despair. In Shelley`s `Ode to the West Wind` I revelled in the wild desire for freedom from stagnation and decay.

My education at Eastry was, by now, more or less in my own hands. Few of my fellows were still there; having achieved as much or as little as they or their families were satisfied with, they had moved on to whatever destiny awaited them. I was not expected to attend the regular lessons and rarely did so. I still had access to the Rev P`s library, and, somewhat reluctantly, acknowledging an obligation to Stephen Roose Hughes, he tolerated me there – but I sensed that he wished to be rid of me, and he generally gave me a wide berth. Sometimes I walked out in the Shropshire Hills and imagined myself a poet, sometimes I studied, but indolence was always a tempting alternative.

I was summoned home from Eastry at the beginning of November on a matter of urgency, the matter being a turn for the worse in my mother`s health. I was now accustomed to travelling by train, from Gobowen to Chester, and then, via Bangor, to Llanfairpwl, a journey which could be encompassed in a day without great difficulty; and so I set out, on that cold wintry morning, trying to distract myself with the passing views of countryside, hill and sea, and trying to hold at a distance the fears which preyed on my mind, but knowing that I would not have been called back without the circumstances being extreme.

Dilwyn was at Llanfairpwl to meet me as arranged. I sought his gaze to read the signs of what I feared, but he did not hold my look.

"She said you were to be sent for," was all he said.

"Is she going to die?" I asked. He did not reply. We travelled together along the darkening road in silence.

There was a fire in the room, which gave it a cheerful aspect; my mother was in bed, Mrs Parry sitting by her. She was asleep, but opened her eyes briefly and smiled as I stood there. Her face seemed softened and somehow younger. Mrs Parry wiped her brow, and then said to me, "best let her rest, now, you`ll see her in the morning."

My first impression was that the illness was not so severe as I had feared; downstairs, however, the doctor, who I had not seen on my entrance, took me aside, and in a quiet voice told me that he held little hope she would survive the week.

I slept in my old room, that night, and just as on the first night, years before, a fire had been set to take the chill off the air. I looked down from the small window towards Moelfre and the sea, thinking, with a heavy heart, of all that had happened in the intervening time, and of the sorrow that was upon the house now.

When I saw her the next morning, however, my mother was able to talk to me for twenty minutes, and, grasping at hope, I tried to make myself believe that the doctor erred in his judgement. She was visited during the day by Stephen Roose Hughes, and his wife, Anne and they sat with her for a half an hour, though by then she had grown tired again. Before they left, he offered me consolation in the usual kind manner and said that we should pray together. I knew from that, more than from the doctor, that there was no hope.

The following day, her eyes had developed a strange glittery expression, and by the next morning, they were all but closed with only a dark glazed expressionless stare remaining. Three hours later, she was dead.

What I felt immediately was a sense of relief, the relief of being rid of the burden of someone dying. Later came a devastating sense of finality – the reality that nothing now could be said, and with it a sense of guilt for all the things I should have said. In one part of my heart I had never forgiven her for marrying Dilwyn, and because of that I had become indifferent to her suffering.

When I tried to explain this to Stephen Roose Hughes he reassured me that in his experience death is often accompanied by guilt on the part of loved ones. "It is," he said, "the tangle of the human heart, and so we must learn that the human heart cannot, without God, and the power of prayer, cure its own ills." He also explained to me what must be done to arrange for her being laid to rest. Dilwyn, at first, as if needing to assert some authority, was insistent that she should be buried in Amlwch where several of his forebears had been interred, but the Rector persuaded him otherwise.

"Let her be buried here," he said. "Where you will be close to her, and she to you, in the church where she worshipped, where her prayers have been spoken."

Dilwyn shrugged and went to the window. "So be it," he said at last.

And so, my mother`s funeral took place in the churchyard of St Galgo. Besides the Rector, his wife and sisters, there was myself, Mrs Parry and Izzy. Dilwyn stood by, but his face expressed no emotion. On our return home, he stood by the fire and I by the window.

"I did love her, you know," he said, after a time.

"Yes, I know," I replied

For a brief moment, the great chasm between us seemed bridged. Then, he set to with a bottle of brandy, whilst I made preparations to return to Eastry.

Chapter 21

It now began to seem a matter of some urgency to organise my studies in a way which would lead speedily to the next phase of my career. I worked hard at my Latin, knowing that to be a weak area, and enlisted the help of the new Classics teacher, Mr Appleyard to that purpose. He gave me Horace`s Odes and Caesar`s Gallic Wars for translation, and agreed to monitor my progress, and though I found the process somewhat dry, the sheer discipline was good for me. I also spoke to the Rev. P, asking him to write letters of introduction to St David`s College, Lampeter, where I hoped to study for a degree before taking orders. This he agreed to do, saying that the early spring would be the best time to pursue the matter further.

It was with some apprehension that I returned to Moelfre in December, partly, of course, because it would bring me back into contact with the still fresh memory of my mother, partly because I found it difficult to imagine how Dilwyn and I would cope together as house mates. It was his home, I had lost the person through whom I claimed it to be my home too, and feared I would feel even more than ever the outsider, and yet it was the only home I had. As with most things, however, it proved less of an ordeal than I feared. Even in the worst situations a kind of ordinariness settles on things after a while. Largely we avoided each other.

I had been home for two days when there was a knock on the kitchen door and Ivor Reece told me that Izzy was there, asking to see me. It was a cold wintry morning with snow on the ground and I had just put a kettle by the fire to heat up.

"Come in," I said. "Come and sit by the fire. You look cold."

"Is he here, the master?"

"No. He`s out. There`s no-one here."

The question had been asked with apprehension rather than curiosity and I could tell from her response that my answer was a cause of relief.

"I`m sorry to trouble you, Master Richie," she said. "But is it possible we may have one or two blankets from our old room. My mother has a fever, you see, and she`s finding it hard to keep warm.."

"I wondered why I hadn`t seen her."

"She`s been ill this last week. The master knows."

"He didn`t say anything. Would you like a drink – something warm?"

She nodded her head, quickly but guardedly, as if acknowledging a forbidden luxury.

"How is your reading coming along?" I asked, trying to be jovial.

"Please, sir, not very well, now that I don`t come here anymore to look at your books."

"You must take some with you," I said. "Would you like to do that?"

Again there was the quick guarded nod of the head. I made her a drink and brought it to where she was warming her hands at the fire.

"I`ve brought some rugs and blankets," I said, later, when she had finished drinking. "I`ll get the trap out and take you."

"No, sir," she said, "I can just as easily walk."

"All right," I said, sensing that not being seen by Dilwyn was her main objective. "But at least let me walk with you and carry them. And here`s an old cloak my mother had for cold weather. I dare say it`s a good bit warmer than that shawl you`ve got on."

"No sir, I`m sure the master wouldn`t approve."

"Nonsense," I replied. "Why, he`s not going to wear it himself, is he?"

We both laughed, and I remembered the old days, when we were still both children, and when our encounters had often ended with her eyes filling with tears.

"And you must stop calling me *sir*, Izzy, I absolutely insist on that."

We set out to walk the half mile to the cottage, and in the bright wintry light, I felt my spirits lifted, acknowledging to myself that, after the gloominess of the farmhouse, it was pleasant to be in Izzy`s company. My spirits were dashed, however, when I saw the cottage to which Izzy and her mother had been consigned. It comprised a single room, ten feet by twelve, with only a curtain, behind which lay Izzy`s mother, for privacy. The floor was stone, with a handful of scattered rushes for cover, and there was a sharp sour odour of damp about the place, clinging and cold.

"Is this where he thinks fit to let you live?" I asked.

"We don`t want to make trouble."

"This is no place for anyone let alone someone sick."

"We have no choice."

"His beasts have better housing than this."

"It`s not too bad except when the weather`s very bad. We make it quite cheerful most times."

I spoke to Mrs Parry who assured me she was better than she had been, though from the sound of her chest I suspected her to be far more ill than she allowed. Then I spoke to Izzy again.

"Do you have any means of heating?"

"There is a stove there in the corner but our wood is mostly gone. I put it on a little each evening to take the chill away."

"Put it on now," I said, "and keep it on. I`ll bring you more."

I returned to the farmhouse. Dilwyn was still out, but I had no intention of asking his permission for what I intended to do, anyway. I filled two sacks from the stable with wood, and told Ivor to make ready the trap. I spoke to Margaret, Ivor`s wife, who had been helping in the house, and filled a casserole with broth, then made up a basket with bread, cheese and milk, adding the remains of a side of ham from the larder. Then, from my mother`s dressing room I took the warmest things I could find, woollens, stockings, skirts, coats and added those to the pile.

Within an hour of leaving it, I was back at the cottage with my haul.

"You`ll get in trouble," Izzy warned.

"I`ll risk that," I said, heedlessly, feeling exhilarated with my morning`s exploits. I helped her to unload the trap, and we stoked up the stove and put the broth on to simmer.

"I`ll call tomorrow and see how she is," I said, finally.

"Thank you, Richie."

I met Isaac that afternoon and told him what had happened. "Take care with Dilwyn," he said. "Some people say he`s letting things slip, and that the drink`s got him. He`s had Lord Boston`s man there, warning him about the rents."

"I`m going to Lampeter College next year," I said. "I`ll get lodgings there and be shut of him."

"I`m going too," said Isaac.

"Away?"

"Yes."

"For good?"

"I`ve got an uncle in Liverpool," he said. "He can get me work on board ship, he says, learn my trade as a mariner, see what I can make of myself."

"That`s great news. When do you go?"

"Just after the new year."

"I`ll give you my address at Eastry. You can write to me there. Tell me everything that happens to you. We`ll keep in touch, come what may."

On my return Dilwyn was waiting for me.

"What`s all this , then?" he asked.

"Are you going to be more specific?"

"Margaret tells me you`ve been giving good food away."

"To Mrs Parry, yes."

"I turn beggars away at the door."

"For God`s sake, man, they are not beggars. We have some obligation to them, and I mean to see they are treated properly."

He looked at me with a grimace of amusement and mockery, as if to say, so you think you are a man, now, do you? And also as if to say, I could crush you in my hand if I chose to.

He scoffed and turned away. Half an hour later he set off for the Talyfron.

The argument did not dampen my appetite for helping Izzy and

Mrs Parry, quite the opposite. I became quite intoxicated with the idea of doing them some good. For the three weeks I was there, hardly a day went by without my stopping by to enquire after Mrs Parry`s health, and on each occasion I found something to take – curtains, some soap and candles, an oil lamp – and in particular, when I had provided the things which I thought would help make them comfortable – books for Izzy. I had my own volumes of Keats, now, bought at a shop in Shrewsbury, and those I had brought home with me I gave to her.

"Byron is my particular favourite poet," I said to her, "but I love Keats and I`m sure you will too. I hope you enjoy them."

"I`m sure I will," said Izzy, somewhat bemused, I think, at my solicitousness.

I went to see them one last time before my return to Eastry. Mrs Parry was much recovered, and was sitting up by the stove. The cottage was brighter and warmer and cleaner, and on the whole, I was pleased with myself at the improvements.

Izzy came to the door with me as I took my leave. "Thanks for your kindness, Richie," she said. She leaned forward to kiss me briefly, and at the touch of her lips on mine I felt such a shiver pass through me, that for a moment I wanted to throw my arms around her and crush her body against mine "And thank you for the books, too," she added, seeming to have no inclination of the effect she had on me.

I mumbled something, and, in my confusion, turned to go.

For half an hour, on my return, I tried to compose a note to send to her, but could come up with nothing better than, *My Dear Izzy, further to our conversation this evening, you may rest assured of my continuing devotion to your mother`s and your own welfare. Richie.*

I then decided that, as a gesture towards Dilwyn, it being my last night at home, I would take the trap to fetch him from the Talyfron, a journey, which, going round by the road, would take me within a few yards of the cottage.

As I approached, I could make out a light behind the curtain, and I pictured Izzy sitting there reading the poems I had given her. It had been my intention to stop, and to leave the note by the door where she would find it in the morning, but at last, the fear of being found ridiculous overcame me, and I drove on, though nevertheless wondering if she would hear the horse`s steps and the sound of the wheels and know it was me.

There was, still, a handful of drinkers in the Talyfron, their faces reddened by the liquor and the fire which had been ablaze all night.

"Come in, lad, take a drop with us," Dilwyn called, his temper mellowed by the drink.

I sat down in the corner and they drew me off a tot of rum. The conversation, which quickly resumed, as if I wasn`t there, was of rents and tithes and other matters on which there were deemed to be wrongs which needed to be righted. I sipped the rum very slowly, trying to give no outward sign to betray the burning sensation I felt with each taste.

"You`re leaving again tomorrow, then," said Dai Hughes, turning to me at last.

"Yes."

"Young Isaac, too, by all accounts. Going to Liverpool."

"Yes. We`re going to Bangor, together, tomorrow morning, with the post."

There were nods. For most of them, references to places outside the island meant little.

"Thank you, lad, thank you, lad," said Dilwyn, as I helped him up to the trap, all animosity now lost in a boozy haze of well-being. We had gone no more than a dozen paces when the sound of his breathing beside me told me he was asleep.

The cottage, as we passed, was now in darkness, and I was glad that I had thought better of leaving the note. The following morning, when I arose early to meet Isaac, the whole business had already begun to seem as insubstantial as a passing cloud.

"That is Porthaethwy, where I used to live," I told Isaac, as we approached the Menai Bridge.

"This is the first time I`ve left the island," he said, as we crossed the strait. "At least, the first by land."

"Are you excited by the prospect of your new life?"

"Terrified to be honest with you."

"There is no need. You have a noble nature," I said, remembering his first words to me, "I`m certain your destiny is to achieve great things."

We travelled together to Chester, and there bade each other a hearty farewell, certain that we would soon meet again to share stories of the new lives we were entering.

Chapter 22

"The Rev P may be a holy man," I said to James Thurbrand, "but I do not believe him to be a good man."

"Don`t forget that he is my employer," he retorted, drily, "I must hear no calumny spoken against him."

"And what about the calumny spoken against him by yourself?"

"Ah, that is a different matter. Anyway, that is in the past and I am a changed man."

"Hence the apple pies that find their way to his larder?"

"The apple pies are entirely of Mrs Thurbrand`s devising. If she has a streak of the Machiavel in her make-up, I cannot be blamed for that."

"So. Is it an act of goodness to send an apple-pie to the Rev. P, if there is an ulterior motive in question?"

"Well, if some pleasure is derived from that apple pie then I suppose some goodness may be deemed to have been done."

"So, do you argue that goodness is an effect produced, rather than an expression of virtue?"

"I argue," said James Thurbrand, "that goodness is the fulfilment of nature."

"Whatever that may mean."

"Whatever that may mean. Indeed."

The conversation took place in his study at Eastry, shortly after my return in January. It had been made known, by this time, that Mrs Thurbrand was with child, and that, it seemed to me, had completed the changes to which he had just alluded. He had become a happier man, a more considerate man, a gentler man. Personally, I rather preferred the man of dark moods and fiery temper that I had first known, but I acknowledged to myself that in talking of the fulfilment of nature as goodness, he was thinking of the fulfilment of his own nature, and that included the prospect of becoming a father.

The topic we were discussing, however frivolously, was one

that had pre-occupied me, to some extent, since Christmas. The action of rescuing Izzy and her mother from the misery in which they were otherwise confined had seemed to me in some ways, in miniature, a model for the work which, as a minister, I intended to profess, and I had derived much satisfaction from it. However, I knew that that was not the whole story. Is it necessary, I found myself asking, in an imaginary conversation with Stephen Roose Hughes, for an act to be selfless in order to be good? I did not know exactly how he would reply, though I knew it would be something to reassure me and alleviate my self-doubt. There can be no harm, I put it to myself, in the pleasure derived from seeing someone else`s suffering eased; I felt, nevertheless, an uneasy sense of prevarication, and I could not hide it from myself that its cause was Izzy. For despite myself, the recollection of that one kiss, and the sudden strange feelings it had inspired in me, formed an image which returned, many times, and sometimes when I least expected it, to taunt me.

I received a letter from Isaac in Liverpool during the third week in January. *Dear Richie,* he began, *just time to let you know that I have secured work as a rigger with the Eagle Line, and hope to be at sea bound for Melbourne on the third next. Greatly excited. Feel my adventure with the world beginning. Write to me before I go, if you can, Isaac.*

I hastily penned a reply expressing my congratulations and wishing him well, though his letter also left me a little dispirited, for if Isaac felt excited about his adventure with the world, nothing could be further from the truth with regard to my own. I resolved, however, to raise the question of letters again with the Rev P. Levison.

I was anticipated, in my intention of requesting a meeting with him, by a message to see him in his study the following morning. I slept that night assured that my own journey was about to reach its next stage, and was outside his study at the appointed time the next day.

"Come in, Williams."

The room still had unpleasant memories of the interview

which had taken place after Simon`s death.

"Sit down."

He was reading a letter in front of him and seemed in no hurry.

"Your fees," he said at last, "have always been dealt with by a company of solicitors in Bangor by the name of Hargreaves and Bentham. That is correct, is it not?"

"I believe so. That is the company to whom my father entrusted his estate."

"Quite so. I have here a letter from Messrs Hargreaves and Bentham to the effect that the trust fund from which your fees have always been paid is now terminated?"

"Terminated? I don`t understand."

"The termination of a trust fund may occur when it is authorised by someone specifically named as a person entitled to do so, or, quite simply, as I suspect to be the case here, when the fund in question has ceased to exist in its own right, in other words, when there is no longer any money in it."

"So what does it mean?"

"It means, unfortunately, that unless you have any other income at your disposal, you are unable to remain a student at this school. Do you have any other such income?"

"No."

"No. Then the only advice I can give you is that you should contact your step-father, who is, in effect, your legal guardian, or speak to Messrs Hargreaves and Bentham yourself to ascertain the full extent of the situation."

"Is that all?"

"If you mean is that the only advice I can give you, then, yes, that is all. If you mean is that the end of this interview, then the answer is also yes, as I see no point in pursuing it further."

The office of Hargreaves and Bentham was in a small side street close to the cathedral in Bangor, and I had vague recollections of being taken there once with my father. A gloomy stairwell led up two floors to an equally gloomy vestibule where an old man with fluffy white hair and pale blue watery eyes asked me to be so good as to wait a few moments until Mr Bentham was ready to see me. As I waited, the old man seemed in a state of perpetual business about the place, tidying here, dusting there, rearranging the papers on a table from one side to the other, humming part of the time and for the rest carrying out a mumbled monologue, the only phrase I was able to pick out, through its repetition, being, very kind of you, very kind, indeed. Finally, without any external prompting, he announced, "Mr Bentham is ready to see you now."

I was ushered into a chamber which, in comparison with the rest of the building, seemed to swim with light. A broad window looked down towards Porth Penrhyn, with its array of masts and spars, and the room was adorned with models of pilot boats, of clippers and schooners, giving the impression of a miniature port here, high above the street.

"My dear fellow," said Mr Bentham, standing to shake my hand, and greeting me as if we were well established acquaintances. "My dear fellow, do take a seat. Now how this came about, you see..." he said, moving from the desk as if to find something in a cabinet, but returning with nothing, "if it hadn`t been for...," he opened a drawer, but still found nothing, "on the other hand, there`s one thing that we can be certain of..."

Mr Bentham, I noticed after a time, had a manner of beginning sentences in a way which gave out a sense of the utmost confidence; it did not take me much longer to notice that his sentences were very rarely finished, leaving an impression of questions left trailing in the air. It was, I suspected, from delicacy of temperament that he had developed this habit, not wanting to disappoint his clients until they had more or less conceded the hopelessness to which he was leading them.

"The Reverend Levison went so far as to say there might actually be no money in the fund."

"Yes, did he really? Yes, yes, well, without stretching a point too far, that does, in fact, seem to be, in some respects, the case."

"In some respects?"

"Yes. You see, the thing is, had your mother made a will in her own right, which I`m afraid to say, she did not, money from other sources, as directed by your father, might have been vired, as we say, to discharge the remaining expenses pertaining to your education, and of course, your own allowance."

"So there is money in other sources?"

"Under the terms of your father`s will, control of the other pots, shall we call them, was invested in your mother. On her death, control of these other pots, as we have agreed to call them, passed to her husband."

"Dilwyn Jones?"

"Your stepfather, Mr Jones, yes."

"Then it is in his power, and his power alone to determine how and even if my education continues."

"The answer to that is both yes and no. Yes, in the sense that he, legally, is authorised to determine how the contents of those pots is put to use or invested; no, in the sense, that those pots, too, are virtually empty."

"You mean that he has spent that money since my mother`s death?"

"In the sense that money has been spent from those pots since your mother`s death, yes, that is true; in reality, the great majority of what was in those pots was spent before your mother`s death, either by her direction or with her agreement."

"So, then, my case is hopeless."

"Hopeless, my dear fellow, is a very strong word."

"Then is there any other word which describes it more accurately?"

"Since you put the emphasis on accuracy, then, no, probably not."

I walked out into the pale sunlight of that February morning with a sense of numbness that was almost like peace. My trunks had been sent on before, by the post, and so I set out walking along the road that leads down to the Menai Bridge on the Bangor side, and came at last to Porthaethwy. It was nine years, almost to the day, since I had departed from my birthplace; now, along the quay, on the high street and in the market field, there was no-one I recognised, and none who recognised me.

So, I said to myself, I have come a full circle, and much as was my expectation, I now have nothing. There was almost a satisfaction about the completeness of it. I have nothing – I owe no-one anything. This is where I begin again.

I wondered, for a moment, if I had enough money in my pocket to take a train journey to London, to see what I could make of myself there. But my better judgement prevailed. Bleak as the prospects it held might be, there was still something that called me back to Moelfre. So, once again, this time on foot, I began that fateful journey.

"I take it you know what has happened?"

Dilwyn shrugged and continued with the business of cleaning a gun.

"It was what she wished," he said at last, quietly, as if speaking from some immoveable bedrock of certainty that overcame moral scruple.

"You mean she wished for my education to be thus terminated? That she wished for me to be penniless, she wished for me to have no prospects in the world?"

"I mean that she wished for this farm to prosper, so that you would have a home. That's what she wished for."

"A home!" I said, bitterly. "Do you call this a home?"

"Take it or leave it. If you can find better, you're welcome to go there."

"If this is to be my home, what is expected of me?"

Dilwyn shrugged again. "Not really something I've thought about. I've no plan to set you out to work in the fields, if that's what you mean. It's as you wish."

Having expended all my indignation, and having no other ammunition to hand, I allowed this to mark the end of the conversation.

Chapter 23

There followed a period of some months during which I settled back, quite easily, into life in Moelfre. I toyed with the idea, for much of that time, that my destiny was to be a poet or an artist, and I began sketching again, and sought ways of expressing the feelings of the heart through the subject matter of the land and nature`s visible forms; and though I learned that solitude can clarify and intensify our understandings and perceptions, I also learned that isolation can leave us without purpose or direction, so that the best of intentions for improvement and application can be left floundering in a welter of indolence.

I spoke, of course, several times, to the Rev. Stephen Roose Hughes during this time. His first endeavour was to repair, as it were, the pathway towards my chosen career in holy orders. "It is possible," he explained, "to be accepted for ordination, in certain circumstances, as a `literate` - that is to say, as one who has achieved a certain standard of education without having progressed to the level of a degree. Because of the poor standard, however, unfortunately, of the ministry in certain parts of Wales, our own Bishop has made something of a point of accepting only those who have achieved the higher levels of qualification. It may, however, be possible to find a diocese where this is not the case and I have friends to whom I can write, if you so wish. The other way forward, as I see it, would be to secure work in a school of some standing, as a junior assistant in the first place, of course, and to progress your career by that means. Many good teachers have entered the ministry, and have made their mark, too. Again, I have friends to whom I can apply, on your behalf, for advice."

"I`m not sure," I replied, falteringly.

"Of course, you need to have time to think. Time to adapt to the blow fortune has dealt you, but I`m sure that you will reach a good decision, and our prayers, here in this house, will be to seek guidance and inspiration for you."

I took time to think, as he suggested, but found that, if

anything, time blurred rather than focused the sense of purpose I needed to achieve, and he did not press me; as the months went by I came to a not unpleasant acceptance of my new Moelfre existence, broken only, from time to time, by moods of listlessness and frustration.

I tried my hand at various things during this time. Notwithstanding Dilwyn`s assertion that he expected nothing of me, I found that there were certain tasks about the farm that I could usefully perform. Alongside the hired men, I could help with the sowing of the barley and the rye, and with the garnering of the crops in autumn; I learned how to set and tie the hay-ricks, and I could drive the cart which often proved useful. Dilwyn acknowledged in his own non-committal way that I was not idle.

What I missed most, at this time, was the comradeship of Isaac, but I visited his mother and father often, and sometimes stayed at the house, when the hour grew late, rather than walk home. Isaac`s ship had exchanged letters with another, homeward bound, off the coast of Africa, and it was with great excitement and pride that his father read out the note Isaac had been able to send.

I had, by now, been out with the fishing boats, too, seeking the shoals of herring and mackerel mainly in the off-shore waters no more than a mile or so off the island, but sometimes further afield. It is no life for the faint-hearted, I certainly learned that! If you stand at Porth Lydan and watch the boats going out nothing is finer: the steady pull of the oars, the swell of the wind in the sails, as the boat makes progress through the waves, rising and dipping on the swell, until it is just a dot on the horizon; but if you go out with them, however, those charming white horses on the waves, so pretty from a distance, may betoken a sea that can throw the boat up ten or twelve feet before it plummets as low again into the trough of the wave, waiting for the evermoving horizon to reappear. For the uninitiated, such as myself, struck with terror, you can only watch the crew and draw comfort that you don`t read your own fear in their faces. Then there are the sudden changes of wind and weather, bringing storms, and the numbing coldness which has to be endured hour after hour. I survived a dozen or so outings without mishap, and tried, in a small way, to make myself useful, but it is a life which only those brought up to it, and for whom it is the only livelihood, can endure for any length of time.

I saw little of Izzy during the months following my return. After her illness, Mrs Parry had returned to work in the kitchen, with Margaret, and Izzy helped occasionally, but she was seldom to be seen out and about in the village, and so our paths rarely crossed.

On one occasion, however, on a day when Dilwyn had set off early to the market at Amlwch, I came across her in my study alcove, reading.

"Keats," I said, recognising the volume. "How are you enjoying it?"

"Very well, though I don`t always understand it perfectly."

"Which poem are you reading?"

"This one? `The Eve of St Agnes`."

"Oh, yes," I replied, remembering the whole business with Hunt and Rossetti, "that`s one of my favorites."

"Can you tell me, what does this line mean?" she asked.

I looked at the line to which she was pointing with her finger, and at the same time she spoke it aloud, *into her dream he melted.* Taken aback that she should choose that of all lines, I turned away to disguise my confusion.

"Well..." I began. I recalled Gabriel`s terse exposition of the line, but felt that I could hardly explain it to Izzy as baldly as that. "It means..." I continued, trying to appear unflustered. Before I could light upon some suitable euphemism or evasion, however, I saw from the sudden transition in her eyes, that no further explanation was necessary.

"Oh," she said, colouring slightly, "I didn`t think of that!"

We both turned away, and nothing more was said on the subject.

As on a previous occasion, however, the momentary incident

returned to take its place amongst the thoughts which now, almost nightly, disturbed my rest. The girls with the coiffured ringlets at the Hanover rooms, Effie and Christina in the tavern in Soho, Miriam with her pale beauty and faraway look, even Mrs James Harbrand, with her pink cheeks and plump bosom; to these were joined the picture of Izzy, her rich hair, her smile, her face caught in the moment of embarrassed recognition, and for many an hour, despite my resolute efforts to dispel them, I suffered the anguish of feverishly conjured images of the coupling of woman and man.

"Much as we may sometimes wish it," said the Reverend Stephen Roose Hughes, in response to the question I had put to him, "we must not expect providence to reveal itself in such simple forms."

Our discussion arose out of a matter which had been touched on in his sermon that morning, and now we were walking through the fields from Penrhos Lligwy where we had been paying a visit to his brother`s church.

"So, virtue is not necessarily its own reward."

"Well, yes, essentially, it is, but not in the sense that we receive a payment from God for virtue in the same way that a labourer receives a payment for his day`s toil. If it were that easy, then everyone would be a saint."

"And wouldn`t that be a good thing?"

"Well, I suppose it would make my life easier," he said, with wry humour. "The point is, I suppose, that we must choose virtue by our own free will, and for its own sake."

"What of the case," I went on, pursuing the topic, "of innocent suffering?"

"Go on."

"Well, last month, for instance, you conducted prayers for the soul of Mrs Owen `s infant son, and you said God`s will be done. So, how is it that God would will the death of an innocent child, and bring sorrow to its parents? Is that justice?"

We had stopped by a stile at the corner of the lane, and sitting down for a moment beside it, he closed his eyes with concentrated thoughtfulness, as if such a question, notwithstanding the theological answer which he could no doubt give me, might test his own faith to the fullest extent.

"We don`t know God`s will," he said at last. "All we know is that in the very darkest hour, in the most terrible of human circumstances, God is there beside us, as he was beside our Saviour on the Cross."

I nodded, accepting the sincerity of his answer as evidence of a wisdom much more profound than my restless questions, and as ever, in his company, I was able to find a sense of calmness that eased my spirits.

"Tell me," he said, later, as we made our way homewards, "have you ever read any of the works of William Wordsworth? He might help you with some of these weighty questions you put to me."

"Wordsworth," I replied shrugging my shoulders, "Isn`t he the poet of nature?"

"Of nature, yes, but not just of its outward and ornamental beauty. Through nature, he attempts to express that which is of greatest permanence, of lasting value and consolation to the spirit."

"I`ve read Byron and Keats mostly."

"Ah, yes, Byron and Keats," he said thoughtfully, but without judgement. "Yes, I remember."

Outside the rectory, as I was about to say farewell, he bade me come inside and wait a moment. He returned with a small volume in his hands. "This is called `Lyrical Ballads`," he said. "It was published some years ago by Wordsworth and his associate, of whom you may have heard, Samuel Taylor Coleridge. It contains a poem entitled `Michael` which I would urge you to read."

"Thank you," I said. "I will return it as soon as I`ve read it."

"No," he replied. "I make a gift of it to you, for if you promise to return it, you will feel obliged to rush through it, out of politeness, and then the objective will be defeated. Here," he continued, "I will write your name inside it and then it becomes yours."

"Thank you," I said. "I will treasure it."

That same evening, I looked proudly in the fly-leaf of the book he had given me. It contained his own initials, *S.R.H.*, with the inscription, *Moelfre, 1853*; and then, in fresher ink, *for R.W., September, 1858.*

It took me some time to become accustomed to the simple direct style of Wordsworth; after the richness of Keats and the extravagance of Byron, it seemed, at first, a waterish diet, so that with some of the shorter poems I felt I had read them without reading anything at all, other than a seeming childish lyric with a moral; gradually however, I learned to recognise the qualities which the Rev. Roose Hughes had recommended.

This was particularly so with the poem 'Michael' he had encouraged me to read. A narrative poem of some length, it relates the story of a rustic shepherd who, late in life, becomes the father of a dearly loved son, who follows his father every day to the upland pasture. When the son, Luke, now grown up, later goes off to seek his fortune in order to pay off a debt which Michael has inherited, Michael asks him to place a stone as the corner-stone of a new sheepfold, as a symbol of their love, and says that he will finish the sheepfold as he awaits Luke's return. Luke prospers at first, sending home glowing letters, but at last word comes back that Luke has fallen in with evil men, and has fled the country to escape justice. Michael goes every day to the sheepfold to remember Luke and the tryst there was between them, and to mourn; the sheepfold is never completed.

A wistful, reflective poem, with a melancholy outcome, it nevertheless seemed to capture the qualities which I most admired in the man who had made a gift of it to me: patience, tolerance, trust in God, even in the face of suffering, an appreciation of simple wholesome living and honesty.

For a time, I rediscovered my enthusiasm for a life dedicated to God and to the service of others, but it did not last; and the more I tried, and the more frustrated I became at my own failure to be like the living example I had before me, the more I seemed to find things in my own nature to pull me further away.

Through the winter months, and into the new year, I wrestled with my conscience and with my recalcitrant impulses, and with an over-riding sense of drifting hopelessly towards a directionless future; and then, in the March of 1859, Izzy`s mother died suddenly, and that event, without doubt, marked a decisive change in the course of both our lives.

Chapter 24

It happened one Tuesday morning, and as chance would have it, I was at home in the house at the time. I was sitting in my alcove reading when Margaret came running through, speechless though evidently in a state of panic. In the kitchen Mrs Parry was lying on the floor, completely still.

"Get a blanket!" I called.

I kneeled beside her, and called her name, but it was already clear that she was stone dead.

"Help me to get her onto a chair," I said when Margaret returned.

"She just said she was feeling a bit queasy and the next thing…"

"Call Ivor," I said, "Tell him to send one of the boys for Doctor Jenkins, and then let him stay with you, here. I`ll bring Izzy. And put the blanket round her, so it seems she was cared for at the last."

I set out straight away for the cottage, muttering under my breath, rehearsing what I was going to say. Izzy was outside the cottage, hanging washing, so I did not have to knock and wait.

"Izzy," I called, "you must come straight away."

"Is it mother?"

"Yes, she`s taken badly. We`ve sent for the doctor, but I fear the worst."

"What happened?" She had already pulled on a shawl and we were making our way back along the path.

"She felt ill, and Margaret sat her down, and called me. We put a blanket round her to keep her warm, but she looked as if she was slipping away."

"She`s been like this before," said Izzy. "I told her she musn`t work until she was properly better. But maybe the doctor will make her come round."

I did not disabuse her of this hope, though I wondered if my intention of softening the shock amounted not to kindness but rather to cowardice.

"Oh, mother, mother!" Izzy cried out when she entered the kitchen, kneeling down beside her. "I believe she still breathes, howsoever faintly. Do you have some salts?"

At that moment the doctor arrived and sent us all from the room, save Izzy. As I closed the door I could see the tears brimming in Izzy`s eyes, just as they had on our first meeting nearly ten years before.

The doctor came out ten minutes later. "I`ve done what I can for her," he said. "The girl, I mean, not the old woman, she was beyond help before I came, as you must know, but you did the right thing. It might be as well now, Master Richie, if you went in to see her. It was you she asked for."

Somewhat hesitantly, I made my way back into the kitchen.

"At least I was here when she went. She will have known that, won`t she?"

"Yes."

"Thank you for bringing me so quickly. Will you help me to do all the things that need to be done?"

"Yes, of course I will."

"I should like her to be laid out at home with me, not here."

"If that`s what you want."

It was a harrowing time. I sat with Izzy in the evenings so that she should not be left alone with her mother`s body laid out there, and on both occasions, the Reverend Stephen Roose Hughes visited too, once alone and once with his wife, even though Mrs Parry was originally of the Roman Church. The burial itself was a simple affair, in the churchyard at Llaneugrad. As with many of the village folk, there was to be no headstone.

"I`ll need to have that cottage, back, then," said Dilwyn. "If she won`t work here, then I`ll have to have it for someone else."

"I don`t think she will," I said. I had never spoken to Dilwyn about the cause of Mrs Parry and Izzy`s moving out of the farmhouse, but now that she was alone in the world I began to worry on her behalf.

"Then let her go whoring in Amlwch," said Dilwyn. "She`ll

not want for customers."

"For God`s sake, man," I said.

Dilwyn grinned as if pleased to have provoked me.

"At least give her some time," I said. "Let her grieve for a while, then I`ll speak to her."

Dilwyn grunted as if this compromise was far from his liking, but he did not press the matter further.

I saw Izzy, without Dilwyn knowing, sooner rather than later. "Do you have a means of securing the door?" I asked.

"For what reason?" she asked.

"Now that you`re alone, it would be well to be cautious."

"I keep a knife by my bed. I wouldn`t be afraid to use it."

"Good for you," I said, "but I sincerely hope you never have occasion to. A bar or a latch would suffice to deter a man the worse for drink."

"Will he let me stay here then?"

"He wants you to work at the house."

She tilted her head sideways, as if considering, but did not answer.

"At any rate, you can stay here for the time being. And if there is any trouble, any trouble at all, promise me that you`ll come to me."

She smiled as if she found my gallantry amusing in some way, and then said, "thank you, yes, I will."

Chapter 25

"Your charity towards Izzy," said the Reverend Stephen Roose Hughes, "has been commendable, commendable, indeed."

"I simply did what anyone would."

"Not everyone. By no means. I know she looks on you as something of a protector."

I was, at first, somewhat flushed with pleasure at this praise, but then he went on, "what I am about to say may seem, in itself, less than charitable, Richard, but you are in a situation where you must take care. Izzy is now a single young woman living alone; she looks to you, as I say, in some respects as a protector and benefactor. It would be wrong for her to develop any expectations which you could not fulfil."

This, I reflected privately, was similar to the imaginary conversation I had had with him whilst still at Eastry.

"I don`t believe I`ve done anything wrong," I said.

"No, of course you haven`t. Quite the opposite. But you have your own way to seek, Richard. Important decisions lie ahead."

"Yes."

"Talking of which…"

He was, of course, right. I had to acknowledge that, even though it seemed harsh to deliberately distance myself from Izzy, which was what I took him to mean. This was perhaps the lesson in the nature of goodness which I had been seeking: to do the right thing, even if your true motives may not be understood; to do good, without receiving thanks, because the person for whom it is intended does not know.

I dwelt on this, in a somewhat melancholy frame of mind, for several days.

It forced me to recognise, once again, that in Moelfre, unless I chose to become a labourer, either a hired man working on the land, or a quarryman, I had no prospect of earning a living. If, as some people believed, I ever thought of the possibility of becoming a partner with Dilwyn in managing the farm, it was only to dismiss it immediately. Not only did I know too little and have insufficient experience, it was gradually becoming clear that what Isaac had said, at Christmas, was true. Dilwyn was, slowly but surely, losing his grip of things. I had seen his ledgers, and even from the simple form of bookkeeping he used, it was evident that the income from market had fallen whilst the rents and other costs had steadily risen.

If there had been a time when people called him `moneybags`, it was a reflection of the fact that he worked, from dawn until dusk, to make the farm prosper; but those times were no longer. Now there were days when he stayed abed until noon, only to return, by mid-afternoon, to the brandy bottle. The yard began to have a look of neglect about it, and if you believed Ivor in his mutterings, Dilwyn was selling off the herd to keep his head above water. One could see a time, in the not too distant future, when Lord Boston would foreclose on him.

After the Reverend Roose Hughes` words of caution I made the effort to avoid seeing Izzy in anything that might seem a personal or affectionate way. When I visited the cottage, I persuaded Margaret to accompany me; sometimes, I sent Margaret alone. In this way, I tried to ensure that she was provided for without compromising her or myself. It was a hard course to take but I believed it to be right, and as the weeks passed by I came to assume that Izzy would see it that way too.

It was perhaps, inevitable, however, that we would meet, at some point, in circumstances which would allow us to be more frank.

It had become my habit to take long walks along the coastal paths, sometimes towards the quarries of Bychan and Red Wharf, sometimes in the other direction, beyond Porth Helaeth to Dulas Bay, as far as Point Lynas.

It was one of those days when a light mist comes in with the tide and stays hovering along the cliffs and the shore; on such days, if you look upwards, you can see the disc of the sun shining above, diffusing its light, and if you stand on the cliff-top overlooking Porth Helaeth, away towards Lligwy, the whole line of the coast is irradiated in a golden mist.

It was towards this point that I was walking when I saw Izzy standing at the cliff-top, gazing out to sea.

"Izzy," I called, as I approached. She did not turn, but as I came beside her, she sat down on a ledge of rock.

"It`s beautiful, isn`t it?" she said.

"Yes, it is."

The tide was nearly at the full, and the waves breaking on the rocks below, threw up a white foamy spray.

"It`s a long time since I`ve seen you out here," I said, after we had watched for a time.

"I don`t come here very often. Just sometimes, when I`ve had a surfeit of my own company at home."

"I know what that feels like," I said.

"Do you?" she asked, turning to me for the first time, and looking at me curiously, as if she had some question or doubt about me in her own mind.

I sat down beside her. "I come out here when I`m tired of trying to work out what I`m going to do with my miserable future."

"Why do you call it miserable?"

"What else should I call it?"

"Is it because you were prevented from going to study for the clergy?"

"Oh, I don`t know. I`m not sure that I really wanted to do that anyway."

"So, what will you do?"

"I don`t know."

"What would you like to do?"

"You`d laugh."

"No I wouldn`t."

"I always wanted to be a poet."

"There`s nothing wrong with that."

"Except that it requires talent."

We started to walk back towards the Swnt.

"What I`d really like – it`s only a pipe-dream, mind you – is to live in a great house, with beautiful gardens and fountains, and be a patron to artists, musicians and writers. Live a comfortable life where everything is in proportion, where people may experience harmony and beauty, and be inspired. I saw the paintings of a great artist once, a painter called Turner, only briefly, but I`ve never been the same since, it touched me somewhere, with a sense of awe and wonder, that is what I would like to foster."

"You`d have to be very rich to live that life."

"Yes."

"But maybe you will one day, who knows?"

"Who knows what will happen, you`re right. What about you, Izzy, do you have any dreams?"

"I used to have dreams but they were only childish fancies. I don`t think of them now."

"Like the unicorns on Ynys Moelfre, there?"

"Yes, if you like."

"Maybe you shouldn`t stop believing in them."

"Well, I`ve never been to the other side, so I can`t say for sure."

"Do you remember that day?"

"You and Isaac?"

"Yes."

We sat down facing the island, now at its smallest in the flood tide.

"I`ll probably go to the hiring fair for the harvest," she said, at last.

"Don`t do that, Izzy!" I replied, recalling what I`d heard of the hiring fairs at Amlwch and Llangefni. "It`s worse than the cattle market."

"I have to do something."

"Why don`t you come back to the farm? At least you`d have some company."

"You mean Margaret?"

"Yes. And myself, too. There`d be time to look at some books, maybe."

"Did the Reverend speak to you?"

"Yes. Did he speak to you, too?"

"Yes. He`s a kind man. He wants the best for both of us."

"Yes. Though it does seem harsh, that we can`t be friends."

I was aware that I had taken the conversation into an area that was, perhaps, all things considered, not wise; nevertheless, when two days later, Izzy appeared again in the kitchen, I cannot pretend that I was not pleased.

And so it was, through the middle months of the summer of 1859, that seldom a day passed by without Izzy and I seeing one another again. Sometimes it was just the momentary exchange of a smile, passing each other in the house; sometimes, when her work was finished, and if Dilwyn was out of the house, she would come to my study alcove, and we would talk about books; often, long after she had gone, I found myself thinking of her still.

The middle of summer was often the best of times on the farm. With plenty of grass in the pastures, the cattle could graze at ease, and needed little tending other than the rancher`s watchful round; the milking and dairy work was started early in the morning and was usually finished by noon, so that in the afternoon, especially on a hot day, there was a lazy indolent mood about the kitchen and the yard.

It was on such a day, towards the end of July, that I set off with Izzy to row around Ynys Moelfre, to make up, as we lightheartedly agreed, for the journey with Isaac from which she had been excluded all those years before.

It was a hot still day, and by three o`clock, when we slipped away from the yard, Margaret was asleep in the chair beneath the pear tree by the kitchen door, and half the village it seemed had gone indoors to rest, escaping the rigour of the sun.

We slipped the boat from its mooring in Porth Moelfre and within a few minutes were out of sight of the village, rounding the headland by Porth Nigwl, and past the slipway of the lifeboat house. There was hardly a breath of wind over the mirror-like surface of the sea, and the boat slipped easily towards the island where even the sea-birds, usually so raucous, seemed drowsy and silent in the heat.

We passed round the seaward side of the island, without discovering, as Izzy noted, ruefully, a single unicorn; but by then a different kind of magic was already upon us, and instead of returning to Moelfre, spurred on by a force as powerful as the sea itself, we rowed on, past the cliffs of Porth Helaeth, towards the beach at Lligwy; and there, where the tall sea grasses made a sheltered bower, that which had been the subject hitherto only of my feverish waking dreams, was realised.

Part 5

Chapter 26

"Hi, mom."

"Saffy! Where are you?"

"I`m back here, with Aunt Liz."

"Did you go to Wales?"

"Yes. Just got back this afternoon."

"Is everything all right?"

"Course it is. How`s dad and everyone?"

"Fine. Did you have a good time?"

"Yes. Probably be going back there next week some time."

"It must have been good."

"Yes, it was. Very interesting. I`ll e-mail dad about it all."

"Yes. I`ll tell him. Have you heard from Charlie?"

"Only that he`s going to the Kruger with Mike and Dan."

"Well, you can`t really blame him."

"I don`t blame him. What do you mean?"

"You know he didn`t really want you to go on this holiday, don`t you?"

"I can`t help that. Anyway, you should be on my side."

"I am on your side. I just don`t want the two of you to fall out, that`s all."

"We won`t fall out. Promise."

***

"Lucy said she`d call you in the week. She wanted to get back. She`s got an essay to finish for tomorrow."

"Right. Typical of her to leave it till the last minute."

"Aunt Liz. Let me tell you something. All students are like that."

"So, how was it?"

"Brilliant. Lovely place."

"They always say the Welsh coast is nice, so long as you get the weather."

"We stayed in a place called Beaumaris, and then drove out over the island to Moelfre."

"I`ve heard of Beaumaris. It`s supposed to be very pretty, isn`t it?"

"Yes, it is. It`s on the Menai Strait. Very unspoilt. Just how you`d imagine a Victorian sea-side resort."

"And what about Moelfre?"

"Just a tiny village, really, built round a shingle beach, quite picturesque, low cliffs all along the coastline round about. Quite a few tourists, I don`t think there`s much else there really, there`s not a lot of development all along the coast. I suppose that`s part of the attraction."

"So, did you find anything out?"

"Well, I think so. It`s quite exciting, really."

"Go on, then."

"Well, I think I`ve found out who S.R.H. is."

"Really?"

"Yes. It`s Stephen Roose Hughes. He was the Rector of Llanallgo, which is basically the local church, in the 1850s and early 60s. Of course, I can`t really be sure, but the initials are quite distinctive, wouldn`t you say?"

"Yes."

"And I suppose – I mean I`m just speculating – but a clergyman would be the sort of person who would have a copy of Wordsworth, don`t you think?"

"Well, yes. I suppose it makes sense. But anyway, how did you come across him?"

"Well, the interesting thing is that he was the Rector when there was this terrible shipwreck on the cliffs at Moelfre in 1859, a ship coming back from Australia."

"Oh, yes, it said something about that in the stuff you showed me from the internet."

"`The Royal Charter`, that`s it. Anyway, hundreds of lives lost, literally hundreds, and they carried the bodies up to the church, and laid them all out there until they could be buried."

"How gruesome!"

"There are still lots of `Royal Charter` graves in the churchyard, and a commemorative plinth, oh, and Stephen Roose Hughes himself is buried there. He was only young, in his forties, but he died just a couple of years later."

"Poor man."

"Anyway, the story was so famous at the time, Charles Dickens went there a couple of months later, and Stephen Roose Hughes took him to see the scene where the ship was wrecked, and Dickens described it in one of his books."

"Really?"

"Yes."

"So how did you find all this out?"

"We were talking to a chap who runs a gift shop there who knows all about it."

"That was lucky."

"The interesting thing is that `The Royal Charter` was bringing huge amounts of gold back from Melbourne – it was a bit like the Klondike there in the 1850s apparently – and there are all sorts of stories about what happened to the gold after the shipwreck."

"Really?"

"Yes. Dickens said there were gold sovereigns strewn on the beach as thick as pebbles, and this fellow in Beaumaris told us there were stories about local people making their fortune and buying up land and property and retiring to a life of luxury!"

"Well, good luck to them!"

"Yes, but what about if, I mean I know it`s only crazy speculation, but what about if our ancestor, Richard Williams, somehow, you know, benefited from the shipwrecked treasure?"

"You mean, that might be how he could afford to build New House?"

"Well, it's an interesting thought, don`t you think?"

"Fascinating. Would it have been legal?"

"Probably not."

"Gosh, how terrible! I think we`d better open another bottle of wine!"

***

From: Saffy Williams
To: Sally Whitelock
23rd June 09

Hi Sal. Went to Wales as planned, cousin Lucy has a mini so transport was OK. Found out that my ancient rel. was probably around when a famous boat sunk near here, hundred and fifty years ago. Met a guy in Beaumaris who told us all this, and guess what, I`ve got a date with him next weekend. His name`s Rob, mid-thirties, a bit raffish, good sense of humour, runs a gift shop and gallery here, and, before you ask, perfectly harmless! It`s not even a date really – he has a boat moored at a place called Traeth Bychan near Moelfre, and he invited me and Lucy to go out on a trip and for dinner next weekend. Lucy can`t make it next weekend, but I said I`d go. It`s no big deal, really, but I know Charlie would be mega jealous if he knew about it. Do you think I`m a terrible person? Tell me what you think! I`ve got his number so could easily cancel. I`m relying on you for good advice! Xxx Saff

Part 6

Chapter 27

As the summer of 1859 slipped towards autumn, I found myself, more than ever, at odds with the world and with myself. About what had happened with Izzy, there was between us now an uneasy silence. The intimacy we had shared, whilst inspiring me at the time with the highest, if vaguest, of aspirations, seemed to leave, in its wake, a void which could not be filled. And in that void, I experienced, more profoundly than ever before, the hopelessness of my situation.

"I see that Izzy has returned to work at the farm," said the Rev. Stephen Roose Hughes, after the service on Sunday, the last of August.

"She was going to go to the hiring fair," I said. "At Llanerch-y-medd, or Llangefni. I was worried for her."

He nodded. "You did the right thing."

"Thank you," I replied, aware of my own duplicity.

"It is almost a year now," he went on, "since your return. Have you thought any more about any of the courses of action we discussed?"

"Yes."

"But..."

"I think I`m not fit, not worthy."

"That`s a heavy charge to lay at your own door. Of what sin are you guilty"

"Sloth," I replied. "And lust."

"That, my dear young friend, is something you share with many men; many good men, too, I should add."

We walked together in silence.

"Would I be correct in thinking," he ventured next, "that the object of these strong feelings is Izzy?"

"Sometimes," I replied. "Sometimes others, in thought."

This, I realised, sensing a relief on his part, was sufficiently ambivalent as to be misleading.

“We must learn not to despise the impulses which God has placed in us, only to use them well. Fire poses great danger yet without its proper use where would we be? But I must be earnest with you, Richard. A young woman without parents must lack the guidance and protection of others more fortunate, and in this sense Izzy is more vulnerable than most. If she were to lose her reputation or gain a bad one, she must slip inexorably lower and lower into misery. I beg you not to put her in this position.”

“No,” I said.

“If, however, you are of a mind, you and she together, then let you be properly married, Richard.”

“But what would I do, to keep her I mean?”

“There is work to be found.”

“Labouring?”

“There is no shame in that, and poverty, so long as it is not attended by hunger or squalor, may well be the best foundation for happiness. But you are young and healthy, there is no reason why you should not prosper.”

This, as I think he could tell, was cold comfort.

“You must think carefully,” he said quietly, his hand on my shoulder, as we parted.

Dilwyn, that day, was in one of his growling moods, and I was glad when he took himself off, early in the evening, to the Talyfron. It was still warm at eight o`clock, though already the evenings were beginning to draw in, and I wondered how few seasons, even how few months, remained for me, for all of us, now, here at the farm. Not many, I concluded; and in my melancholy mood, I wandered back up the lane to the church and to my mother`s grave. It was less than a year old, but already the moss and the weather were taking their toll, and some of the older monuments were worn and pitted so that barely a word could be read; and if one considered that loss of clarity as a sad reminder of time`s power to erase every trace of what we have been, there were, too, all the countless others whose resting place, like Izzy`s mother`s had never been marked. Such a perspective, I concluded, as I stood there until the gloom finally descended to surround me, made nonsense of the petty travails of our daily lives, and nonsense, too, it seemed, of the dilemma in which I found myself entangled.

When I returned to the house, I shackled the horse to the wagon and set off towards the Talyfron. Out in the bay, there were the lamps of a dozen boats, changing their lobster pots and bringing the catch which would be taken, still live, to Amlwch the following morning. Outside the Talyfron, some of the carousers had spread across to the shingle, sitting on upturned boats and baskets, smoking their pipes.

Dilwyn was inside, half senseless in the corner chair, and it took three men to help me drag him to the wagon. The cool air revived him a little, and, sitting beside me as we climbed the hill he mumbled an animated discourse, but the meaning, whatever it was, eluded me.

The following day, notwithstanding, he was up early, and, according to Ivor had set out for the market in Amlwch with one of the bullocks bred in the spring. It was a sturdy animal, fit and spirited, and it would bring a good price, no doubt, though from the twist of Ivor`s mouth, I could tell that he did not approve. There are many factors which affect the well-being of a farm: the weather, the price of winter feed when the crops don`t do well, sickness in the herd, the work of poachers and predators; but most of all, a farm needs breeding animals to ensure its future prosperity, and when the breeding animals are sold, it is a sure sign that all isn`t well.

Dilwyn returned in the late afternoon, and that evening, Lord Boston`s man called. They took some port together, and spoke amicably enough, but the talk was of arrears, and when Dilwyn pushed the bag, containing the proceeds of his day`s sale across the table, it was clear that it was only part of what was due.

For ten days after that he stayed sober as a judge. Setting out from the farm in the morning, on horseback and with his long coat and wide-brimmed hat, he recalled the imposing figure I had first seen in Porthaethwy ten years before, though now the grizzled hair and the network of red veins lining his face belied that recollection.

It was a mild September, carrying with it, for me, the nostalgia of leaving for school, though it was pleasant enough to feel the season changing, and to have things, at least seemingly, back to normal at the farm. I spent a week with Ivor bringing in the hay, and tried to put at the back of my mind the other questions which were troubling me.

I was in the study alcove one morning when Izzy came through.

"I`m sorry," she said, hurriedly, "Margaret sent me to…" and without finishing her sentence, she turned to go.

"Aren`t you going to say good morning?" I called.

She turned and looked at me sharply as if to say something pointed, then just shrugged. "I thought you were busy."

"Is everything all right, Izzy?

"Yes. Why shouldn`t it be?"

There was, in her manner of saying this, something which was at the same time both obtuse and vulnerable, and I realised that she was harbouring some disappointed expectation which she was too proud to confess.

"I`m sorry if you think…"

"If I think what?" she said cutting in sharply. "If I think what?"

It was my turn to shrug my shoulders.

"You mean you`re sorry if I think you`ve been ignoring me? If I think you don`t respect me, if I think you despise me for giving you what no girl should give outside wedlock? Is that why you`re sorry?"

"Izzy, it`s no such thing. But you must see that it`s not easy for me either."

"I have to get back," she said. "Margaret will be coming to see where I am."

"I`ll speak to you later," I said, but she was already gone.

I tried to seek her out during the rest of the day, but she was always busy in the kitchen or in the yard within earshot of Margaret.

That day, after a fortnight of sobriety, Dilwyn set out for the

Talyfron early in the evening. I deliberated with the idea of walking across to Izzy`s cottage to see her, and then decided to wait until I took the wagon down to pick him up, thinking that perhaps I would catch a glimpse of her, and would have the chance to say enough to clear the air a little.

As I approached, turning into the lane that ran past the cottage I saw that she was already there, by the wicket gate.

"I was hoping you`d come past," she said.

"I`m just going to pick him up."

"I wanted to say sorry for my outburst, you know, this morning."

"It`s all right," I said, "there`s nothing to apologise about."

"I just wanted to say, though, I know I don`t have any claim on you, that`s all."

"I`m sorry if I`ve disappointed you, I just don`t really know what to do for the best."

"No need for you to think you have to do anything. I`m all right."

"I do care about you, Izzy, I want you to know that."

She shrugged. "There`s no reason why you should be interested in me."

"Why do you say that?"

"I know you`ve been let down in your expectations. When you talk about the people you`ve met and the things you`ve seen, who can blame you for wanting something better?"

"No-one`s better than you, Izzy. It isn`t anything like that. I just have no way of being independent, not anything I can see, now, anyway. That`s what makes it difficult. Do you understand that?"

She nodded. "You should go away from here," she said, "make a start somewhere else where you have no ties. Look at you, even going down to pick up Dilwyn and bring him home drunk, when he`s the reason you`re in such a position, to start with."

"It`s not as simple as that."

"Maybe not. But you`ve nothing to thank him for, if you ask

me, or anybody for that matter."

"Perhaps you`re right. I do it because it`s something my mother once asked me to do."

"I know."

It was my turn to shrug.

"You`d better be going, Richie," she said, at last.

She patted the horse`s neck and then stood back. I pulled on the rein and the horse walked on.

As the wagon made its way slowly down the hill I thought about what she had said. Of course, it was true, in part at least, that I had not altogether rid myself of the cherished notions which had planted themselves in the mind of an impressionable child on his first visit to London: sophisticated young women who mixed with artists; pampered girls with their tumbling ringlets and powdered bosoms, who adorned the Hanover Rooms; goddesses from the realms of poetry – it was from this gallery that I had created my idealised woman, a woman who never did, nor ever could, exist. It all belonged, unlike Izzy, to a world of fantasy.

Inside the Talyfron, a game of cards was reaching its conclusion. At the other corner of the fire, where he customarily sat, Dilwyn was slumped on the floor, unconscious.

"Let him sleep where he lies," said the Landlord. "The dogs like some company when it gets colder."

There was some laughter from the card players. I turned to go and rode back up the hill alone. Izzy was still there, in the shadow of the house. Seeing me approach, she stepped forward into the moonlight.

"Is he not with you, then?"

I shook my head.

"I was going to wave to you as you passed," she said.

I offered her my hand, and pulled her up onto the seat beside me.

"I should have brought my shawl," she said.

"It`s not far," I replied. "Draw close to me if you`re cold."

That night we stayed together, sharing a bed as man and wife, and in the honeyed darkness of midnight, and again in the misty wakefulness of dawn, I made such promises as, in my situation, only a fool, perhaps, would make.

Part 7

Chapter 28

My name, unless I choose, or am persuaded, to publish this manuscript under a pseudonym, is Sophia Davis, and at the beginning of our voyage, from Melbourne to Liverpool, August the 24th, 1859, I have reached the age of nineteen years and four months. As I fully intend this diary to be the promising start of a celebrated literary career, I mean to include not only incidental description of geography, food and nautical detail, and other such things proper to a sea voyage, but observations of my fellow passengers in which few may hope to escape the satirical sharpness of my pen.

My prime objective as a writer will be to expose the delicious follies of our company, for I`m sure there will be many, for the benefit of society, and I hope for my own, as I intend to profit greatly from my labours, and to retire from them an independent woman well before I reach the advanced age of twenty five.

I am, I feel obliged to point out, a seasoned traveller. My family came to Australia, from Bristol, in 1853, when I was thirteen years old. My father, a banker - seeing no greater contribution to humanity than to put his humble banking skills at the service of the goldminers of Ballarat, a sacrifice by which he also hoped to grow considerably richer than he was before - brought his family, that is to say, myself, my mother and my sister, here with him, and, even at the tender age of thirteen, one does not undergo such a journey without ingesting a considerable slice of what might generally be called life

I am not, therefore, one of those delicate creatures, who, coming out to Australia for the first time, expect to take tea on the vicarage lawn; nor, however, am I one of those who think it natural to arm wrestle with men in public houses, and drink with them, glass for glass, until one or the other of them slips under the table.

These are my credentials, and I have no doubt whatsoever that they will meet with the approval of a readership which, if it did but know it, is eagerly awaiting the emergence of my as yet unwritten draft from the printing press in London.

August 25th, 1859

We have been aboardship, here in Port Philip, for two days, and having seen our own luggage hauled aboard, we have had little entertainment so far other than to watch other people having their luggage hauled on board, too.

Melbourne, my father commented, is greatly changed since our first arrival here, six years ago; to which, the only possible rejoinder – and my mother did not disappoint in this respect – is that it has not changed enough! Having made his assessment of the city, and having deposited us here, father then made his way back to his office. He is not, you will have gathered, travelling with us, though a considerable part of his increased wealth is. His purpose in remaining here, of course, is to increase it further, and he is happy to do so; ours, in going, is to decrease the amount which will arrive with us in England in pursuit of our own happiness, so I do not doubt but that a fair equilibrium will be kept.

My mother is eager that my sister, Florence, and myself, having suffered the privations of colonial existence these six years, should now have the full advantages of English life; by which she means Bath, Tonbridge Wells, and London, of course, with the ballet and the opera and the meeting rooms, and the receptions, and the calling cards, and the scandal, all of which she has missed, especially the scandal, and all of which, she is convinced, will improve us greatly. Florence, she says, would have been married two years now in any civilised country, and Sophia, she says, can only have any sort of hope at all if regrafted where the softening influence of cultivated society may render some benevolent change.

However, there is no doubt that father is right in his assessment of Melbourne. Where once there were muddy horse tracks, rutted with carriage wheels, and buildings thrown up overnight, made of wood and corrugated iron and any other material to hand, now there are wide streets and raised pavements, with shops and business premises that exude commercial confidence, and the suburban residences have gardens and orchards, and sheltering trees so that I am sure as much peacefulness may be enjoyed there on Sunday mornings as in any rural cottage in Somersetshire.

"I shall not be at peace until I have seen you safely on board," said my father. His anxiety in this respect may well explain why this obligation was fulfilled two days early, though to judge from his self-satisfaction, it might have been thought that an extra degree of safety had been conferred on us by his alacrity.

And so we find ourselves here, observing the busy activity of the harbour. The tug boats, commented my sister, are like little fat bailiffs going smugly about with cigars in their mouths. The simile is perhaps a little strained but I see fit to include it anyway. Any further felicitous expressions will be included but not acknowledged. Leaving aside the tug-boats, however, we are too far from the waterfront to be privy to anything of real interest, tearful partings, for example, or even more promising, angry partings, anything that might tend to the kind of petty human interest that I intend to be the life blood of this diary.

August 25th, 1859

A sudden influx of fellow passengers today, so many that I will be hard pushed to get to know all of them, and so I will have to be judiciously selective about those I choose for my satirical purposes.

I will confine my study of the passengers in steerage to a minimum; this does not reflect any social prejudice on my part, and I am sure that their lives and dramas are every bit as colourful and lurid as those in First Class, it is merely that the usual regulations aboard ship prevent any degree of intercourse between us, and I would be loath to make things up. In the event of insurrection or mutiny, I shall of course reverse this decision.

This afternoon we witnessed – and here I must remain utterly serious – the loading of the gold! Weighed in the bank, witnessed and signed, it was then loaded into chests, and locked, signed and witnessed; then, taken to the dock, under guard, it was loaded into tugs, signed and witnessed, then brought to the ship, under guard, hoisted aboard, and loaded into the strong room astern, signed and witnessed again, and finally signed for as all present and correct by the captain himself. The amount of paperwork involved is, I imagine, almost as heavy as the gold itself, but there we are – we must not have any part of our wealth spirited away by anyone who has not signed for it or been witnessed doing so.

When I asked the captain how much there was altogether he tossed his hand in a gesture of inconsequence, and said, in the region of four hundred thousand pounds. Very inconsequential, indeed! At least, I hope father is able to rest easy now that his portion of it is safely aboard.

August 26th, 1859

We are under sail at last!

When I say that we are under sail, I mean that I think we are under sail, for the ship is in open water, and it is moving through it, though smoke is also coming from the funnel which may mean that our engine and not our canvas is the means of our propulsion.

For those amongst you, my dear readers, who are not familiar with the modern nautical technology, I shall explain. The ship we are on, The Royal Charter, is a steam clipper. This means that she has sails, which do very well when the wind is blowing, and an engine, which does very well when the wind is not blowing, so that, between the two, our general expectation is to do very well indeed.

There. I hope that explanation is not too rigorously scientific.

A touching scene! The last of our arrivals yesterday was a Mrs Rose, who came aboard with her brother Mr Pratt. There was much fuss of the sentimental kind before the brother departed again for the harbour. There is, unless I am very much mistaken, a story to be ferreted out there!

We saw our last of land at about eleven o`clock this morning, and the next time we touch dry land is expected to be late in October when we reach Liverpool, though there is some talk of making a brief landfall in the south of Ireland, which will suit some of the passengers. Apart from that, however, we will not go into port at all – such is the self-sufficiency of our vessel!

We are to travel via Cape Horn, which, despite its ferocious reputation, is apparently the quicker route for homeward travel to the northern hemisphere, on account of the trade winds. This is in contrast with our outward voyage, six years ago, when we came down the coast of Africa and through the Indian Ocean. This means that we leave Australia in a different direction from whence we arrived, though, the earth being round, we trust, all should come right in the end.

August 27th 1859

Our dinner last night was to be the first at which the collective company was to be assembled, though, owing to the sea-sickness, there were a number of gaps at table, and my Mrs Rose, with whom I was hoping to begin cultivating a confidential friendship – for she is not much older than myself – was one of them.

I have made a friend, however. Jane Fowler is seventeen, full of youthful brightness and enthusiasm for life, and I intend to make her my protégée. Her sister, Edith, is a sweet young thing of six or seven, who has a devoted nurse, Emma Calf, who repeats everything that is said to her, nods vigorously, and then laughs in a rather horse-like manner at every opportunity. They are travelling with their father and mother.

During dinner, Mr Fowler was in conversation with Mr Gapper, a farmer from New Zealand, whom he was keen to quiz about the Maori wars of the last decade. Mr Gapper, who is in his thirties, I would say, is a tall man with an athletic physique, and when standing, he leans slightly towards those he speaks to, as if in quiet deference to those smaller than himself. He is returning to England to purchase agricultural machinery, and seems to be a great enthusiast for the future of New Zealand and the opportunities it offers to men such as himself.

We also have a Scots family, Mr and Mrs Russell, and their two little girls Catherine Margaret, aged ten, and Elspeth, aged two. They are an engaging family, who dote on one another; the parents are attentive to the girls in a way which might, you could be forgiven for thinking, make them selfish and spoilt, though in fact nothing could be further from the truth: they are perfectly well behaved and charming. I`m sure Florence and I were never so appealing as children!

Indeed, we are very much a ship of comfortable families returning home, rather than brave pioneers, setting out to try our mettle at the very edges of the known world.

August 28th

Trouble aboard ship! The reason for Mrs Rose`s absence from dinner last night was not the sea-sickness but apparently a consequence of having been waylaid and importuned by certain rascals from steerage who attempted to persuade her to sup with them in the nether regions of the ship. She was rescued, it seems, just in time, by Mr Gapper, the New Zealander, but was too discomposed to appear at dinner. Unfortunately no clear description of the offenders was to be had, so they have gone unapprehended, though the captain has made it known that anyone caught at this sort of behaviour will be clapped in irons for the duration of the voyage.

Talking of which, it is rumoured that we have at least one lunatic aboard who is kept under lock and key below to prevent his distress being spread amongst the ship`s company, but as yet I have no further detail to corroborate this.

But back to Mrs Rose. Mother commented that a woman who travels without a companion must ever be aprey to those who would take advantage of her, especially, she might have added – though in fact she did not – a young and pretty woman. But the question is, why is Mrs Rose travelling without a companion, and why was it her brother and not her husband who accompanied her to the ship? These questions, and many more, I will make it my business to answer.

I feel at this point that I ought to describe the sea, but, there being really very little to say that has not been said already, I feel it sufficient to refer my readers to other sources.

August 29th, 1859

We are, it has to be said, very comfortable. Our quarters are spacious and light, tastefully furnished and generally well appointed so that, as father said when we embarked, it is rather more like being in a superior hotel than aboard ship, and, for once, mama did not disagree with him. It is certainly a great improvement on our outward journey, when we were always cramped, frequently damp, and consequently generally very bad tempered. There is a dressing table with a mirror, where mama has plenty of space to prepare her coiffure, comfortable armchairs, an escritoire where I sit at this very moment at my usual labour, and a closet with a porcelain washbasin, and marble fixtures. We also have the luxury of a bath reserved for our own use, quite a contrast to our previous voyage!

A corridor with prettily embroidered hangings, and stained glass windows separates us from the Grand Saloon, and this cloister, as it might be described, provides us with a convenient promenade when the weather outside is inclement. The Grand Saloon, where our meals are served, is a luxurious room, a hundred feet long, as I would guess, though one of the masts, called the mizzen, I am told, extends through it at the lower end. Along each side, tables form a continuous line, with upholstered banquettes facing each other, and in the middle a carpet of red and gold, with gold fringes and tassels.

There is also the Ladies` Boudoir, a very pleasant room which runs across the ship at the stern with several windows which look out over the sea, and the ship`s wake, providing refreshing ventilation in the warmer weather; this room serves also, we are told , for dancing and other entertainments, though we have not seen anything of this kind yet.

Amidships, the main deck, somewhat lower than the poop deck and the forecastle, and thus rather more sheltered, is the busiest area of the ship, and it here that passengers of all classes frequently mix, for it is where meat, bread, milk and other provisions, including wines and spirits may be purchased. This area also contains the stables and the pens where livestock is kept, an assortment of geese, turkeys, chicken, pigs, sheep and cows, some for milk and some for the slaughter, so that there is always a supply of fresh meat.

The kitchens are also to be found in this section of the ship, and there is great activity thereabouts all day long, with a score of stewards and cooks hastening about their business. Adjacent to the kitchens are the main offices of the ship, and accommodation for the engineers and officers, as well as access to the engine compartments and the hold.

In calm weather, it is possible to promenade the whole length of the ship, from aft to stern on the port side and then back on the starboard side. The poop deck at the stern, however, is reserved for first and second class passengers.

This will be an ideal place from which to observe whales, porpoises, flying fish, albatrosses and all the other creatures that must find their way into this journal. Indeed, if I do not see them I will be tempted to invent them, for I would be loath to disappoint my readers.

The weather so far has been very pleasant indeed. On our journey six years ago we travelled, in effect, from one summer to another summer; now we going from one winter to another, though the south Australian winter is quite a different thing altogether! Secretly we are looking forward to an English winter especially if there is snow for that is a commodity we have not seen these six years. It is one of the many things which, when he created Australia, the Good Lord omitted to include.

We have heard, from travellers arriving in Australia, that during our absence, and largely influenced by the Queen Consort, Prince Albert, a custom of bringing living trees into the house has become popular as a means of celebrating the Christmas festival. Father is firmly of the opinion that this `Prussian frivolity`, as he calls it, will be nothing more than a passing fancy, but nevertheless, we are looking forward to seeing it.

August 30th

The fine weather continues.

We have passed Tasmania – Van Diemen`s Land, as mother calls it still - off the extreme south east tip of Australia, and are now making our way towards the south and the east, skirting the lands of the Antarctic, towards Cape Horn.

I took a turn about the deck for a good twenty minutes this morning on the arm of the Captain, Mr Taylor. He is a florid, bustling man, with a hearty laugh and a determined manner. He extolled the virtues of his ship – it seems he was a passenger himself when the ship had her maiden voyage five years ago, under the captaincy of Mr Boyce – and assured me that he expects to be `on the leeward of Mrs Taylor in Liverpool` after sixty days and an uneventful journey. When I said that I hoped the journey would not be entirely uneventful, he smiled and said that he hoped a little in the way of music and dancing would prove an agreeable entertainment once we had passed by Tierra del Fuego and Cape Horn.

Besides Mr Taylor, we have two other Captains aboard, Captain Adams and Captain Withers, both travelling as passengers. Should we encounter any nautical difficulties of an exceptionally testing kind, I am sure that the heads of these three gentlemen, put together, will be more than a match for them. It is, perhaps, a little disconcerting that both the additional captains are with us following somewhat unfortunate circumstances, Captain Adams having lost his ship off Buenos Aires and Captain Withers having lost his off the Fiji Islands, but I am sure that a captain may well lose a ship without it being entirely his fault, and so I will be optimistic. We are, after all, on the Royal Charter!

I meant to discover more about Mrs Rose but in my preliminary study of fellow passengers I have been preoccupied by Mrs Woodruffe, who is quite the beauty of the ship. She is what my father would call, if he were here, a `handsome woman`, for she is tall and slim, though with a well defined bosom, and features that might be described as statuesque. She is related to Mrs Foster, who is also her companion on board, and she is taking her young children, two boys, back to England to be settled in school. She is, I suspect, a woman of some spirit, and I like her for it. This morning, at breakfast, at the utterance of some pompous absurdity from Mr Parker [of whom more anon] I caught her eye, and saw a fine look of amusement there, so that we nearly both burst out laughing.

Mrs Foster is a jolly woman of fifty who is the proprietor of the Shakespeare Hotel in Manchester, and this is her second voyage on The Royal Charter this year, having come out in the spring to assist her husband in the setting up of a third hotel in Melbourne. Mrs Woodruffe is married, if I understand it correctly, to one of Mrs Foster`s nephews, and he too is engaged in the trade of hospitality which prospers well in these new territories, and, as Mrs Foster points out, is like to continue to prosper when the gold runs out!

But, to Mr Parker! A fine example, if ever there was one, of the English gentleman, who, having travelled about the dominions, knows a thing about the world, though to hear him speak you could be forgiven for concluding that the more he has travelled, the less he has learned! He describes himself as a financier, and has had some dealings, he says, with my father`s bank, and if we are to judge from his own boasts, he has done rather well from his three years in the colony. His wife is a quiet, seemingly timid woman, who closes her eyes for long periods when he is speaking, though when she utters his name, usually with a rising intonation which is followed by a distinct exclamation mark, he responds, rather like a dog who has undergone many years of strict training, promptly.

August 31st[th]

I have considered including our positions of latitude and longitude each day because, according to my protégée, Jane Fowler, it is the done thing in such diaries. I do not wish to deviate from convention lest it be taken as a sign of arrogance, but as these nautical bearings mean absolutely nothing to me, nor, I dare say, to many of my readers in years to come, I have decided to run the gauntlet, and omit them.

At dinner tonight, the discussion turned to the merits of our ship, and though someone has reputedly heard Captain Adams saying that the positioning of the masts is not entirely to his liking, the general opinion was of approval.

"Sixty days to Australia, sixty days back! Whoever would have believed it?" said Mrs Woodruffe, casting a glance towards Captain Withers, as if to convey the meaning that he alone might be responsible for such technological advancement.

"But why not fifty days or thirty days?" said Mr Russell.

"It will never come to that," said Mr Parker, sagely.

"You think otherwise?"

Mr Parker made a sagacious grunt to indicate that he did.

"What about a ship powered entirely by steam?" asked Mr Carew.

"Nonsense," said Mr Parker. "Think of all the coal she must carry. What room would remain for the cargo or the passengers?"

This was considered by some a rather witty proposition and Mr Parker spent a few moments acknowledging the mirth he had caused. "Besides," he continued at last, resuming his sagacious tone. "The wind is free. Don`t forget that. The wind is free!"

With this, Mr Parker evidently considered himself to have had the last word, and though, to judge from the looks of one or two others, there might well have been other words to follow it, the general agreement was to let the conversation move on.

After dinner, those of the gathering who were so inclined retired to the Ladies` Boudoir, where, at Mrs Foster`s instigation, we were given an impromptu recital by Mr Judd, `Piping Judd` as he is generally known in the ship`s company. His official duties on board are amongst the most menial, and he has no musical training whatsoever, but he has the most remarkable ability to play by ear, and has a repertoire which includes almost every operatic aria that anyone proposes. And all this on a mere tin whistle! He is, also, the most genial of characters and his merriness infects the company.

"A very pleasant evening was it not?" said my mother when we returned to our quarters.

"Mrs Foster is a very jolly woman," said Florence. "I quite like her."

"Mrs Woodruffe flirts wickedly with Captain Withers," I said.

"Indeed," said my mother, "the poor man`s head is quite turned."

"Mr Gapper was very attentive to Mrs Rose," said Florence.

"He saw that no-one else included her in the conversation," replied my mother. "He is quite the gentleman in that respect, despite his background."

"What do you mean by that?"

"Well, he has been a farmer these fourteen years, has he not? And in New Zealand, too. So many men lose their manners in such circumstances."

September 1st

We are racing through the southern seas under full sail, and there is not a finer or more bracing experience to be had!

We have fallen in love, each of us, with the sails. Jane has fallen in love with the Mizzen Royal Staysail, I have fallen in love with the Main Top Gallant Sail, and young Catherine has fallen in love with the Jib Topsail. It is a good thing that we have fallen in love with different sails for we all have it in us to be passionate mistresses, and any jealous rivalry would be like to end in poisoning or bloodshed!

But we all agree together to be in awe of the mariners who live most of their lives above. We watch them climbing the rigging, in all weathers, until they are tiny specks no bigger than insects high above, and then, shinning along the spars, where they hang above the ocean without a trace of fear, whereas we, watching them from below, feel a lurch of the stomach at every move. Mr Suaicar, the boatswain`s mate, and Mr Rodgers, whom everyone calls Joe, are particularly agile and fearless and we admire them greatly. They are both of Malta and it seems the men of that island are prepared for a life at sea as if by an instinct they are born with. Then, of course, there is our own dear Isaac, from the coast of Wales, whom we admire just as much.

Isaac it was who taught us, at our request, the names of the sails. Isaac is on his third voyage home, he tells us, and he has an open face, and a shrewd twinkle of the eye so that we are never quite sure whether or not he is sporting with us, and that, of course, is an uncertainty by which any charming female may be pleased to be flattered! He is not supposed to talk to us, and has to keep a weather eye open for the Captain, or other Officers, having been reprimanded once for telling us of a whale that followed the ship for four days, and advised to get on with his duties, or risk being keel-hauled, but he is quick-witted, and can usually be up from the deck forty feet into the rigging and out of harm`s way, at the drop of a hat, and so we do not fear that he is in any real danger of suffering this fate; besides, we would intercede most vociferously, all three of us, on his behalf, and I believe that would be a fair test of the authority and resolve of any Midshipman!

The admiration of our bold seamen is not universal, however. I now present a transcript of a conversation overheard by myself between Mr Parker and Mr Eltham on the above topic.

"Do you not applaud the skill of the men aloft, Mr Parker?"

"A Barbary Ape might do the same, for that`s all the skill required."

"But an ape acts from instinct, surely, and therefore without fear. If not their skill you must admire their courage. Take Mr Rodgers, for example."

"Let me tell you something, Eltham. The African and the Indian are children by nature, but as faithful as the dog and brave as the mastiff. The Mediterranean races, by contrast, are quintessentially sly, and above all cowardly, mark my words, cowardly. Put him in a situation where true bravery is required and he`ll fail you every time. Mark my words."

"Indeed."

"Indeed. You may take it from me"

This phrase is Mr Parker`s characteristic way of concluding a discussion, calculated to precipitate resigned agreement on the part of his interlocutor. We are now seven days out, and I doubt if Mr Parker has yet conceded a point in conversational differences of opinion; at the end of sixty days, it would not surprise me to learn that this record is still intact.

September 3rd

The weather has turned cold and I have been abed two days with the rheum. Yesterday we ran through a squall, and the ship lurched forward and then lurched backwards, and tipped constantly one way and then another, so that all those who had not yet been tested by the seasickness were driven to the limits of their tolerance. I include myself in this. Just as I was priding myself that I had as good a pair of sea-legs as any old salt on the main, I succumbed to the green complexion and found my way to the rails just in time. The sea was grey and hostile, like furrowed and splintered metal, and the spray slapped into my face with a stinging effect which despite the unpleasantness went some way to revive me. Later, however, as other symptoms prevailed on me, I was forced to take to my bed. To be sick on land is one thing; to be sick aboard ship, and in bad weather especially, is another, and I should be surprised if the noble poet Dante has not reserved it as a punishment in a special circle of his Inferno.

We are informed that the weather will continue to grow less clement as we make our way, by degrees, closer to the pole in order to plot our course around the tip of South America. I took a turn around the deck with Florence this afternoon to break the monotony of being confined in quarters, but there were few others about, and I find myself somewhat dispirited about the chances of finding interesting material for my diary. I fear that the Captain is right, and that apart from the usual round of maladies, the voyage home will be disappointingly uneventful.

September 4th

Very cold. Sharp blustery winds. A little hail and sleet from time to time. There is an outbreak of sickness in steerage, apparently, but nothing contagious according to the surgeon. We are taking our meals in our cabin, however, as a precaution, and only leave it for the briefest of walks on the poop deck for fresh air. The Ladies` Boudoir has the windows closed and the shutters fastened. No-one goes in there at the moment.

In the depths of the southern winter, we are told, ships have been known to be lost several days in the encroaching ice fields, which may resemble vast white plains, or snow bound coastlines, with their own bays and headlands, and mountains beyond. In such a landscape, said Captain Withers, who was telling this tale to Mrs Woodruffe and myself, one might imagine Dr Frankenstein`s creation taking flight from his hated maker. This romantic notion, a reference to Mrs Shelley`s novel, which I have been forbidden to read and which, consequently, I know from cover to cover, had the deepest effect, it seemed, on Mrs Woodruffe. With eyes which expressed boundless wonder, she replied, "It is very much to be hoped, Captain Withers, that you will never attempt such an escape." To which the valiant former captain of the `Victoria` much affected, replied, with a slightly uncomfortable catch in his throat, "No, indeed, ma`am, no indeed." It was at this moment, catching only the briefest of glances from the corner of Mrs Woodruffe`s eye, that I detected, once again, the evidence of skilfully repressed laughter. But Captain Withers, I fear, is smitten!

September 5th

I found, occasion, this morning, to speak briefly to Mrs Rose. She is, as I conjectured from my first impression, a very pretty woman, small and neat, with dark hair, and a slight chin which adds very much to her femininity. She has been suffering from the same ailment which afflicted me two days ago, and so this is why, she said, she has been very little abroad since embarkation. She did not, alas, allude to the contretemps with the fellows from steerage, or Mr Gapper`s bold intervention, so I am no wiser on that score. She is not, I suspect, a woman who volunteers information easily.

"We are travelling on to Bristol," I said, using a ploy which I have sometimes found successful whereby a piece of information given may prompt a reciprocal response.

"I am travelling back to my father in London," she replied. I smiled with bland expectation, not wanting to say anything at all that might prevent further elaboration on this, but, much to my frustration, no such elaboration came, and at the very moment when I might have used a different tactic to press a little harder, Mr Gapper himself appeared.

"Miss Davis," he said, "Mrs Rose. I trust you are both feeling much better."

September 6th

The weather is much clearer today, with sunshine and good visibility, though still very cold. In the distance, ice-bergs can now be seen each day, though looking hard for any length of time, the eye can start to play tricks, and one imagines seeing all kind of things. Isaac, in one of his cheekily stolen moments off duty to talk to us, tells us that this is pretty much the utmost limit of the ice-bergs and that what we see now are merely the remnants of what were once much mightier masses of ice. In winter conditions the crew have to stay aloft all night to warn of the presence of these mountains of ice as, apparently, they present a great danger to shipping. In response to Catherine`s question as to whether penguins might be seen on the ice flows, he told her that if she looked very carefully and very diligently, she might well observe one or two of those same creatures eating their fishy dinners – and then he was off up the rigging like a gazelle.

Our main meal today was excellent. The stewards, having sensed, I think, some despondency amongst the passengers on account of the poor weather and sickness, have gone out of their way to provide a dinner which will bring good cheer to the participants. Because I have not yet, despite my promise, furnished an account of our fare I will do so now.

The dinner is served to us on silver plate, and the fare for today included, after an excellent soup to start, for the main course, roast beef, boiled mutton and mutton cutlets, roast chicken, chicken curried, tongue, roast pork and apple sauce, with vegetables to select from, potatoes, carrots, rice, and cabbage. For dessert we were presented with rice pudding, fruit tarts, plum pudding [with brandy aflame] and sago pudding. Beside all this, there are wines and cordials as requested, and the breakfast provision is equally lavish. Indeed, there is hardly an hour of the day when it is not possible to satisfy one`s cravings for food and drink, and for many passengers it is the chief means of staving off the anxieties or, indeed, the boredom, of the voyage.

September 7th

According to the Captain, we are averaging ten knots, or about two hundred and fifty miles a day, so he is pleased with our general progress. We have only had to use the engine alone [or the `screw` as they call it] twice. We should round the Cape in about another five days.

Catherine is mortified because of Isaac`s mockery vis-a-vis the penguins. Unfortunately, she did not pick up the light heartedness of his suggestion straight away, but watched intently for a good half hour, and later told her father of the vigil, and he could not help but laugh outright. She has threatened to report the matter to the captain, but we have told her this will not do, and when we explained to her the horrible nature of such nautical punishments as keel-hauling, and tarring and feathering, she was sufficiently impressed to agree to desist. Nevertheless, she is carrying her ten and a half years very heavily today, and it will be a good day or two more, I am certain, before the wound is fully healed.

The Ladies` Boudoir is open again, and it is warm enough to be pleasant sitting there, at least during the hours of daylight. We have resumed saying prayers there in the evenings, and tonight we had a musical interlude in which Mr Bartel, a musician from Prussia, entertained us with a piece from Schubert.

Our prayers are conducted by the Reverend William Vere Hodge, about whom several tales circulate, none of them very complimentary. Depending on whom you believe, his wife left him several years ago in charge of their six children in order to visit a relative in Hobart. Despite his having travelled half way round the world to find her, she steadfastly refused to return with him, and when his impatient Bishop finally summoned him back, two months ago, he was forced to plan the journey alone. He is a thin creature, not especially tall, but seeming taller on account of his lack of substance, with a pointed nose, red at the tip and constantly sniffing, and he wears a worn black frock-coat, always buttoned fully to the collar.

He conducts prayers without great enthusiasm, and in conversation is acutely sensitive to anything that might be deemed a slight, so that people are very much on guard not to offend him; when he departs, however, it is open season, I am afraid to say, and the taste for wicked innuendo which some members of our company enjoy is fully exercised.

I personally feel sorry for him, not so much on account of the treatment he receives here, but on account of the six children who, I presume, are still waiting for him at home. What on earth can he tell them about his exploits to recover their mother that will leave him, or them, with any dignity? Wicked as I am myself, when I picture their poor expectant faces, I am moved to tears of pity, though I have to confess that one night abed, when I had been contemplating this sad picture for some considerable time, I was forced at last to stick a handkerchief in my mouth for fear that a sudden stray gulp of laughter would awaken my mother and my sister!

It was after prayers last night that some of the men began talking of the matter of *natural selection* as propounded in various forms and by various learned men, but none more controversially than by Mr Darwin, who has published several treatises on the topic, and who, apparently, according to the latest news from England, is to publish a book later this year which will put the whole matter to the public once and for all.

To what extent our manners are changed aboard ship may be evident from the fact that, at home, at the very mention of such a topic, the ladies would be invited, for their own tranquillity of mind, to leave the room forthwith. Last night, however, no such distinctions were made, though I can well see why they might be, for I have never known a topic to cause such extreme or such violently held opinions.

Some are so scandalised that they will barely open their lips lest, against their will, some foul expletive should emerge; Mr Fowler, normally a quiet and unassertive man, expressed the view that if the authority of God and Divine Providence stood to be challenged by this, he would defend that authority and that providence to the death for his children`s sake; Mr Parker, never a quiet and unassertive man, taking up the controversial issue at what he deemed an intellectual level, asked why it was, that if he, Mr Joshua Parker were to be proved the descendant of a Barbary Ape, the other Barbary Apes had been allowed to be so lazy as to remain exactly as they were. My mother, putting an alternative, and I think very ladylike construction on the matter, said that she didn`t mind at all being descended from an ape so long as it was an ape with good manners and a large pocket-book.

At last it was Mr Gapper, who, having listened to everyone else quietly and attentively, said that he, for one, would welcome the publication of Mr Darwin`s book, not because he believed in it one way or the other, but because it would give him the opportunity to form his own opinion. This, everyone seemed to agree, struck a sensible note on which to conclude the debate, and we continued, for some time, but in very jolly spirits, to discuss lesser matters.

In bed later, however, and, as is sometimes the case, less jolly than in company, I began to wonder if, like Frankenstein`s poor monster, we are all creatures in an alien world where the very best our creator can do is to regret the very act which brought us into being. I must have slipped in and out of sleep several times, waking on each occasion with the same monotonous sense of oppressed nerves, and then, just at about the time of first light, I was aware of the sound of a woman`s voice, singing. Perhaps because it appeared to come from quite a distance away, the voice had a strangely ethereal quality, and was very soothing to my rumpled spirits. I listened for some time, dismissed the thought that it might be a mermaid, and then, putting on my coat and bonnet, went to the door and then along to the end of the corridor where, to one side, the steps lead down to the third class and steerage berths.

The door at the top of the stairs had been left open, and from there the sound of singing was louder; it was an intermittent song, as if it belonged to someone who was busy at something else, and was singing unconsciously, and I thought it must be a woman from steerage doing some routine morning task. I wanted to go down and see her, and tell her how much her singing had cheered me with a sense of the simple ordinariness of life, but I dared not go down. Instead, I sat down on the topmost stair, and listened from there.

I was disturbed some time later by a voice which I thought to be that of one of the stewards, but when I looked up it was Mr Gapper, and for a moment he seemed as discomposed as I about being there.

"I couldn`t sleep," I said, at last.

"Nor I. Would you care to take a walk on the deck?"

He offered his arm and I took it. The sea had become still overnight, and apart from a constant low moan from the main sails, the ship was as quiet as I have known it.

"I was thinking of what we were talking of last night," I said.

"Ah that!" he replied.

"Does it not worry you?"

"The only thing I know for certain," he said, "is that life will go on, come what may. That`s enough for me. You have your whole life ahead of you, nothing anyone can say or write should prevent you from enjoying it."

I doubt if this constitutes a complete rebuttal of the anxieties that will no doubt arise from Mr Darwin`s theories, but in the circumstances, I was heartened, and when breakfast time came, I was in possession of a very healthy appetite.

By the time breakfast was finished, the screw had been lowered and the engines started up, and we cruised for four hours under steam, until the wind picked up again in the afternoon.

September 8th

I wish now that I had taken the opportunity to question Mr Gapper a little more closely. How like a woman to assume the position of weakness! Instead of seeking reassurance over great questions of existence, I should have been probing! After all, he, too, was up and about at an unusually early hour of the morning, was he not? Is there a tale thereby, and did I miss my opportunity to winkle it out?
I must do better!

This afternoon, we are speeding under full sail with a strong following wind, and Captain Taylor says we shall round the Cape within two days. Amongst the passengers, though little is spoken aloud, there is an unmistakeable tension. The skies are ruggedly grey and inhospitable, and the ship moves through a relentless swell that sends waves crashing over the bows, but so far no storms of the fearsome sort travellers frequently report in these notorious seas.

September 9th

We have rounded the Horn and are now on a steady course northward through the South Atlantic. As the momentous event happened in the middle of the night, there was nothing very momentous about it at all, and now that the danger is past, I must admit to feeling somewhat deprived. I had hoped to catch at least a fleeting glimpse of Tierra del Fuego, which I consider one of the most romantic names ever appointed to a place, and to have experienced one or two moments of extreme terror at the ferocity of nature to report to my grandchildren in years to come. However, perhaps in time the memory will fade and become inaccurate, so that what I remember will be as my imagination prompts, and then what a tale I will have to tell!

Plenty of people about, promenading on the deck, albeit in their top-coats for the weather is still fresh with a sharp wind from the south. Mrs Fenwick and Mrs Woodruffe walked out together with their children, all very properly turned out, and very well-behaved, too, I must say. Later they made a group on the poop deck with the Fowlers and the Russells, and a pretty sight it was too! Mrs Woodruffe seems in every way a sensible woman and an exemplary mother, though I doubt her husband would entirely approve the sport she has at Captain Withers` expense.

There was, no doubt, after the apprehension of the last few days, a sense of relief, as if we are on the homeward run, which is hardly the case yet, though according to Mr Bane, the Third Officer, it will not be many days before we begin to experience the more temperate climate, and I must admit that I too shared the holiday feeling.

Amongst the men, there was some talk of hunting, for albatrosses have been sighted apparently, though I saw none, and I certainly hope they steer clear of us. I have no desire at all to see wanton bloodshed, and though I`m not superstitious, `The Rime of The Ancient Mariner` left a deep enough impression to make me wary!

In the afternoon, we had coffee in the Ladies` Boudoir, and Mrs Foster suggested that we should have some amateur dramatics! She was supported by Mrs Woodruffe, and by Jane Fowler, but most of the company demurred, including myself, Florence and Mrs Rose.

When the coffee was finished, Mrs Rose accepted Mr Gapper`s arm for a walk on the deck. He is becoming quite her chaperone!

September 10th

Fine weather, though still a cold wind from the south; we are told, however, that we must not complain as this is the wind that will hurry us onwards. A school of porpoises followed the ship for two hours this morning, and these creatures seem to radiate such a gleeful pleasure in their own leaping and diving that they remind one of children playing. Almost the whole ship was out to see them at one moment or another, and children were hoisted on parental shoulders to get a better view.

Mrs Rose, in the company Mrs Fenwick and her children, though with the faithful Mr Gapper close to hand, as ever, laughed aloud – quite the most animated I have ever seen her. The voyage seems to be having a good effect on her spirits.

Mr Gapper continues, on the whole, to make a good impression, I think. Mother, having conceded him to be a gentleman, and of good manners [despite his profession!] has half an eye for him as a suitor for Florence, I rather think. Florence, though acknowledging him handsome enough – and we are all agreed that a man does not reach the full maturity of his attractiveness until his mid-thirties at least - says that she cannot really imagine herself following a man half way round the world to the Antipodes when she has just travelled half way round the world to escape from them. Mother, in turn, finds this an incontrovertible argument. For myself, I would like to think that I would travel anywhere with the man I loved, so long as I loved him well enough; the difficult thing is finding such a man. And then, of course, there is the question of him loving me as well in return, for I would be loath to commit myself to such a bargain, unless on equal terms.

I was very much affected as a child, I remember, reading of the history of Grace Darling, the heroine of Longstone Lighthouse fame. Having become a figure of national celebrity for her deeds on the stormy sea whereby many lives were saved from the foundering ship, the HMS Forfarshire, she was besieged with proposals of matrimony, but died before she ever had the chance to take any of them up. To a child of eight, this was a very sad story, indeed, not least because of the thought that, had her health not let her down so vilely, she could have had the pick of the pack!

After lunch, we had an interesting talk with Mr Carew, who is travelling with his infant daughter, and her nurse. Mr Carew is a Magistrate of New South Wales, and he tells us that the law as applied in Australia is very different from at home in England. "The model is basically the same," he said, "but the conditions of life are very different, and so are people`s expectations. There are certain things that just won`t wear, out there, and the differences will grow, as people put down roots and insist on having their say."

"A colony," interjected Mr Parker, "which had convicts for its first immigrants is bound to have a certain view of the law, no doubt!"

"Indeed," said Mr Carew. "And a colony of men and women who have endured much to carve out a new life for themselves, will stand for no nonsense!"

Had he concluded by saying, "You may take it from me!" the pleasure of my afternoon would have been complete!

September 11th

We passed the Falkland Islands, just visible on the port bow this morning. These territories have been under British sovereignty, Captain Taylor informs us, since 1833. It is a small colony of sheep farmers, mainly, though the islands apparently have some strategic value because of their position. The life there is very hard.

Mrs Woodruffe is insistent that we all make preparations to take part in the amateur dramatics. Brandishing a copy of Shakespeare, and having established that the bookshelf in each cabin contains the like, her plan is that short scenes from the plays should be rehearsed, monologues, duologues, even songs, to be performed in the Ladies' Boudoir, in two to three weeks' time. Costumes to be improvised from our own wardrobes.

"She's a very difficult woman to say no to!" remarked Florence, when she had left us.

"Then don't say no," replied mother. "Say yes, and *mean* no. That's the way I've always dealt with your father's whims. It never fails."

However, despite our protests, silent or otherwise, the project has created a sense of excitement, and I was amused to discover Florence, this afternoon, leafing through 'Much Ado About Nothing' in search of suitable material.

Now that the weather is turning a little warmer, many of the male passengers from steerage bring cages on deck with parrots and cockatoos and other exotic birds, to let them have the benefit of the fresh air. Some complaints, of course, from other passengers about the raucous noise they create, but I rather like the little splashes of colour they make in the midst of a world of grey seas and grey skies. Great excitement is caused when one of these birds escapes and takes refuge in the rigging, and the sailors have wonderful sport helping to retrieve them. Apparently, these birds are brought largely as an investment rather than as a pet, as they will fetch a very good price if brought back to England in good health.

I learned today that the reason sailors have tattoos on their body is that, should they be drowned and their bodies washed up, the tattoo will be a means of identifying them. It was Isaac who told me this rather ghoulish piece of information. He himself has a small dragon tattooed on his forearm. It is, he says, the emblem of Wales.

There was a heavy shower this evening and when it had passed, the wind had deserted us, for the sails barely stirred at all. The Captain looked on with some consternation, and said that if it does not improve by morning, he will order the screw to be lowered and we will proceed by steam until we again meet favourable conditions. Some people say he is under great pressure from the Eagle Line to achieve the passage in less than sixty days, as the last return voyage of The Royal Charter was delayed by almost a month. The competition with other shipping companies making rival claims is intense!

September 12th

I rather think that we have a romance on board!

Amongst the groups of people from steerage gathered around the shops and the caged birds this morning was a very pretty girl of seventeen with very long dark hair, taken up under a neat hat, with a calico blouse, black shawl and dark plaid skirt. Also in the crowd was Mr William Bane, our Third Officer.

Later in the day, the two were seen together, walking arm in arm, towards the forecastle, and then back again; and if I am any judge of faces and expressions, it was a case of much ado about something!

I am very pleased about this. So far my diary has been starved of this most precious commodity! I am so looking forward to all the delicious gossip it will provoke, and for my own part, I intend to watch them with the eye of a hawk!

September 13th

Her name is Maria Lundy, and she has been two years a nurse with a family in Dalhousie, not far from Melbourne. The family being now about to move to Sydney, she was given the option to have her passage paid, and to return, with references, home to

England. She is making her way back to her sister-in-law, who lives in Durham.

There! You see I have not been idle!

Unfortunately, I cannot take the credit for this information. It was Jane Fowler, who, seeing the opportunity to walk beside her on deck this morning, made friendly overtures and came into her confidence to this extent. Mr Bane, she said, had been very kind in helping to secure more comfortable accommodation for herself and her companion when their berth had been subject to the effects of flooding from one of the upper decks.

She was eager to point out, Jane reported, that on the journey out the family travelled first class, and she is somewhat sensitive about the lowly status conferred on her by the present arrangements.

There will be more to report anon, I hope!

Florence has suggested that she and I perform the duologue between Rosalind and Celia from `As You Like It` for the amateur dramatics. I agreed that this was a good choice and have elected, since I am two inches taller than her, to play Rosalind and thus dress up as the boy, Ganymede. Mother has some long hose which can be adapted and the rest, I think, can be improvised quite easily. Now that the choice has been made, I am growing quite enthusiastic. After breakfast we rehearsed, with mother as our audience and critic, and did very well. The extract is not too long and I already have my first twenty lines or so by heart.

Jane, following our lead, has said that she would like to do Hermia from `A Midsummer Night`s Dream`, but she says she does not know where she will find a Helena since the latter must be considerably taller than herself. We said that we would try to find her something else equally suitable if a Helena does not materialise. I think she was rather hoping that I would take on the part.

September 14th

A beautiful morning, almost like an April day in England, cold in the wind, but very pleasant in the shelter, an open sky full of clean sunshine, but with great clouds, like sculpted monuments, on the horizon.

We had a meeting of what has been christened `The Thespian Committee` before lunch.

I`m not sure whether this should be a cause for celebration or not, but Mr Parker has agreed to perform Antony`s oration over the body of Julius Caesar; there were some suggestions, not uttered in his presence, that he might otherwise be in many ways suited to Falstaff, but I suppose we should be glad that one of the men has agreed to take part at all. They are, almost to a man, stubbornly reluctant!

Mrs Russell has said that she will try to persuade her husband to do either Macbeth or Benedick, and that if successful, which she doubts, she will take on Lady Macbeth or Beatrice accordingly.

We are getting somewhere, at least, and the more people say they will join in the more the impetus gathers, and we hope, by this means, to put on a full programme. Needless to say, Florence and I, alongside Mrs Woodruffe, have become movers and shakers in the enterprise, though, curiously, Mrs Woodruffe has not taken the lead by declaring what part she is going to play. Perhaps she has some secret up her sleeve.

Mr Gapper, though declining entirely to take a part, has said that he will assist in the construction of a stage, and in the fitting up of some kind of moving curtain so that we may begin and end our scenes with at least this theatrical convention in place. Mrs

Rose, I fear, is very timid. Whenever the topic is mentioned, she shrinks away as if she wishes she were anywhere else, and when pushed, as was the case when Mrs Woodruffe spoke to her this morning, she appeared to become almost tearful. I felt quite sorry for her, but there was no need, as Mr Gapper, her Knight in Shining Armour was soon upon the scene administering his usual discreet support!

September 15th

It is all change! I am now going to play Helena so that Jane can be Hermia. Florence is going to change from Celia to Rosalind so that Mrs Rose can be Celia. And here, to quote Peter Quince, we may have a play fitted! The idea occurred to me that I might play against Mrs Rose, with the hope of sounding her out a little more about the exact nature of her circumstances, but it did not quite work out that way. Florence is by no means such an inquisitive creature as myself when it comes to these matters, but I will just have to hope that she may glean something about that interesting lady!

September 16th

We came into one of the sitting rooms just off the Saloon this afternoon and into the midst of a very interesting conversation.

"Of course," Mr Carew was saying, "the situation in the colonies is different in this respect, that emigration to them, by whatever means, is often a great disrupter of family life at home. This is particularly the case with felonious deportation, as the party concerned not only forfeits his liberty for a certain period of time but also the freedom to bring his family with him, whether he might wish to or not; but also, if we take the case of mining, how many men come to the colony alone in search of their fortune, and how many return to their families? For every man returning home in this ship, either to stay in England, or return with his family, I warrant there are ten who abandon their obligations and stay to make a new life here."

"And how does the law stand?" enquired Mr Gapper, who made up one of the company along with Mrs Rose, the Reverend Vere Hodge, Mr and Mrs Russell, Mrs Foster and Mr Parker.

"This is my point. Common law has it that if a spouse is not seen or known to be alive for seven years, then the remaining partner may remarry. This is called *presumption of death*. Where things become complex is when the missing partner returns after seven years. And it has also been known that the *presumption of death* has been made several years in advance! The reality is that throughout the colony there are in fact bigamous marriages which, if proved, would be felonious."

"Or adulterous ones," said Mr Parker.

"Or, indeed, adulterous ones, in which the offspring, should there be any, stands in forfeit of the legal entitlements of legitimate issue."

"But the law on divorce has changed, has it not?" said Mr Gapper.

Now, I happened to glance towards him at this moment, and what caught my attention was not the expression on his face, which gave away little other than detached interest in the topic, but the look on Mrs Rose`s, a kind of tension in her half-glance towards him, which made me suspect, rightly or wrongly, that he was asking the question on her behalf. After this, as far as was possible without seeming rude, I made it my business to study her changing expressions.

"Yes, indeed," Mr Carew continued, "and in England, the case is clear. Under the Divorce and Matrimonial Causes Act, passed by Parliament, two years ago, a man may sue for divorce on the grounds of adultery, without petition to Parliament itself. This then becomes a case for the courts to decide."

"And a woman?" said Mrs Woodruffe.

"A woman, however, has no legal recourse."

"Even in the case of adultery."

"Even in the case of adultery."

"What about desertion?" said Mr Gapper.

"Desertion does not constitute a case for divorce, unless, as I said, after seven years, the *presumption of death* may be invoked."

"It does seem rather harsh," said Mrs Woodruffe, in a tone of high amusement rather than serious concern, "that a woman may not sue for divorce on the grounds of adultery, when her husband may. Is there one law for men and another for women?"

"Well, indeed , that is, in effect, the case. In many respects, the law treats women differently from men, there`s no getting away from it."

"In Scotland," said Mr Russell, "the case is somewhat different. The law in Scotland does not admit that when a woman marries she ceases to become, in her own right, a legal entity."

"The point we`re missing," said Mr Hodge, coming into the conversation for the first time, "is the principle of the sanctity of marriage in the eyes of God."

"Don`t talk to me of the sanctity of marriage!" said Mrs Foster, in jocular fashion. "If you`d seen some of the things I`ve seen, the sanctity of marriage wouldn`t trip so easily off your lips!"

"Surely, Mr Hodge," said Mr Gapper, "if the vow of marriage is broken by one party, the other party should no longer be held by that vow. Isn`t that a matter of simple natural justice?"

"The vow of marriage," said Mr Hodge, "is made to God, not simply to another person. The trouble with our liberal age is that we try to pass laws that permit us to do just as we like."

"In my experience," said Mrs Foster, "people do pretty much what they like anyway."

"The point I`d make," said Mr Parker, "is that an adulterous wife may bring spurious offspring into the family who may carry off the titles and estates!"

"I can`t imagine," said my mother, "why on earth any woman should wish to commit adultery in the first place."

"Well," said Mr Parker, in the peremptory tone of one summing up a discussion in which he has lost vital interest, "I don`t pretend to know anything about your sanctity of marriage, Mr Hodge, and I don`t pretend to know anything about your Divorce and Matrimonial Affairs Act, Mr Carew, but I do know this – if you don`t keep things tight, if you don`t keep a tight rein on things, I say, things go to pieces, and I defy anyone to contradict me on that. As soon as you give people an inch, they take a mile, as soon as the gate`s left open the horse bolts, and what you`re left with then isn`t worth having. That`s my opinion, and if anyone here thinks they have a better opinion, they`re welcome to it, but I`ll stick to my own, thank you very much."

There was a small round of polite, and, I suspect, largely ironic applause.

"Mr Parker," said Mrs Woodruffe, "you cannot imagine how avidly we are looking forward to your `Friends, Romans, Countrymen`!"

I am convinced, however, that Mr Gapper`s interest in the legal niceties of marriage and divorce is more than one just of passing curiosity. Has Mrs Rose taken him into her confidence? If, as we all suppose, but are too polite to say openly, Mrs Rose`s being despatched home to her father is the consequence of some marital difficulty or breakdown, has Mr Gapper become her guide and councillor? Or is there some warmer interest than that? Is Mr Gapper curious to know not only where she stands, but where he stands, too?

I have spoken of this to no-one, not to Florence or my mother, not even to Jane; I would not be true to myself, however, or to my mission as a diarist, if I did not record it here!

September 17th

Some drunkenness and fighting last night in steerage. We were aware of a slight disturbance at about eleven o`clock, but it was short-lived. Isaac tells us that it was two men, normally the best of friends, arguing over a woman. The Captain sent a half dozen of the crew down to separate them, and it was soon settled.

There are certain stages of the journey, Isaac tells us, and certain conditions, when such squabbles are more likely to take place than others. On the last outward journey, things were particularly bad because of short rations; this is difficult to imagine when one considers the lavish provision we have each day, though I suppose any sort of delay will soon put calculations out. Dampness, as a consequence of flooding, which percolates to the lower decks, is another such condition. A third provoker of arguments is drink, in itself provoked by boredom and idleness, and always worse when the weather is `slow`. So, there we have it.

I must admit that I am growing very fond of Isaac. If the world were a different place, I would certainly marry him, and be a-waiting, every time he came home from sea, to let him have the leeward side of the bed. Ah, me! If the world were a different place!

Let me not forget to record that Mrs Woodruffe has at last unveiled her great secret. She is to give us Cleopatra`s lament from Act 4 of `Antony and Cleopatra`.

September 18th

The weather grows warmer each day and we are making our way steadily towards the infamous doldrums. I can well recall, on our own outward journey, six years ago, we were becalmed for eight days, with hardly a breath of wind, at the hottest time of year. There was great sickness aboard; indeed, six passengers were buried at sea in a period of ten days, which more than compensated for the new arrivals, including a set of twins, who joined us during the voyage.

Great news! Captain Withers has volunteered to play the dead body of Antony to support Mrs Woodruffe in her rendition of Cleopatra`s lament.

September 19th

Felt a little unwell this morning and so stayed in bed until ten o`clock, missing breakfast. In fact it was rather pleasant to have half an hour or so alone; the fact is that on a voyage such as this, one tends always to be in company, which is all very well most of the time, but can become an annoyance.

I took the opportunity to learn some of my lines for Helena, at the height of her bedraggled confusion in the Athenian wood, and tried to think of some ways of enacting the character to bring out the comedy most effectively. She is, I think, something of a misfit; someone who does not meet the normal conventions of female beauty; a gentle soul, basically, who can become vituperative when threatened, or misunderstood. I much sympathise with her!

Feeling refreshed after my lie-in, I went on deck and chanced to meet with Maria Lundy, just taking her leave of Mr Bane who was about to go on duty. I introduced myself, and we walked together for a time. She is a very pretty girl indeed, though at every turn of the conversation, I noticed, she betrays a sense of injured pride, rather like the shepherdess convinced that she is, in truth, a princess.

"Mr Bane, of course," she said, confidentially, "is a very junior officer, I am well aware of that."

This remark was really a propos of nothing, and it had no sequel; she seemed merely to wish me to acknowledge that her own aspirations, in a just world, would be of the higher rather than the lower order. In fact, it had the effect of making me despise her just a little, for William Bane is a courteous and thoughtful young man, always kind and well-intentioned, though I can also understand why he is so infatuated with her! Men do not always see what we women see!

This afternoon, Mrs Woodruffe tried out her lament of Cleopatra for the first time with Captain Withers as her body. So successful was the rehearsal that Mr Parker has now asked Captain Withers to play the dead body of Caesar, too, to add verisimilitude to his own performance in the funeral oration.

September 20th

We find ourselves in an absolute calm. The sails have been furled entirely, and we are proceeding by steam alone. As we sit in the Ladies` Boudoir, with the window shutters open, a trail of black smoke drifts behind us, growing progressively thinner with the distance. Mrs Fenwick expressed the opinion that if all the ships crossing the ocean were powered thus, the air over the sea would be as thick as a London fog.

Mrs Fenwick is, as we have noted before, something of a worrier! There is always something, it seems, to trouble her mind, a concern for the children`s health, an anxiety about her husband`s well-being, a fear that this may happen when they arrive in England, or that may happen in Australia because of their absence. To talk to her is sometimes quite exhausting because of the multitude of things which queue up in her mind to be fretted over.

Having managed to reassure her on the subject of the ever blackening skies, I found myself thinking that ocean travel would be much less romantic without all the billowing, and whooshing and whispering of the big sails, and all the craftsmanship that goes into their management, but perhaps, indeed, such a day will never come. As things are, the Captain is concerned that if the engines are run for anything more than a few hours each day, we will run short of fuel, for, certainly, no coaling stops are scheduled anywhere in our journey.

September 21st

Oppressive heat until noon! A painted ship upon a painted ocean;

it could well have been the sea that Mr Coleridge imagined for punishment of his Ancient Mariner! Then the sky darkened and there were flickerings of lightning across the horizons. This lasted for an hour, and then the wind started to blow up, and the crew were up in the rigging unfurling the sails.

What followed was the worst storm we have had so far, with the ship tossed like a cork, it seemed, on monstrous waves, and with rain hurtling down like rods of steel. The mariners were constantly at work during this time, even in the worst of the weather, trimming and fighting the sails, as the wind shifted in direction and intensity. Captain Taylor, however, coming into the saloon to reassure us, seemed quite elated with the events.

"She`s riding well, ladies, have no fear, she`s riding well. We`re on the move. Fear not, the storm will abate, and dinner will be served on time!"

At this particular moment – quite apart from the fact that food was very far from our minds – this seemed an idle boast, but it proved to be the case. After two hours, we had sailed out of the worst of the storm, and the stewards were calmly swabbing away the excesses of water that made their way into the internal passages, and the tables were being prepared.

I am pleased to say that I was not one of those who were revisited by the seasickness, but despite its promptness, dinner this evening was a very muted affair, and all plans for rehearsal were set aside for the day.

It is not uncommon, Mr Stevens, the Chief Officer, told us, for men to be lost to the sea in such weather as we have seen today. Once overboard, he said, there is no hope for them at all, even if they can be seen, they will be dead within minutes.

The very thought makes me shiver. It could be Isaac, Joe, Mr Suaicar – any one of them. We watch them, day by day, and think how fine and free it must be to be up there, above the elements, but all the time death is just a slip of the hand or foot away!

September 22nd

The wind has lessened today, though we still make good progress, and the breeze is sufficient to mitigate the effects of the sun`s heat. Mr Bane has supervised the erecting of a sun shelter on the poop deck, and as we sat there this afternoon, Mr Judd entertained us with three arias from `The Magic Flute`, including Papageno`s song which suited his tin whistle perfectly, so that he had us all laughing with the impudent little trills he added between the lines.

I had a short rehearsal with Jane afterwards. She looks the perfect Hermia, and she reads her lines pleasantly, but those she has memorised come out so slowly and ponderously, and with so much screwing up of the face in frustration, that I fear much of the character and emotion is lost. Mr Parker, evidently experiencing the same problem of memory, has asked if we might actually read our lines from a script, but Mrs Woodruffe has absolutely forbidden this. Her only concession is that we might each have a prompter in the wings to assist us in the event of complete blankness of mind. I am to be the prompter for Florence and Mrs Rose, which suits me quite well as I have already memorised a good section of their lines!

Their rehearsal went satisfactorily. Florence is very amusing as Rosalind, playing the youth Ganymede, and does it, I`m sure, far better than I would ever have done. Mrs Rose speaks the lines very fluently, though with the occasional wobble of nervousness in her voice, and she has yet to develop her gestures and expressions to a sufficient degree, but she improves all the time. Mr Gapper certainly thinks so, as he watches each attempt with great patience and applauds heartily when it is concluded.

September 23rd

The weather continues hot, and though the ship`s progress remains satisfactory, there is a mood of languor which seems to have affected everyone on deck. Our pavilion continues to provide shelter from the sun through the hottest part of the day, and it is very pleasant, though we have been too lazy to rehearse today.

September 24th

Slept very little last night because of the heat. Florence was the same, and we chatted for a while in our dawn whisper until mother complained that we had woken her too, and then we all tried to go back to sleep. Whilst we were talking, Florence and I were speculating about what lies ahead when we reach England. We are to spend some time in London before returning to Bristol, and great excitement surrounds both those events, as occasions long looked forward to. Beyond that, however, the future is shrouded in a mist, and excitement vies with apprehension as to which is the stronger.

By mid-morning the air was so thick and grey we could hardly see from one end of the ship to the other, and then, shortly after noon, a heavy shower set in which lasted two hours, and left the air much cooler and cleaner.

Tonight we have promised ourselves an early night in order to catch up on the rest we missed last night.

September 25th

Woke up early this morning, feeling much refreshed, and bathed whilst mother and Florence were still asleep. On deck, I met with Miss Lundy, who came towards me and took my arm as if she had been waiting for me.

"I must beg your advice, Miss Davis," she said, as we walked on, "for I`m sure I really don`t know what to do!"

"What on earth has happened?" I asked, responding to the apparent agitation in her voice.

"I have received a proposal of marriage from Mr Bane," she said, in a hushed tone, as if it were something mildly shocking.

"I`m afraid, Miss Lundy," I replied, not knowing quite how to reply, "that my advice will avail you little, for I have never been proposed to in my life and am therefore the most inexperienced of advocates."

"Do you think it would be very heartless to reply with a summary rejection?"

"Is that in fact how you intend to reply?"

"It is how I am inclined."

"Then the sooner you tell the gentleman, the kinder you will be to him."

"Yes," she said considerately, as if she had expected a rather different response from me. "Do you think," she continued, after we had walked a few steps further, "that Mr Bane would be a very poor match?"

"By no means," I said, trying to avoid straying into considerations of rank, "I think him to be a very personable gentleman, and no-one can deny that he has a pleasing face: a very promising combination of qualities most people would say."

"Do you really think so?"

I began to understand that she fully intended to accept his proposal but wanted someone else`s affirmation.

"If I thought," she went on, "that his prospects were secure, I would have no difficulty in tying my future to his, but a seafaring life, well, it is so fraught with uncertainty, is it not?"

"Mr Bane is a very diligent and capable young man, I`m sure," I said. "I have no doubt that he will prosper."

"Do you really think so, Miss Davis?"

Once again, I felt that I had given her the satisfaction of providing exactly the answer she wanted.

"Miss Lundy, I hope you won`t think the question impertinent, but have you considered whether or not you love Mr Bane?"

"I think I love him as well as I could ever love anyone," she replied, though without, it seemed to me, great conviction.

Later, seeing Mr Bane in the Grand Saloon, I felt somewhat compromised by the confidence Miss Lundy has entrusted in me. Nevertheless, I could not help but wonder if he has yet had his answer; if, under his officer`s uniform his heart is swelling with pride or expectation. Poor man, is he so blinded by her charms that he does not see the person beneath? But then, who am I to moralise?

Apparently, it is the custom to have certain rituals performed on board when the `Line` is crossed. I remember some such thing happening on our outward journey, but the recollection is vague. At the time, the concept of a `line` was somewhat obscure to me, and not seeing one actually marked across the sea, I lost interest!

However, the Captain is anxious that any such ceremony should not delay the progress of the ship. We are, it seems, exactly on course to reach Liverpool by the last week in October, the 26th of that month being the sixtieth day of the journey, and he is very keen to meet that deadline.

September 26th

The performance has been set for next Saturday, which is the second of October, so after a rather lethargic few days, rehearsals have resumed with a new sense of purpose. We are all busily sorting through our trunks to find suitable clothes to adapt for our costumes.

Florence and Mrs Rose [we have learned that her name is Rachel] went through their scene twice, and I only had to intervene once as the prompter when Mrs Rose jumped ahead by several lines. Apart from that the scene is beginning to come to life quite nicely.

My own scene with Jane was a little flat because Jane is not yet fully recovered from a cough which developed after the last storm, but I am confident that we have enough time to bring our contribution up to standard. The Purser, Mr Redfern has offered to print a programme of the events and has been going about making sure he has our names spelt correctly.

When the rehearsal had finished, we sat and watched for a time as Mr Gapper set about constructing his device for opening and closing the curtain, until at last only Mrs Rose and myself remained, and I took the opportunity of asking her if she pleased to take a short walk around the deck.

"You must miss your brother a great deal, do you not, Mrs Rose?" I began, still hopeful of teasing some morsel of information from her.

"Yes, indeed," she replied.

"Did you travel out together, I mean when you first went out to Australia?"

"Yes."

"And does he plan to stay there long?"

"There are some business arrangements from which he must extricate himself. With Mr Rose."

"I see. They were partners?"

"They both put money into a venture, yes."

We walked on towards the fore deck, and I waited for her to continue. We passed Mr and Mrs Russell, and their two little girls, and stopped to pass the time of day, then walked on again.

"And when matters are resolved," I said, hoping to resume the conversation, "between Mr Rose and your brother, will Mr Rose join you in London?"

"I`m afraid I don`t know what his plans are."

"Forgive me. I didn`t mean to be impertinent. I hope I haven`t offended you."

"I am not offended. But you must understand, Miss Davis, the subject of my marriage is painful to me, and that is the reason I do not readily speak of it."

"I am truly sorry," I said. "I give you my word that I will never raise the subject again."

"Thank you. And I would be grateful if you would not repeat this conversation to any of our companions."

I gave her my assurance that I would keep her confidence, but almost immediately wished that I had not been so absolute about not raising the subject again. After all, having volunteered as much as she did, she might easily have been led to say a little more! I know it is wicked to be so inquisitive about other people`s private life, but to get so close and not get to the very bottom of it, is frustrating in the extreme!

September 27th

This morning at eleven o`clock, we crossed the line. Great hilarity when two of the ship`s boys were head-shaved and then thrown – protesting but nevertheless thoroughly enjoying themselves - into the sea. Then, one of the ratings, got up as Neptune, trident and all, was lowered and brought back on board. This, it seems, is the traditional way of propitiating the forces of the deep!

Almost everyone was on board for this, and there was great mixing of the passengers as if on a festive day. Amongst them, I saw Mr Bane and Miss Lundy in close conversation, no doubt on the subject of their nuptials!

September 28th

We rehearsed the entire programme this morning, though there was a problem with Mr Gapper`s curtain, and the rope will need to be replaced with some type of yarn that will not snag so easily. Apart from that, all was satisfactory, though a degree of nervousness is creeping into some of the performances now that the real thing is so near.

Returned to the cabin just before lunch and found mother in an emotional condition.

"I do sometimes miss your father so much."

"So do we all. I expect he misses us too just as much."

"I have a terrible fear that I will never see him again. It`s so real, such a real conviction that he will die or I will die, and then there will be so much that I never had a chance to say."

By this time, she was in a full flood of tears, seeming quite inconsolable. I put my arms round her and rocked her slowly, as one might a child, until the sobbing lessened.

"It won`t be long," I said. "Eighteen months, two years, he said so himself, enough time to see everything settled, and then he will rejoin us in England."

"Two years, yes, he said so."

"In the meantime, we will go to London, as we said, then refurbish the house, and time will pass by so quickly we will hardly have time to think, and then we will all be together again."

Gradually, she became pacified, and, reassured by my picture of the future, she began to elaborate on it, with increasing cheerfulness, herself. "The garden will need a great deal of attention, I`m sure, and I always thought a summer house would be rather nice."

Later, I mused on the effect of soothing words, but in consoling her I seem to have had the opposite effect on myself. What if, after all we have invested in it, this journey turns, in the event, to disappointment? What if two years turn to three, and three to four, and still father finds reason to stay in Australia? What if we end up as ladies living a comfortable but retired and dreary life in the suburbs of an English city?

September 29th

I have banished the melancholy fit! It is all too easy, in the confined world of a ship, with the same company and the same daily round, week after week, for one`s thoughts to get stuck in the gloom! So, away with it! From now on, be my thoughts happy, or nothing worth!

I was cheered, immediately after breakfast, at the sight of Mrs Woodruffe, with Captain Withers on one arm, and Captain Adams on the other, strolling on the upper deck amidships. The glorious thing is how finely she mocks them, each one as proud as a peacock to have her on his arm!

Mother, too, is much more cheerful today, I am glad to say. She made no reference to yesterday`s little upset, so I am sure that it is now out of her system, too. After our turn around the deck, she went to join Mrs Foster, Mrs Russell, and Mrs Fowler for a rubber of whist. All seems to be well.

If I was wondering how long it would be before I was to be treated to another instalment of Miss Lundy`s saga, I was not wondering long! She was hovering by the shops amidships, with a basket on her arm, as if much preoccupied with her purchases, though no sooner had she caught sight of me from the corner of her eye than she hurried to my side.

"Am I to congratulate you yet, Miss Lundy?" I asked.

"Pray, Miss Davis, I beg you to keep your voice as low as you may," she replied. "It is not yet official."

"So," I whispered, "am I to take it that it is unofficial, then?"

"It is not to be made public until we arrive back in England," she said.

"I see. Well, I`m sure Mr Bane has very good reasons for preferring a measure of discretion."

"Oh, I assure you, Miss Davis, it was not Mr Bane`s decision, but my own insistence."

"Really?"

"Indeed. I have no wish to be the object of idle curiosity. None whatsoever, I assure you."

It was, perhaps, this note of emphasis which led me to suspect that the opposite might be true, but I maintained my own discreet silence.

"I have told no-one of this but yourself, Miss Davis. You must promise me you will repeat it to no-one."

"You have my word, Miss Lundy."

September 30th

After our rehearsal this morning, Mrs Woodruffe suggested that our woodland scene between Hermia and Helena would benefit from having a Lysander and Demetrius present, to make it clear to everyone in the audience what the argument is all about. This, of course, makes perfect sense, but, as was pointed out, we have very few young men to choose from, and no-one had an answer to that.

The weather is very pleasant, having turned a little cooler, but still very fine. Last night Florence and I watched the stars and tried to remember all the constellations of the northern skies. It made us feel that home is getting closer.

October 1st

We have a Demetrius and a Lysander, but not without drama of another kind!

It was at dinner last night that Mrs Woodruffe announced that she had obtained the Captain`s permission to approach Mr Stephens and Mr Bane with a view to their taking part. On the understanding that they would have only to stand in the appointed place, and say an absolute minimum of words, they both agreed and after an impromptu rehearsal was called, it was agreed by all that with a little guidance from Mrs Woodruffe about how they might manage their facial expressions, those two worthy gentlemen will make a great addition to the scene.

Perhaps I, more than anyone, should have foreseen the problem that might arise, but I am sorry to say that I did not.

It was only this morning, when I received a note from one of the stewards asking if I would be so kind as to grant Miss Lundy a few moments` conversation that I began to sense that something was wrong.

"Miss Davis," she said, when I met her, and evidently very much upset, "I have taken you into my deepest confidence – and now this! Miss Davis, I shall never, never forgive you."

"What on earth can you mean, Miss Lundy? How can I have offended you?"

"Do you deny that you have enticed Mr Bane, my fiancé, into playing a part in a love scene with you?"

"I assure you, Miss Lundy, that I had nothing whatever to do with his volunteering to make up the numbers in the scene you refer to…"

"Then you admit," she interrupted, "that such a scene is to take place, and that you and he are to play the part of lovers!"

"It is an entertainment, Miss Lundy, a frivolous piece of make-believe, nothing more."

Instead of reassuring her, however, this might have been a confession of guilt, for she let out a muffled sob, and then turned and fled.

At first I was so incensed by her behaviour that I resolved to do nothing to reconcile myself to her. Then, as my mood settled, my resentment was replaced by pity. Her jealousy, I realised, is not a matter of Mr Bane`s or my affections, but of her own exclusion, and the bitter feelings such exclusion causes her.

I made my mind up, before taking any advice that might persuade me otherwise, to seek her out.

The stairs which lead down to steerage are the ones where I sat that morning several weeks ago to listen to the singer. It leads immediately down to a long corridor with a plain red carpet and doors each side which I think are mainly the second class accommodation, though I have heard it said that there are larger cabins there, with vents and portholes which are also for the first class.

The next flight of stairs takes one lower again, and here, immediately clear to view, a very different world exists. Close to the foot of the stairs where I stood were portholes which gave a kind of twilight illumination, and several lines of washing hung across from bulwark to bulwark, catching the slight breezes and airs from the ventilation hatches. Beyond, stretching away into the gloom, were cabins and compartments, some defined only by curtains and rugs, around a seeming maze of corridors, with, here and there, hammocks stretched between timbers. There was a musty smell of dampness mixed with smells of cooking and drying wool.

A group of men, sitting around the bottom of the steps, interrupted their game of cards to take me in, and I sensed that some jocular or ribald comments might soon follow.

"I`m looking for a Miss Lundy," I said. "Maria Lundy."

There were some comic murmurs and sucking of the lips, as if I were asking some task of considerable difficulty, though it was also clear that they knew who I was talking about.

"If any of you can direct me to where I might find her, I should be very much obliged."

"Well, now..." said one of them, a small man with a wiry frame and full white whiskers. "What do you think, Matty?"

"I don`t know, John. I don`t know."

"If you`re just going to jest with me," I said, deciding to take the offensive and not appear a shrinking violet, "please continue with your game of cards, and I will find her myself."

"Not sure why anyone`d want to go seeking that firebrand!"

said Matty, making them all laugh.

"You`d better ask young Robby, here," said John, "he`s been sniffing around her skirts enough, and getting the sharp edge of her tongue for his trouble."

Young Robby did not reply, or laugh with his companions, but made a surly toss of the head.

Finally, it was Matty who stood up, and pointing away behind him, said, "Go down Elizabeth Street here, as far as Victoria Square, then turn right into Swanston Street, and there you might find her at number fifteen."

At first, thinking he was still mocking me, I decided to walk on, anyway, then realised that there were signs indicating the places to which he referred. I passed a group of children playing a game of chase, and two middle aged ladies standing by a doorway with their arms crossed, who watched me as if they thought I was up to no good. At the corner which turned into `Victoria Square`, an open area of perhaps fifteen feet by twenty, a mandolin player was sitting on the floor picking out a tune, and he stopped and drew his feet in to let me pass.

There were several passageways which led off from `Victoria Square`, and I had to go round twice before I found the sign on which was written `Swanston Street`. I made my way to the doorway which was marked with the number fifteen, and knocked. A man sitting on his haunches on the opposite side of the passageway called across, "can I help you dearie?"

"Thank you, but I don`t think so."

"Are you sure I`m not your man!"

"I`m looking for a young woman."

"Now that`s a right pity, that is!"

At that moment, the door opened and the face of an old woman, with bedraggled hair, appeared in the gap.

"I`d like to speak to Maria Lundy, please."

"What if she`s not here?"

"I was told she was. Is she here?"

"What if she don't want to see no-one?"

"What is it, Mrs Barratt?" came Maria's voice from inside.

"Someone here wants to see you. I told her you don't want to see no-one."

Maria's face appeared at the door. "All right, Mrs Barratt," she said. And then, to me, "I'll get my coat."

Through the door, as I waited, I saw a dormitory with four or five beds down each side, two cabinets at one end, and a small table with chairs in the middle.

"You see how we have to live," said Maria.

"Are you coming over to see me tonight, Maria?" called the man opposite.

"Shut up, Sam Compstall!" she replied, in a shrill voice. "Or I'll have you up before the Captain."

He held his hands up in a gesture of resignation, and laughed, but it was clear that Miss Lundy knew how to protect herself.

"Come in here," she said after we had walked back past 'Victoria Square'. The compartment had an oven , and tables, and was obviously where the women in steerage prepared their own food.

She turned to look at me.

"Is it not enough," she said, "that you have made a fool of me already, but now you seek to shame me by coming to see me where all the disadvantages of my situation are most obvious."

"I do not seek to shame you, Maria," I said, "but I have come here to apologise to you most sincerely for an oversight on my part which I know has been most hurtful to you, and to tell you that if there is anything, anything at all, that will compensate for my insensitivity, tell me what it is, and it will be done."

She turned away from me.

"You have already explained," she said. "I accept your explanation."

"If you would like me to cancel the performance, I will do so."

"No," she said, in a flat and rather miserable voice, "what

would be the point of that?"

"I truly believe that Mr Bane was coerced into taking part in the performance, not by myself, but by Mrs Woodruffe, and that he only agreed as one carrying out a duty, not for any pleasure he hoped to derive for himself."

"Yes. I know. Thank you."

"Then you will accept my apology?"

"It is I who should apologise," she said after a moment. She turned towards me. "For the petty spitefulness of my behaviour. For my shallowness. Oh, I know it, Miss Davis, but I am made so miserable by the limitations my station has set on me, that sometimes I`d rather not live."

By this point, she had grown so upset that I could think of nothing else to do but to take her in my arms, and try to persuade her that any course of action linked with this latter wish was strenuously to be avoided.

We parted on amicable terms, and I was glad that I had gone.

Later, after our final rehearsal, Mr Bane approached me discreetly, and touching my arm, said, "Thank you."

October 3rd

Our revels now are ended! And very sorry we are about it, too!

The evening was a great success, much greater than anyone had dared to expect, and now that it is over, we all have an empty feeling, as if nothing in our lives will ever be so exciting or intense again!

The entertainment began with a piece of music which Mr Bartel had composed especially for the occasion, one which combined comic and solemn elements, and which gave the proceedings a very dignified and formal introduction. The audience, which numbered sixty or more of our fellow passengers, clapped appreciatively, and then, without a hitch, the curtain opened.

Standing in the wings, shoulder to shoulder, the tension was unbearable, and we all felt that Mr and Mrs Fowler, going out as Lord and Lady Macbeth, were like lambs to the slaughter. Their performance, however, was very creditable indeed, and was well received, the applause continuing for a good half minute after the curtain closed, just enough time for the dead body of Julius Caesar to compose himself on the stage, and then it was the turn of Mr Parker to give us the oration of Mark Antony.

This was a very fine performance indeed! Mr Parker rose to the occasion by producing a tremendously bombastic style of delivery which none of us had hitherto witnessed. Indeed, so loud was his utterance, that, as mother later commented, had we opened the doors, it might well have assisted the sails and hastened our arrival in Liverpool by a good few hours! But it was truly impressive, and would certainly have held the audience in complete awe, had he not, unfortunately, at certain key moments of alluding to Caesar`s merits, pressed his hands, with some force, into the midriff of the recumbent corpse, causing its head and feet, by reflex action, to jerk upwards. This was greatly appreciated by the spectators who cheered him to the rafters on the completion of his speech, so much so that Mr Parker insisted that Mr Gapper allow him two curtain calls, which we all approved of heartily.

Next, Mrs Fowler gave a lovely rendering of Portia`s speech `The quality of mercy is not strained`, and then Mr Carew, a late recruit to the company, entertained us with John O`Gaunt`s `This precious stone set in a silver sea`, which filled everyone with nostalgic thoughts of home.

Mr Bartel then provided a short musical interlude, and those who had now completed their performance made their way out to swell the numbers of the audience.

The second part of the entertainment began with Florence and Mrs Rose`s scene from `As You Like It` and so nervous was I on their behalf that I forgot that I was meant to be prompting them, and then nearly flew into a panic trying, in the dim light, to find the place they had reached in the text. However, my concern was quite unnecessary as they flew through it without a hitch, gaining warm approval from the audience.

As they came off I gave Florence a hug of congratulation and saw that Mrs Rose was receiving a similar hug from Mr Gapper. "I was *so* nervous!" I heard her say.

By now Mr Stephens and Mr Bane were ready and Jane and I prepared to set about one another as Hermia and Helena. I was wearing a pair of mother`s heeled boots, and Jane a pair of flat slippers so that the difference in our height was emphasised as much as possible, and this was a cause of great amusement to our audience. I made myself as clumsy and awkward as I could in all my movements, and flailed my arms in an ungainly way to express my exasperation at being suddenly the amorous object of both of the young men. After trying to plead for her loyalty, came the moment when Hermia turns on Helena, and Jane was suddenly like a woman possessed. So convincing was her acting, that I fully believed she intended to scratch out my eyes, and the audience howled with laughter as she rushed towards me, nails held up like weapons, and I picked up my skirts and ran away.

There was a fine round of applause, and as Mr Gapper reopened the curtain, Jane and I stepped forward to take our bow, with Mr Stephens and Mr Bane just behind us.

The high point of the evening was Mrs Woodruffe giving her lament over the body of Antony – which was a triumph! She had let down her hair, which gave an altogether different aspect to her face, and had made a gown of a soft gauzy material which helped to give great pathos to the character. When she came to the climax of her speech: `*for his bounty, there was no winter in it; an autumn `twas that grew the more by reaping*` the whole audience was enraptured, and Captain Withers, untroubled by the prodding he had earlier received at the hands of Mr Parker, made a very dignified body, well worth the praise he was receiving.

When the performance was completed, Jane and I went up onto the poop deck. We were both in a mood of high elation, and we talked of the evening, and about how wonderful it must be to be a great artist capable of holding an entire audience spellbound. We agreed that Mrs Woodruffe was an admirable performer.

"Who do you think she was thinking of?" said Jane. "You know, when she was doing her speech about Antony – do you think she was thinking of someone real?"

"I don`t know. Her husband, maybe?"

"Yes. Though I know if I had a husband as marvellous as that, I wouldn`t leave him in Australia."

"Perhaps she was just thinking of Captain Withers!"

Jane snorted with laughter.

"If Mrs Rose had done that speech, you know who she would have been thinking about?"

"Mr Gapper?"

"You think so too?"

"I`m not sure."

"Oh, I do. Absolutely. She`s head over heels in love with him, if you ask me, and he with her. You only have to see them together."

"He did give her quite a hug after her performance."

"And that wasn`t the only one either. I was watching them."

At this point we were joined by Mrs Woodruffe herself.

"Hello!" she said. "What are you two up to?"

"We were just saying how splendid everything was!"

"And now it`s all over," added Jane.

"Well," said Mrs Woodruffe, "we shall have to find something else to put in its place, shan`t we?"

October 4th

Mother has changed her mind and says now that we will go first to Bristol and settle in there before going to London. I don`t quite know what has brought about this change of mind, but she seems determined. It is slightly disappointing to Florence and me, but it will be nice to see the house again.

This evening, a most splendid sunset, like molten gold poured along the horizon. So beautiful, and yet over so quickly!

October 5th

It has been decided by the Thespian Committee that we shall have an evening of dance and music, and suddenly the mood of despondency has been lifted. Mr Bartel will be the main organiser, though it is agreed that the event will be quite informal. If the weather remains fine, it will take place outside, on the poop deck.

We are now sailing towards northern waters, and in England, we imagine, the leaves will be changing colour as autumn draws on. Here, however, it is warm and the skies have been beautifully clear for three days or more, with just enough wind to keep us moving nicely. The captain is ever watchful of our progress, however, and Mr Stephens told us that he calculates, day by day, how much coal may be burnt, so that we will still keep a reserve for unforeseen circumstances. As the coal stocks diminish, we are told, the ship will ride higher in the water, though at present this is not discernible from the deck.

October 6th

I do sometimes regret that moving to Australia six years ago interrupted our musical education. Until then, both Florence and

I had regular lessons, and had become quite proficient, but the journey provided an excuse, I`m sorry to say, for avoiding the tedious business – so it seemed at the time – of practice, and in Melbourne there were few music teachers. Seeing Mr Bartel play makes me wish I had continued to develop my fluency. As it is, when I sit down at the piano now, my fingers feel like lumps!

Perhaps it is not too late, however. If I resolve, once we are settled in at Depleach Road, to practise for at least an hour a day, perhaps I can make up the lost ground.

For our musical soiree, however, I think both Florence and I will be content to play a supporting rather than a leading role!

October 7th

Another glorious sunset, though the days are growing shorter.

Spoke to Mrs Rose this afternoon, over tea. She enjoyed the theatricals, she says, though she is glad it is over. She seemed relaxed, however, and there is something about her, a freshness and bloom about her cheeks, perhaps, that is very different from five weeks ago. Perhaps Jane is not altogether wrong in her surmises!

October 8th

Passed through several hours of squally weather this morning, with the ship pitching and rolling violently; the ranks at breakfast were much depleted due to the sea-sickness. By noon, however, we had sailed through into calmer waters, though still with a following wind which pleased the Captain. On the whole we have been very lucky so far on this journey; people can tell far worse tales of sickness, violent weather and deprivation than we have had to experience.

The Captain, according to Mr Stephens, sleeps little, even when conditions are good. He is on tenterhooks about getting home within sixty days, and is, therefore, ever-watchful.

Conversed at some length with Jane Fowler later in the afternoon. If we get home on the 26th of this month, it will be her eighteenth birthday the day after we disembark. Like many of us, she is beginning to think of what lies ahead when we resume our lives in England.

"What do you think of the prospect of getting married?" she said.

"The prospect is all very well," I replied, "it is the reality on which I have yet to make up my mind!"

"It must be a very fine thing to be in love, though," she mused. "I should like to be in love, just to see if what the poets write is true."

"The poets usually write of unrequited love," I said. "That I believe is the most intense form in which the condition may be experienced."

"I shouldn't like that. Obstacles I wouldn't mind, but the passion would have to be felt with equal intensity on both sides, I believe, to make it worthwhile."

"Have you noticed," I said, "that a great many novels lead up to the point of marriage, but never really delve very much into what lies beyond?"

"My mother has always brought us up to believe that certain aspects of marriage are only of pleasure to a woman insofar as conception may follow."

"Yes, so has mine, but I tend to believe that there is rather too much evidence in the world to the contrary to make it as simple and clear-cut a matter as she would have us believe."

"Sophia!" said Jane, with a slightly shocked though thoroughly approving giggle.

"Well," I retorted, "we girls who have a touch of Australia in our make-up are perhaps a little less squeamish than our thoroughbred English cousins in acknowledging such things!"

"If I had to be married," said Jane, "I would choose Mrs Russell as my example."

"Not Mrs Woodruffe?"

"No. Mrs Woodruffe is very beautiful, and very accomplished, but we have no full picture of her domestic life. The Russells, however, are as close as I have ever seen to a truly happy family. She has two sweet children and a husband who dotes on her completely."

"Yes. She is very fortunate in that respect."

"What concerns me most, however," she continued, "is the business of childbirth. Who can look forward with unalloyed pleasure to an event which by all accounts is likely to be exquisitely painful, and from which even recovery itself is a matter of some uncertainty?"

"Quite so! And then the drudgery which follows! For it is one thing to hold a pretty child on one's knee for half an hour, but beyond that, the occupation must surely lose its attraction very quickly."

"There are nurses, of course."

"Yes, there are nurses. Have you spoken recently, by the way, to Miss Lundy?"

"Yes, but I promised her confidentiality."

"Oh, well, in that case."

"Though I don`t expect she would mind me telling *you*."

"I wouldn`t expect you to break a confidence, Jane."

"Well, it`s nothing really. She`s engaged to Mr Bane."

"Really, Jane, you have taken me completely by surprise."

"You won`t repeat it to anyone will you?"

"Absolutely not," I said, "You have my solemn word!"

October 9th

Our concert is to be on Wednesday. We have been trying to persuade mother, who has a very pleasant singing voice, to contribute a song, but she absolutely refuses.

October 10th

The Reverend Hodge conducted a funeral service this morning for one of the steerage passengers who died suddenly yesterday, Mrs Finnerty. The doctor says it was heart failure and that nothing could have been done. She was in her sixties. Very sad, however, to have survived so much of a journey such as this, and not reach home. It is a reminder to us all how fragile our safety is, and how unpredictable our health.

October 11th

The evenings and early mornings are growing cold, with a slight hint of frost. The days, however, are still gloriously warm and sunny, just like the Mediterranean in Spring, according to Mrs Woodruffe.

Walked for a short time with Maria Lundy on deck this morning. Her opinion is that Mrs Finnerty died not from heart failure but as a consequence of the filthy conditions and dampness in the living quarters of some steerage passengers. The doctor, she says, is under pressure from the Captain because the Eagle Line does not want anything to become public that might show the ship in a bad light.

October 14th

Our evening of music and dance took place last night, and it proved to be a memorable occasion. A beautiful sunny afternoon turned into warm gauzy evening with a lovely rich sunset, and later the sky was black and soft as velvet.

Mr Bartel gave us pieces from Handel and Purcell in the Saloon, and then we moved up onto the poop deck, and Mr Judd performed a medley of the tunes that the sailors sometimes sing carrying out their work, and there was much joining in when it came to the chorus sections.

The dancing came later, with a variety of sets that had almost everyone up on their feet, not least myself and Florence. We danced until we were breathless!

Mr Gapper proved to be a very keen and agile dancer. He danced first with Mrs Rose, and then with Florence, and Jane, and with myself. It was Jane`s opinion that Mrs Rose encouraged him to dance with other partners in order not to draw attention to his fondness for dancing with her, and there may be some truth in this, though if it was an attempt at concealment, I have to say that it was not entirely successful!

There was a break for refreshments at half past eight and then we began again. First of all, one of the mariners Tom Smart sang `The Bay of Biscay` in a rich baritone voice, and then Mr and Mrs Russell together sang an old Scottish song, `Will you no come back again?`, and then we had `The Rising of the Lark" and `The Bonnie Mary`, and finally, Isaac, our own Isaac, sang an old Welsh song `Ar Hyd y Nos`, in his light tenor voice, and without any accompaniment, so beautifully, that he made us all cry!

Afterwards, the dancing started again, this time with the emphasis on the jigs and the reels, and all the merriment of the highland dances.

We all joined in with careless abandon, even mother agreeing, at Mr Carew`s behest, to make up one of the number for one dance. The high point for me, however, was seeing little Elspeth Russell, standing on a chair, watching the dance and trying to clap along with it, her eyes expressing a bright and burning pleasure of excitement. Oh, if only in my writing, I could evoke such delight in living as shone from that child`s eyes, then, I would be able to say I had achieved something worth leaving behind for humanity to peruse!

At the end of the evening, our fiddler played a beautiful, mournful Irish lament – a simple tune, full of the yearnings, it seemed, of parted lovers, or lonely people far away from home. Many people had brought out their coats by now, as the night grew colder, and we sat huddled as he played, listening to the plaintive notes rising to join the wind in the sails. I glanced towards Mrs Rose and Mr Gapper, sitting close together, her shoulder overlapping with his, his cheek almost touching her hair, and to the Russell family, and the Fowlers, Mrs Woodruffe, Mrs Foster and the whole company who have lived together for all these weeks, and I felt that the moment was very special, a moment that should be preserved forever in art or poetry to remember us all!

October 16th

I begin to realise how sad I will be when this voyage is over. We will all go apart and never meet again, and I shall spend the rest of my life wondering what became of everyone!

I am also, however, beginning to plan my own life, and to look forward to all the things there are to be done when I reach England. I suppose, at the end of a long journey like this, everyone feels themselves to be arriving at a crossroads, with choices lying ahead, perhaps marvellous choices, who knows?

It is a wonderful thing to feel optimistic about the future, and it is a feeling I would wish for everyone in the world. As we begin to count the days to our arrival, I find myself making such resolutions and promises to myself more and more. It is almost as if there were a new person waiting on the quay at Liverpool, and the moment I step off the ship, I will become her!

Oh dear! I find I am getting more serious day by day. Perhaps there is something in the ship`s diet that does not quite agree with me!

October 24th

After several days coming up through the Bay of Biscay we are now level with the Channel and should make landfall on the south coast of Ireland tomorrow. Everyone is wearing their warmest clothes and we have been putting extra blankets on the bed at night. The weather has been misty with almost constant showers. There is, however, now a sense of excitement running through the ship about the prospect of getting home before the end of the week. We have all been packing our trunks and making ready to decamp!

October 25th, 1859

We came out of Queenstown yesterday afternoon, and made our way across the Irish Sea overnight in a stiffening breeze, as far as Bardsey Island, off the Welsh coast, where we picked up men from a steam tug, to give them passage back to Liverpool. At four this afternoon, in poor visibility, we came level with Holyhead, and later, the crew fired a gun and a rocket, for the Pilot, but none has yet answered. Nightfall has brought no abatement of the weather, and the gusting wind, at times, is truly terrifying; even the crew say they have never witnessed anything like it.

It is a great comfort to know that we are so close to home.

Part 8

Text Message, from Saffy Williams to Sally Whitelock [Cape Town] 27th June 2009
Bn out sailn. Grt weathr. Goin 4 dinr 2nite. Rmantc? Mmm…dont no! Wsh me luk! Wll tel all wen I get bck. Saff.

Part 9

Chapter 29

My twentieth birthday, the 25th October, 1859, fell on a Tuesday, and it was on that day that Izzy told me there remained little doubt but that she was with child. It did not surprise me, for though we had been cautious with regard to other people`s knowledge of it, we had not lacked occasion for the further continuance of our pleasure, nor, for good or ill, had we let any scruples stand in our way.

So I was not, as I say, in any way shocked or dismayed by the news; it simply added a new aspect to what had become the life I had embraced. Softened, as it had been, for nearly a month, in its own misty glow, it was now a life which beckoned hard decisions.

"Promise you won`t abandon me, Richie."

"You already know better than that," I said, holding her in my arms to reassure her.

"What will we do?"

"We must get married," I said, "and I must find work."

She did not question this or pursue it further. It was left to me to settle on the details of a plan.

"Will it be all right?"

"Yes, of course it will."

Once out of her company, however, some of my initial

confidence deserted me. I walked out on the cliff top beyond Porth Helaeth. It was a low sky, rugged and louring, driven on by blustering winds, a sky full of disturbance, with a fast moving sea beneath. I went as far as Lligwy, looking down from the cliff path to the place where, on a hot still day, just three months before, we`d first lain together.

The first thing necessary, I decided, would be to see the Rector, the next day if possible, to ask him to marry us and arrange for the banns to be read for the first time the following Sunday. It was not a meeting to which I was looking forward, especially if he questioned me, as I supposed he must, on what exactly had led to the decision; once it was known, however, that we were betrothed it would take away the stigma of any speculation that might arise about Izzy`s condition.

Beyond that, I still had no precise idea of what we were going to do. I had just enough money, I calculated, to take us to Liverpool or Manchester, to pay for lodgings for a month, perhaps, sufficient time for me to find work on the docks, or in a factory. It was vague, however, and I had no idea what we would do if any of my margins of calculation were inaccurate. I had heard tales of the misery into which people could be sucked if they fell into the traps which lay waiting in the city.

From Lynas Point, by mid-afternoon, a darkness like premature night was spreading under the sky, bringing with it squalls of hard rain. I turned and began to make my way back but by the time I reached the outskirts of the village I was already soaked through to the skin.

"Richie, what are you doing out on a day like this?"

The call came from Isaac`s father, standing at the door of his cottage at the top of the village, smoking a pipe, and watching the progress of the weather.

"Just taking some fresh air," I replied.

"Fresh air!" he retorted, laughing. "I don`t know about that, but there`s foul weather on the way. If this wind gets any worse, there`ll be trees down and we`ll all be watching our roof-tops."

"Have you had any word from Isaac?" I asked, after he had

invited me in to dry off.

"Only from Melbourne. They were due out the end of August, should be back in Liverpool by the end of this month now, give or take. They say sixty days but it`s often a bit more coming back."

"Will he be able to come back home this time?"

"That`s as maybe. Depending on how soon they`re off again. So long as he`s well, mind you, and happy doing what he`s doing, that`s all right by us."

"Here," said Mrs Lewis, bringing in a pile of dry clothes. "You put these on. They`re Isaac`s and you`re as near in size as will do. Leastways we can try and stop you catching your death of cold."

I changed into the dry clothes and came back to the fireside.

"What are your plans going to be, then, Master Richie? Is it true that you`re still thinking about going off to college?"

In other circumstances, I might have prevaricated, as I had done in most conversations about this topic over the last year, but now there seemed little point. If I managed to speak to the Rector the next day, it would not be long before the news reached the village.

I began tentatively, but gradually let the whole story unwind, and felt better for getting it off my chest for the first time.

"It`s nothing new," said Mrs Lewis. "There`s many a one in this parish born just on the right side of the vestry!"

"Will you stay living with Dilwyn?" said Mr Lewis.

"I think not," I replied. I confided in him my fears about the farm, and he nodded as if the question had only been asked to see if I was as aware as everyone else.

"I was thinking of chancing my luck in one of the cities, Manchester maybe. They say there`s always work there."

They both inclined their head as if to conceal, as politely as they might, the deep concern this gave them.

"Well, our Isaac went to Liverpool, of course," said Mr Lewis, as if in mitigation. "But, then, he had his uncle to go to. It always helps if you know people somewhere."

I stayed with them until the mid-evening, sharing their meal, and then prepared to go. Outside, though, the rain was lashing down on the street, one way and then another, in gusts, as if the wind couldn`t make its mind up which way to blow.

"Come back in," said Mrs Lewis. "Or are you after seeing the lass tonight?"

"No," I said. "I told her I`d call tomorrow. She`ll not be expecting me in this."

"Then come back in by the fire, and rest here tonight. You know there`s a bed you`re always welcome to."

Mr Lewis and I went out to the back to look out over the sea. At the edge, fifty yards off, only the harsh white spindrift was visible; beyond that all was black. There was only the boom of the wind in the distance, and its buffeting about the house.

"The pilot boats were out earlier," said Mr Lewis. "There`ll be no landing for them tonight. They`ll have to seek the open sea for refuge, nothing else for it."

I slept that night in Isaac`s room, and from what I remember of it, I slept well. There is something about being warm abed, whilst the wind is roaring about the house, that is strangely comforting; you little think of those poor souls who may be out on the sea, in peril of their life, and, of course, none of us knew how near such poor souls were, that night, and how great the peril was they were to face before we opened our own eyes safely on another morning.

Of the events of that dreadful day, the 26th October 1859, the years have not sufficed to lessen the horror that surrounded them; and yet, even days later, like a poor witness in a courtroom, I could not say with precision that this happened now, and this then, or that one thing was a consequence of another.

The first cry came just after dawn. There were voices and shouting in the street outside. Then, Isaac`s father was shaking me by the shoulder. "Wake up, Richie, wake up! That was Thomas Hughes, he`s just come from Mesech`s cottage, there`s a ship on the rocks."

I pulled on my clothes and followed him out of the house. Mesech Williams` house was on the rising ground, between Porth

Helaeth and the top corner of the village. Mesech was on a ladder, he told us later, trying to protect his roof from the wind, when he saw the ship foundering on the rocks below.

It was not uncommon, at certain times of year, and in certain kinds of weather, for ships to get into difficulty on our stretch of coast. Ynys Dulas, out in the bay, had been set up with a tower and a beacon, there were the lights at Lynas Point and Penmon, our own lifeboat house, and there were many tales of mariners thrown up on the shores, or pulled from the sea, or drowned, and the old men said the sea-bed up and down this side of the island was littered with wrecks.

What no-one, myself included, imagined, when we hurried along the path from the village to Porth Helaeth to witness what Thomas Hughes had described as a ship on the rocks, was the sheer size of the vessel in question. Three hundred feet from bows to stern, she was greater by far than any vessel anyone amongst us had seen before, and with her masts, shattered or axed away, lying in the boiling surf to landward in a ruinous mass of timber, spars and rigging, leaving only broken stumps protruding from the deck, she made an awesome sight.

Later, they said that she had come aground in the sand at three o`clock in the morning, in pitch blackness, with the storm roaring about her, and that aboard the panic was quelled when they said that as soon as daylight showed them the coast they had struck they would be able to walk ashore. Those who fondly awaited such a providential outcome must have felt their very souls wither when that light first glimmered to reveal their true plight.

From where we were standing, on the hillside above - and we were a crowd that grew with each minute - the hull was hardly a stone`s throw away, but if she had come aground in sand, the sea, with the tide turning to the flow, had thrown her towards the bottommost of the several ragged terraces of sharp rock below our vantage point, and there, pounded by every monstrous wave that broke over her from the seaward, or swirled round her to thunder onto the rocks to the landward, she lay helpless like a great beast caught in a trap

Of what was happening on board, we could make out little. The light, even now, as day came on, was little more than a dull muddy gleam, and the air besides was full of the rain and the sea-drift discoloured with the churned sand it carried, that swirled here and there in the high booming winds. She was listing away to seaward, so it was only when the huge waves broke on her and tilted her towards the rocks, that we caught glimpses of activity there, and that through a mist of swirling air.

That there were five hundred souls aboard no-one could have guessed; as with so many aspects of that terrible scene, it was only what we discovered later that put it into its true perspective

Half a dozen men by now had edged their way down to the level below where we were standing, for though it seemed there was nothing they could do, the instinct to take risks and help was greater than the evident hopelessness.

At some point, I can`t say how long exactly, we became aware of some activity amidships, and peering through the murk, I could make out a man, with a rope around his waist, climbing over the rail; it seemed he was going to let the others in a small group lower him into the raging water below, but then, after letting him down a yard or two they pulled him back. This man, who I later learned to be George Suiacar, the boatswain`s mate, and one of the survivors, anxious, I think to let people know that he had not backed off from fear, told that he had been commanded back because of the danger of being sucked under the ship at that point amidships.

This group of men then tried to throw the rope towards the shore, and seemed to be shouting towards us, exhorting us to try to pick it up.

The rocks below the cliffs are treacherous at the best of times, slippery with seaweed and pitted with fissures and trenches in which even a sure-footed man may easily break a leg at the least slip. Nevertheless, those who had gone first made their way further down towards the crashing surf, now growing ever nearer as the tide came in, step by step, and others followed.

The rope thrown from the ship was flung back like cotton

thread in the wind, but as we watched, someone called out and pointed towards the bow of the ship, pointing away towards Lligwy, and there, climbing out along the flying jib boom, another figure was visible, clinging and hanging as he went hand over hand towards the very edge, which tipped with his weight towards the water, until, finally, he let go and plunged into frenzied waves beneath.

It was at this point that I remember Izzy being at my side, clinging to my arm.

"I couldn`t find you," she said. "Margaret said you didn`t come home last night, and then…"

"Shush," I said. "I`m safe, unlike those poor souls."

As the enormity of the spectacle came home to her, she grew silent and clung closer to my arm.

All of our eyes were on the spot where the solitary figure had plunged into the sea. There were false cries of `there!` and `there, now, do you see him?` but I truly believed him already lost. Then I found myself crying, `there, look, now!` and surely enough, twenty yards from where he had disappeared, his head and shoulders were momentarily visible before he was sucked back again towards the hull of the ship.

This happened two or three times. Each time, somehow, miraculously, he reappeared, and now the line of our own men from the village, edged towards the point on the rock below nearest to where he had last been seen, each man clinging on to the next, hand to hand, so that they formed a ragged human chain.

If, in the ensuing days, there were times when I felt my own spirit wither at the horror of that day and its consequences, the sight of that chain of men, risking everything, was enough to make the heart, swelling with pride, reclaim itself.

The next wave threw the swimmer along the rock shelf to within ten feet of them, and as he clung on with his fingertips against the backdraw of the surf, inch by inch, the foremost man came towards him, then dragged him to his feet just in time for them to cling to each other as the next surf broke over them. We fully expected, when the fiery surf receded to see an empty space where both of them had been standing, but the chain held firm, and within seconds they were dragging him up to safe ground, and unfastening the rope which was tied about his waist.

"Man ashore!" came the thin cry from aboard, and we could make out a scurry of men to the point forward where the rope was being paid out. Meantime, ashore, the men below us were securing the rope to a rock and pulling it in, and the desperate bold swimmer was being helped to the cliff-top.

He was dark skinned and dark haired and some said he was a Spaniard, for when he spoke, it was with a heavy foreign accent which few of us could understand immediately, and besides he was shaking and chattering with the cold; later, when he had been persuaded to be taken off to have his lacerations tended to, and when we saw him in the village, we found out that he was of Malta, and that his name was Joie Rodriguez, though his shipmates, he told us, had already familiarised him as Joe Rodgers, and this was the name that was to appear in the newspapers when the story of his heroism was told in the weeks to come.

On the cliff top, still rapt with the drama that was unfolding before us, we now watched as a thick hawser, linked to the rope, was drawn across the gulf between the ship`s deck and the shore, and to that, on the deck itself the apparatus of a harness or boatswain`s chair.

Now hopeful that we would quickly see a full rescue operation take place, it was with some consternation that we witnessed, amongst those clustering at the bows, what seemed to be an altercation. A female, so it seemed – for all the figures we had seen heretofore were men, and evidently men of the crew – was being exhorted to climb into the harness, whilst about her men were gesticulating angrily.

I was distracted from this by a sudden cry from Izzy by my side, which nearly curdled my blood. "Look," she sobbed. "Look there, it`s Isaac!"

I strained my eyes to see, at first with disbelief, for I could not comprehend how, in the conditions, she could be so certain of detail, and hopeful that she had merely succumbed to a momentary attack of hysteria, but then, even before I had pinpointed his face amongst those on deck, it all fell into place: this was the ship, returning from Australia which Isaac had written to his father about; this, it dawned on me for the first time, was The Royal Charter.

And with that knowledge, my gaze automatically sought out and confirmed his face, standing off slightly from the group who were arguing on the foredeck. It was Isaac.

What happened next, or soon after – for as I have said, the exactness of events and their sequence was soon lost in the overwhelming shock of what went on over many hours – was that which was feared most by those who understood the coast well enough to know the full devastating power of an unleashed sea with a full gale coming in over the tide.

The ship, which had been listing and tilting all the while with the great rollers that burst over her, sending foam shooting a hundred feet in the air, now, seemingly on a single huge wave, was lifted and thrown onto the jagged edge of the rock plateau, and a second and third wave, following hard on, smashed her relentlessly against it; it was as if the sea, a wild predator, was now homing in, remorselessly, for the kill.

I heard a gasp from all who stood around me as the iron casing of the hull amidships split suddenly like the casing of a nut, and a whirlpool of seemingly boiling water and surf burst in. Within minutes, the ship was broken entirely into two parts. Those within the stern section able to get on deck had now lost - short of throwing themselves into the sea, which many of them did - all means of escape to safety; those trapped below – and we were to learn over the next few days as the cargo of their bodies made landfall up and down the coast, how many they numbered – were already dead.

On the foredeck now, there was frantic activity; first one man and then another made the perilous ride on the harness; swaying violently with the wind, the sagging hawser was aprey to every exploding wave, but foot by foot they made their way, and the hands of the village men, waiting on the rocks, plucked them to safety. A fourth man set out and plummeted almost immediately to his death in a violent tug of wind. A fifth was more lucky. The sixth was Isaac.

I felt tears streaming down my face as his familiar form, clinging bravely to the rope, launched from the deck. Then, as if the sea had saved its utmost fury for the homecoming of its local son, he was lost to sight in an explosion of wild surf; as it subsided momentarily his figure was seen again still clinging to the rope. A second wave, as violent as the first encompassed him once more and the swaying rope was lost to view; again, he reappeared. He was so near to the shore now, some said afterwards, that he was able to call out to his father, who was one of those in the chain below, and to hear his father`s reply. Whether or not that is true, I do not know, for Isaac`s father spoke never a word of it after; what I do know is that when a third wave had expended its fury, and receded, the rope was empty.

I heard those around me gasp, and I heard Izzy`s scream, and it was too much for me to bear. I broke away from Izzy`s clasp, and began to scramble down the path towards the rocks. In my moment of madness, I wanted to lose my pain in action, regardless of the danger, to do something to offset the helplessness of standing as a spectator seeing these sights.

"Get back you fool!" shouted Robert Hughes.

"I can help. I`m not afraid."

"Get back. Can`t you see, you`ll make it worse for us all."

"We`ll end up rescuing you!"

They pushed me back, and those on the top helped me back, sympathetically.

"Don`t risk yourself, Richie, it`s not worth it."

"We know you`d do it."

"Come here!" said Izzy. "Don`t ever do that again!"

At the stern of the ship now, people were gathering, if that word can describe the panic and confusion amongst them – small groups, parents and children hugging each other desperately and fighting the wind and the lurching of the deck. Several were hurled headlong into the sea; some clung to the rails in a last helpless effort to preserve themselves; at least one child that I saw was thrown into the sea and then thrown back by the counter wave onto the deck where she slithered grasping for some safe holding.

Those with more control began to lower themselves and those dear to them, by whatever means they could down into the waters below, which was now a seething cauldron, a chaos of spars, tangled rigging, shattered timbers, boxes and other detritus released from the innards of the ship, in which the living, amongst those already dead, struggled and gasped for survival.

One sight in particular caught my attention, a man and a woman, standing together, his hands under her elbows as if giving her instructions, then helping her to take off her boots and outer garments, as he did his own. Then, they held each other in a fast embrace for ten or fifteen seconds before he lowered himself into the water, urging her to jump towards him, which she did. Then, with his arms fast round her again he grasped a broken spar which floated nearby and pushed away.

But this was a small detail amidst the desperate turmoil all around. By now the sailors who had survived the perilous crossing on the harness were on the rocks below, alongside the men of Moelfre, and whereas before all eyes had been on single individuals attempting to get ashore, now, with each surging wave, three or four bodies were being thrown onto the rocks with all the pounding force of a hammer on an anvil. Some lay immediately lifeless until the drag of the surf sucked them back; others grabbed at any holding they could find, and crawled, inch by inch, until another wave crashed on top of them, or until the failing strength of their desperate fingers met the grasp of those who risked their own lives to save them.

Those who were brought clear, some of them already half dead, were handed up towards us where we stood on the path above.

"Come on, then, now you can be of some use!" one of the men called. I joined a group who supported the poor creature who had just been half carried, half dragged up from the rocks.

"Take him to my house," shouted old Gwyllm Evans, "My daughter will take care of him,"

The poor man was groaning in terrible pain, his forehead smashed on one side, and blood obscuring the place where his eye had been. I pulled one of his arms around my neck, Dafydd, on the other side, did the same. We struggled with him fifty yards up the hill, as far as the stile where the path splits, going one way to the village, the other to the Swnt.

"Did you see Isaac?"

"Yes."

"Terrible, terrible," said Dafydd. "Do you think..."

Before he could finish his question, a terrible noise came from the mouth of the poor soul we were carrying, and from limpness of his dead weight, we knew immediately he was dead.

"What shall we do?" asked Dafydd.

"Carry him to the village?"

"What`s the point?"

"We can`t leave him here."

"Why not? We can`t do him any good now. There may be others."

"All right. Let`s lay him down here. Cover his face at least."

Dafydd kneeled and took off his neckerchief to put over the man`s face. "Do you see there, Richie," he said, "he has a purse about him? Do you see that?"

"Leave it," I said, appalled.

"I didn`t mean steal it," said Dafydd. "Though there`s others who will."

"Just leave it," I said.

"It might tell us who he is."

"Leave him. It`s not our business."

"All right," said Dafydd. "Come on, then, let`s get back."

When we returned, half a dozen more had been pulled off the rocks, four of them already dead; of the two survivors, one had sustained no injury at all, as it seemed: the other, around whom a small crowd of villagers was gathered, I recognised as the man I had observed entering the water together with a woman twenty minutes before.

"Come and talk to him, Richie," said one of the group, who spoke only Welsh, "He needs tending. See if you can make him see sense!"

"Please, please!" the man shouted, struggling with those who were trying, for his own good, to restrain him. "I must go back. I have to find her."

I went to kneel beside him. "There`s nothing you can do down there, now," I said. "Look, it`s wild. Those men down there know what they`re doing. Leave it to them. You`re hurt."

"Just shaken," he said. "Just shaken. I`ll be all right in a moment."

"Your shirt has been ripped off your back. Your shoulder is bleeding, see. It needs to be cleaned and dressed. Let me take you back to the village, get some dry clothes at least. Then, if you wish, I`ll bring you back. Maybe by then there will be news."

"Yes, all right," he conceded, standing, and lurching, so that I had to catch him from falling.

"She was with me," he said, appealing to me out of his distress, as we stumbled along the path, his weight heavy against me. "I held her in my arms."

"I know. I saw you."

"A wave came over us, but I didn`t let go. I promised her I wouldn`t let go."

"My name is Richard," I said, trying to distract him from his anxiety.

"Richard," he said vaguely.

"Yes. What`s yours?"

"What?"

"Your name?"

"Edward," he mumbled. "Edward Gapper."

Chapter 30

In the village, those who had not gone to the scene of the wreck were waiting in the street by doorways, waiting more news to add to what had already filtered back.

"Is it as bad as they say?"

"Is it true about Isaac?"

"It`ll be the death of his father."

"His mam`s with the neighbours. She was in a dead faint when they told her."

"We don`t know he`s drowned yet, do we? He`s a good swimmer."

As I came towards them, with Edward Gapper leaning against me, I wondered if they would still think this if they had seen, as had I, the tumultuous violence of the sea and the wind not half a mile away.

"He needs somewhere to rest and his wounds tended," I said.

There was no shortage of offers to assist. I took him into Mary Davies` cottage, where he sat by the fire. He was mumbling and chattering by now, a little deliriously, repeating what he had said to me on the cliff path. "My wife," he kept on repeating. "Not now. Not ever. I promised to hold her."

"What`s he saying?" asked Mary, who spoke not a word of English.

"He`s lost his wife," I said. "Down there, at the wreck."

"Poor man!" she said, pulling a blanket around him.

I stayed with him for half an hour. At first he was insistent that he was fit to return with me in a moment`s time; eventually, he fell into a sleep.

I ran back to the cliff top, passing others on the way, carrying the injured and the dead towards the village. At the scene itself, the tide had now risen three quarters to the full, and the air was thick with shreds of wool, released from the ship`s cargo, blowing here and there with the rain and sleet. As I reached the cliff`s edge, I saw Izzy, helping a man to his feet who was wrapped in a blanket which had been sent down, with dry coats and shirts, from the village. Seeing me, she broke away and came towards me.

"Have you heard what they`re saying?"

"What?"

"They say it`s a treasure ship," she said.

"What do you mean?"

"Carrying gold. From Australia."

"Gold?"

"Yes. Great bullion rooms full, that`s what they`re saying."

"Who told you that?"

"I overheard them. That man over there. He says he lost twenty sovereigns, ripped from him, in the water, but the main part of his fortune is on the ship."

At this moment in time, I thought perhaps Izzy had heard something and was exaggerating, and gave it little more thought, though it was not long before this and similar tales were being spread at large amongst the villagers.

Soon after this, the Rector, Stephen Roose Hughes appeared, hurrying down towards the cliff top path, a small group of villagers gathering round him as he approached, talking, pointing, gesticulating. When he arrived at the brow of the hill overlooking the scene he stopped, and the group around him, as if in awe of his response, grew silent and melted aside.

I saw the scene as he saw it, at that moment, and it was a picture someone might have painted from a nightmare of hell. The two parts of the ship had now turned away from the shore, and were sinking. A few figures on the decks were still gripping the rails or huddling together helplessly, as the waves ripped past them. One of the boats, now loose on the seaward side, was tossed extravagantly high by successive rollers, and was then thrown upside down, its occupants tossed out and lost. To the leeward, the space between the broken hull and the rocks was a chaotic jumble of wreckage, masts, spars, barrels, rigging and bales of wool, amidst which the living bodies fought frantically amidst the corpses of the dead, whilst still the surging waves exploded around them. This was what the Rector saw, and whereas earlier, the terrible nature of the drama had been mixed with the excitement of escape and rescue, now there was only the certainty of death happening before us on an unimaginable scale.

He stood there for a moment, a single forlorn figure blasted by the wind, seeming every bit as helpless and vulnerable as the rest of us, his eyes charged with some terrible question, as if reaching to the very bottom of his faith, to a place he had never been before, to test what was there.

"What shall we do with them all?" someone asked.

The Rector, coming to from his reverie, looked around as if to take some bearings, and then said, "take them to the church."

At the full tide, only the tips of the broken masts showed above the water, but though the weather continued foul for the rest of the day, the crowd did not diminish, waiting for the tide to go out again; if anything, with stories getting back to the village that it was a treasure ship that had been thrown up on the rocks, it increased.

As the waters receded, the crowd was joined by people from further afield; Mr Smith, who was Master of the Customs House at Beaumaris, together with a Mr Wagstaffe, a councillor, they said, from Liverpool, arrived in the early afternoon, and the word spread that Mr Smith had made it known that, by virtue of his position, he was to be regarded as the Receiver of the Wreck.

The hull of the ship, now in three parts, was visible as jagged iron plate from which sections had been wrenched by the action of the tide and which now lay strewn on the rocks, with twisted and mangled railings, and with the other wreckage which had been floating on the shoreward side of the ship as it went down. There was at least a dozen bodies, some of them tangled in with the jetsam, and many more were discovered in concealed positions when the searching began.

Izzy and Dafydd and myself released the body of a young woman, and Izzy tried to make her decent, for the waves had stripped off much of her clothing, before we took the poor creature up to the cliff top.

"If there is anything that might help identify her," said the Rector, giving us his instructions, "make a note of it and tell Anne who`s waiting at the church. She`ll tell you what to do there, until I get back."

He went off to another group, and Dafydd and I looked at each other. "We`ve got a hand cart in the yard," said Dafydd, "if we can get her up to the village."

"She`s hardly any weight at all," I replied. "We should be able to manage that."

"I`ll stay here and see what I can do," said Izzy.

Dafydd and I set out. It took us twenty minutes to get the girl to the village, then Dafydd found his handcart, and we set off up the hill.

"Do you think we`ll get anything for this?" said Dafydd.

"You mean pay? Trust you to think of that!"

"I know it sounds bad, but you have to think, see, Richie, I`d be working if I wasn`t doing this."

"Not on a day like this, you wouldn`t. There`d be no boats going out today, wreck or no wreck."

"Well, no, not today, maybe, but it`s still work this, after all, and those left there will be helping themselves to the gold, won`t they!"

I laughed. "I don`t think it`s as simple as that, Dafydd. Let`s just get this done and then we can go back and see what`s happening."

At the church, however, we were delayed longer than we thought. Anne Hughes and her sister were there to meet us, and two or three bodies had already been brought to the church and left.

"How many more do you think there`ll be?"

It was clear that whatever message they had received had not prepared them for the scale of what had happened.

"Quite a lot, I think."

"Hundreds," said Dafydd.

Her mouth grew taut, and then her eyes closed as if on a grim silent prayer; then, she sucked in a deep breath, and prepared for action. "We'd better move the pews then, I suppose. Lend us a hand, boys, they're too heavy for us to do alone."

So we stayed, and moved the pews to one side to make a fair sized space; then, we laid the girl on one side, next to another woman, and the two men on the other side, and the Rector's wife and her sister covered them up with sheets. One of the men had on a gold watch and there was a belt round his waist with pouches that were filled with something; I saw Dafydd eyeing them curiously and stealing a sideways look at me, but he realised, as much as I did, that here, of all places, was no place to satisfy such curiosity.

More than an hour had elapsed before we completed our return to the scene of the wreck. All the bodies at first visible had now been removed to the cliff top and were awaiting transportation to the church, others, trapped in the accessible wreckage on the foreshore were proving, in some cases, more of a problem, for some were in a state of severe dismemberment and there were many who lacked the stomach to approach them, let alone work at their release.

Mr Smith, the Receiver, had, by now, made his way down to the widest flat shelf of rock, and was trying to marshal the scores of people who were scouring and searching the shore like ants.

"What's he doing?" we asked Izzy.

"He says anything that's found has to be given over to him.

He's giving out receipts."

"He could do with a dozen helpers, if you ask me," said Dafydd.

"There was a dreadful scene here, just after you went," Izzy continued. "That man over there, do you see him?"

"The one lifting the child?"

"Yes. He found his one child, but his other daughter's missing, and his wife. He was screaming and howling, and foaming at the mouth. Beside himself, he was, until the Reverend Hughes calmed him down a bit."

The man was now sitting, cradling the dead child in a blanket, and swaying from side to side, his hair blowing loose in the wind.

"Have you seen himself up there?" said Izzy, taking my arm and drawing me away to one side. On the cliff top, mounted on horseback, and in his familiar hat and long coat, was Dilwyn Jones. "He`s been patrolling up and down for over an hour, now. Had a word with the man down there, he did. Shouldn`t wonder if there isn`t some funny business going on there."

"Richard!" came the Rector`s voice. "This is Mr Russell." He took me over to the man holding the dead child, and continued quietly. "He needs to be taken to the village now. Take him to Robert Lewis` house."

"Isaac`s father?"

"Yes. He knows. I`ve spoken to him and he`s gone on to prepare his wife."

"What about, you know, the body?"

"Let the child stay with him."

I helped the man up by his arm. He came quite placidly, seeming grateful for my care, but the walk to the village was one of the hardest half hours I have ever lived through. At first, he talked to the child in a soft wheedling voice, the way a mother might talk to a suckling child, stroking her hair as we walked, and then he grew angry, muttering curses. "There will be repercussions," he said to me directly. "Mark by words, by God, there will be repercussions, if I have anything to do with it!" and then, he began crooning to the child again. This went on until we arrived, and I was thankful that the Rector was not mistaken, for Isaac`s mother and father were there to meet him, and glad I was, I must say, to have him off my hands.

Such afternoon light as still remained was now fading, and by the time I reached the site of the wreck again, it was growing too dark and too dangerous for anyone to remain on the rocks longer. A party of coastguardmen from the Mersey Guardship had arrived as evening was falling and they set up camp, to watch over the remains of the wreck, just as the last remnants of the village were leaving.

I walked home with Izzy, and we lit a stove in her cottage,

and heated up some broth, and sat together until we were warm, though hardly a word was exchanged between us. I thought that she would want me to stay, for company, at least, after such a harrowing day, but at eight o`clock, she said that she was going to go to sleep. When I asked if she wanted me to stay, she demurred. "Go down to the Talyfron, Richie," she said. "Find out what is happening. Call on me early. There may be a lot for us to do tomorrow."

Chapter 31

In the Talyfron that night all the talk was of gold; as many different sums were put about as to the total of bullion on board as there were men to utter, repeat and exaggerate them, and as many men again who knew of this law or that law which said who owned it if it fell on the land, or who owned it if it fell in the sea, or who owned it if it stayed in the sunken remains of the ship.

"And who owns it," asked someone, "if it be found on the person deceased?"

"Well, it still belongs to them, until it be found out who they are, see, and who their kin is, and then it belongs to them."

"And what if it can't be found out who they are?"

"Well, then, that's as may be."

"Or, to put another case, if their kin died with them likewise, for from what I've heard there were families enough, mother, father and children together all went down with that ship, who does it come to then?"

"Well, that's as may be, too."

"In that case it must be determined if there are other kin elsewhere to whom it should rightfully come."

"Ah, but, then, see, to go back, if it can't be discovered, from the effects of the water and the rocks, and such like, who they are, how will it be possible to find out if they have kin elsewhere?"

"In that case, it probably goes to the Queen."

"Hardly seems fair, does it, you know, her having so much already?"

So the conversation went, ebbing and flowing one way and then another, as the liquor flowed. The company was joined, later, by Mr Foster, the ship's carpenter, and Mr Suaicar, the boatswain's mate, who I recognised as the man who had been lowered towards the water just before Joe Rodgers had made landfall, and who subsequently had been prominent amongst those working down on the rocks to bring people in. There were also, it became clear, as the room swelled both in number and in the volume of noise generated, several reporters from the newspapers of North Wales and Chester trying to get a slant on the story for publication the next day.

"Is it correct, then, as I understand, that no officers of the ship survived?"

"Barring a miracle," said Mr Foster, "we must believe that to be true."

"And is it correct, as I`ve been told, that not a single woman, nor yet a single child survived?"

"Women and children were below," answered Mr Suaicar. "And when the ship broke in two, you see, they were in aft of ship, wrong part."

"The wrong part of the ship?" questioned the reporter, though whether incredulous or simply finding it difficult to follow Mr Suaicar`s foreign accent in the noise of the room, I do not know.

"The line, you see, how say, the hawser, was at bows. If they could have been there, could have been saved, but ship broke."

"And how, may I ask, were you saved?"

"Same. By hawser to shore."

"So, let me make sure I understand this, you were in the *right* part of the ship. Is that correct?"

"Is correct," said Mr Suaicar, though I fear he did not fully understand what the reporter was leading him to say.

"There was some delay, we`ve heard, between the hawser being attached and anyone using it as a means of escape."

"Is correct. Mr Bane, officer, Third Officer, he is trying to persuade Miss Lundy to go first on the hawser, but she is afraid. Won`t go. Mr Bane arguing with riggers, saying passengers must go first."

"I see."

As the night grew later, and as the liquor continued to flow, the mood became argumentative. There was speculation: was the Master drunk? Someone had heard someone say so. Would it not have been wiser to seek refuge or make out to the open sea – or was the ship in such a great hurry to be back in Liverpool within sixty days that sound judgement had gone out of the window? Not necessarily my opinion, sir, but anyone with ears may hear what people say, even if they say it in a whisper!

In a crowded room, full of people speaking different languages, it was not surprising, after such a day, that there should be misunderstandings, or that feelings should run high.

Why had the pilot not answered the signal from the ship when she was off Point Lynas, the previous night? asked one of those rescued who would hear not an ill word of the master, Captain Taylor. Why had no-one heeded the flares which had been set off through the night, or the shot which had been fired off until the guns were too wet for the powder?

And what about the looting of the bodies, asked one of the reporters, looking round and shrugging his shoulders, for was it not something that had been said, however erroneously, and was it not better to clear the air? No-one answered. For those who understood it, the imputation was beneath contempt; though it was perhaps as well, for his own good, that many didn`t.

In his usual corner by the fire, Dilwyn Jones did not pre-occupy himself with any of this speculation about what had happened, or recrimination about who might be to blame. Sharing his bottle affably with Mr Smith, the Receiver of the Wreck, he was much more intent on discovering what was going to happen next.

I drank two glasses of rum, witnessing all this, enough to warm me through, and soften some of the terrible images of the day which still lingered in the nether regions of my mind. Then I walked home, following the uphill track where earlier the labour of taking bodies to the church had taken place, until I came again by Izzy`s cottage. The light was out, and I had no intention of disturbing her. As I passed, however, the latch opened, and her figure appeared in the shadowy slot of the door.

“Richie,” she called, in a light whisper.

“Are you still up?”

“I couldn`t sleep. I keep seeing it all again.”

“Would you like me to stay?”

She nodded her head.

As we lay together, I wondered at how the simple business of seeing the Rector, to talk about the banns, the business intended for the day, had become now a matter of seemingly infinite difficulty.

I dreamt of the face of the man who had died on the cliff top, his brow and eye smashed, and woke several times with a sudden start, grasping my way back to the ordinariness of the night. Then, the image came into my sleep of strong rooms split open, and gold pouring out into the sea.

When I awoke with the first light, Izzy was no longer there.

Chapter 32

The first bodies to be washed up on the beach at Porth Moelfre had come in with the tide overnight, and were lying on the shingle, covered by oil skins and strips of old sail, waiting to be carried away. The question was silently asked, and met with a brief shake of the head: none of them was Isaac.

I went straight on to Mary Davies` cottage on the rise of the hill to enquire after Mr Gapper. He was sitting in the parlour, making a statement to a man from the newspaper.

"No," he was saying, "I never knew Captain Taylor the worse for drink."

"Is it true that the Captain refused to take refuge in Holyhead?"

"I believe the Captain said he would not divert course simply to see The Great Eastern which was moored at Holyhead; I was never aware that there was any advice to take refuge there."

"The wind changed, I believe," he went on, in response to another question, "after we had rounded Point Lynas, to blow from the north east. An attempt was made to anchor the ship but the anchor chains snapped, first one then the other, in the early hours of the morning, and then the ship drifted towards the shore like a log."

"Is it true that the passengers were kept below, almost up to the point where the ship broke in two?"

"Yes. We believed that when dawn came we would be able to walk to the shore. The women had dressed their children. We were waiting below and then there was a tremendous crashing noise."

"Was that when the ship hit the rocks?"

"Yes, it must have been. The hull shuddered, and people were thrown this way and that, and the children and women were screaming. It was then that the Reverend Hodge took control."

"There was a clergyman present?"

"Yes. The Reverend Vere Hodge. He had always seemed,

to be honest, a rather meek and ineffective individual during the voyage, but for those few moments he was magnificent."

"In what way?"

"He calmed everyone down, and led us in prayer. He asked God to bring us to safety, or if not, to prepare us for death. The panic subsided. Then we started to go up onto the deck."

"Thank you, Mr Gapper."

"How are you?" I asked when the reporter had gone.

"Better," he said, "much better, thank you. The Rector came to see me last night. We talked for a while and said prayers."

"No further news, then?"

He shook his head. "I`m under no illusions that there will be any more survivors."

I nodded agreement.

"But if you will wait a moment for me to get ready, I would be grateful if you would accompany me to the scene. I should like to see it again myself, and perhaps look for her amongst those who`ve come ashore during the night."

The night`s tide and weather had further reduced the visible sections remaining of the hull, but there was still a profusion of tangled wreckage on the rocks below, spreading a length of over a two hundred yards; and inevitably, more bodies to be brought to the cliff-top.

A hundred villagers, and more besides, from where I do not know, had been out since the first light, and though it might have been the motive of adventitious gold that had lured them there, their activities, more than on the previous day, were being monitored by the coast guards, under the direction of Mr Smith, who now had a voluntary right-hand man, it seemed, in the figure of Dilwyn Jones.

I cast my eye along the rocky platforms but I could see no sign of Izzy.

"She was here before," said Dafydd, "but someone said some more bodies have come up towards Lligwy and a few of them went off to see what help they could give."

I walked along the path with Mr Gapper, going through the

grim business of looking at each face in turn to see if it was the woman he was looking for.

"No," he said. "No, not yet. By God, this is a harrowing business."

"How many were there," I asked, "altogether?"

"I don`t know," he said. "Five hundred, I`d guess, if you include the crew. I can`t be sure. Some people got off at Queenstown on Monday night."

"And there are forty we know to be saved."

Neither of us uttered the grim piece of arithmetic which followed.

"It seems so placid now," said Mr Gapper. "I can hardly believe that such a storm should catch us so near to home. What`s that place there?"

He was pointing towards the shingle beach of Porth Helaeth. I told him its name.

"If we had come aground there," he mused, "not two hundred yards further, we should have walked ashore, every man woman and child."

I remembered Isaac`s words, back in the days of our childhood friendship: "Porth Helaeth, that`s the place to go and watch when there`s a really big storm blowing!"

"I`ll walk up to the church," said Mr Gapper, at last. "Is it easy to find?"

I gave him directions.

"What was she like? I mean, what should I look for if we find more?"

"Just in her twenties," he said. "Slim, dark hair, about so long – just to her shoulders." He shrugged and I realised that most of the features of a loved one that would be dearest would be those already vanished from a body in the sea for more than twenty four hours.

"A ring?" I asked.

"What? A ring. Oh, yes," he added, almost as an afterthought.

Another person who had been examining all of the bodies

was Mr Russell, the poor man I had accompanied as he carried his drowned child to the village the previous day. Now in a calmer frame of mind, he was casting his eye along the reach of the bay, evidently looking for further sea-borne corpses.

"I suppose," he said to me, "there must be places, inlets and coves the tide favours more than others. "

"It depends on the wind," I said, "but they were saying before that some came ashore further up, near Lligwy."

I pointed out the direction.

"Would you be so good as to accompany me?" he asked.

"May I ask," I said, as we walked along, "how old your other daughter might be?"

"Ten," he replied. "Ten years old."

I hardly knew what else to ask him. In the circumstances, ordinary conversation was impossible. He was, however, seemingly still quite glad to talk to himself.

"They say Mr Bartel has survived. That`s good. Good. His music will go on, hmm? We had dancing, you know, oh yes."

"On board the ship, you mean?"

"Oh, yes. Yes, indeed. My daughters loved watching the dancing. Could hardly contain themselves for want of joining in. But the Davis girls, oh, they were dancers, my word. And then, Jane Fowler is missing, too, and all the women, of course. All of them. Mrs Woodruffe, too, beautiful woman, with children, too, what a waste, what a waste!"

"It must have been a terrible ordeal."

"We were all in the saloon," he said. "Captain Taylor said we were on the sand and all would be well. We were told to stay below. Do you think he knew?"

"I can hardly say."

"Surely something could have been done. The children were terrified, you know, terrified."

When we came to the cove, before the line of the cliffs cuts back towards Lligwy, I saw Izzy and a small group of women from the village standing by two bodies. Mr Russell hurried on ahead of me, but I could tell from his immediate reaction that neither of them were his.

"It`s a man and a woman," said Izzy. "This girl is from the farm up there on the hill. Her father has a cart, she says. We can borrow that to take them back."

I nodded and went to look at the bodies. One of them was a big man, still wearing his buttoned top coat, and one boot. The other was a young woman who lay wrapped in a sheet the girl had brought from the farm."

"Is there anything to identify them?"

"The man has a pocket book. I don`t know what`s in it. The woman had hardly anything on. But she has a ring."

I looked closer, remembering Mr Gapper`s description: in her twenties, slender, dark hair to her shoulder. It could have been her.

"It`s Mrs Rose," said Mr Russell. "I don`t know who the man is, though I`ve seen him. I think he was in steerage."

"We`d better get them back," I said, disguising the disappointment I felt that I was not able, as for a moment I had thought, to put Mr Gapper`s mind at rest.

We fetched the cart, and with the help of the farmer`s lad, managed to take both bodies back to the village by the Lligwy track that ran at the back of the headland. The hill up to the church was too steep, however, and so we left the man by the corner, with Izzy to watch over him, and with the burden lightened, were able to push the cart up the track with relative ease.

As we approached the church, Mr Gapper hurried towards us. I stepped forward, to anticipate the disappointment of his sad expectation. "I`m sorry," I began, "but I`m afraid it`s not your wife."

He stepped past me and uncovered her face. "It`s her," he said, his voice tremulous, as he took her cold hand from under the covering, and pressed it to his lips. "It`s her."

Chapter 33

By the following day, the Coastguards and had been joined by the English Militia and Marines of the HMS Hastings from Liverpool, and the area along the coast where the Royal Charter had gone down was sealed off. There had been three arrests of people caught in possession of coins or other effects pilfered from the scene, and they said the English newspapers, ignoring what the folk of Moelfre had done for the living and the dead alike, were only interested in what they called `such savagery`.

Twenty or so villagers were employed by Mr Smith to continue the search amidst the wreckage on the rocky platforms, and in the gulleys and crevices. They were given arm bands to wear, to identify them, and they were watched like convicts to ensure that anything found was handed over. Meantime, the village was filling up with `foreigners`. The newspaper stories had aroused interest up and down the country, it seemed, and visitors flooded in to satisfy their curiosity; and, of course, there were the relatives of those who had perished, most of whom, arriving in the throes of their grief, were directed immediately to the church of St Galgo.

There were, by the Friday evening, upwards of thirty bodies laid out on the church floor, and more were taken to the churches of Penrhos Lligwy and Llaneugrad, nearby; as the number of bodies coming up from the sea each day increased, and as the villagers, most of them now eager to return to their usual work, grew more reluctant to spend whole days about the lugubrious business of manhandling corpses and transporting them to the churches, the Rector offered, from his own money, small payments to encourage their help, and commissioned those who were able to begin the process of digging graves and making simple coffins.

Mr Gapper and Mr Carew, another survivor, now waiting in the village until the inquests and the enquiry began, agreed to be stationed at the church, to help identify those who had been their fellow passengers.

"Mrs Woodruffe," said Mr Gapper, indicating one of the women who had already been laid out in the church when Dafydd and I first went there, a woman with striking features, though her temple and the side of her left eye were bloody and bruised, as if from a single blow

"That`s Sophia Davis," said Mr Carew, indicating a tall slim girl, about the same age as Izzy. "I saw her with Jane Fowler just after the ship split. They were both thrown overboard by a huge wave. Before I jumped myself I saw them floundering in the water below with a hundred others."

"That`s little Ida Fowler, and her nurse beside her. They say they were found together on the beach. The nurse must have held onto her until the very last."

"Florence Davis, Sophia`s sister."

"Mrs Foster."

"Mr Parker."

"Mrs Fenwick."

But the process of identification was not always so easy. Some of those who had been dashed onto the rocks had suffered terrible disfigurements, with, in some cases, limbs severed entirely, and injuries to the head and face of a kind to sicken even those of the strongest stomach. Those who were now being brought out of the water after two and three days presented other problems of identification, for the sea itself, and indeed, the creatures who live in it, are no preservers of the beauty or dignity of the human form.

The Reverend Stephen Roose Hughes, as if drawing from some deep well-spring of faith, met each challenge and encounter with a spirit of purpose and compassion; if, on the cliff top that morning I had seen the spectre of doubt or despair in his eyes, there was no trace of that now. With his wife, and her sister, the business of noting every detail of possible identification was carried out meticulously; some carried purses or pocket books, others might have a locket or a ring; for many, those who had entered the angry waters with nothing, or who had been stripped by their fury, it was a question of noting perhaps a birth-mark, or the almost invisible trace of a long healed scar, anything that a loving relative could affirm before being taken to see the mortal remains.

After the day`s heavy work was done, the Rector retired to his study to begin answering the scores of letters which came in, some from the bereaved who were unable to make the journey through age or ill-health, some who merely sought news of relatives known to have been aboard but so far unaccounted for.

"I marvel," said Mr Gapper to me, as we stood by the churchyard gate as evening drew on, "I marvel how any one man copes with this day in day out, with no end in sight. It would drive a normal being to despair, or to turn his own heart to flint, but with him neither. The strain must surely tell at last."

The expectations of those arriving in the seemingly unending stream of the bereaved were sometimes pitifully wide of the mark; there were some who believed, against all the evidence, that their son or daughter, or brother or grandchild would suddenly appear, smiling and unharmed; there were others who believed that the features of their lost ones would somehow be beautified or rejuvenated in death. It took only one pace through that church door to disabuse them of any such cherished notions, and there were some who could bear to step no further.

Not least oppressive was the odour of death which grew each day until it became a pervasive stench. Pitch buckets were lit, and burned slowly by the door, but they could only mask the scent of putrefaction filling the little church, which was, to many people, as obnoxious as the hideous images of death which met the eye.

Chapter 34

Isaac`s body came in with the tide on Sunday morning, drifting slowly into Porth Moelfre on a gentle flow as if the sea, ashamed of its anger, now offered him peacefully back to the home of his ancestors. The men of the village said he had probably been caught in the local currents around Ynys Moelfre and had been kept there, delaying his final homecoming.

His body was lifted onto the shingle beach, and I was sent to bring his mother and father. They came slowly down the hill, stern faced and silent, but with the dignity of people who were carrying out a task that they had rehearsed in their own minds many times. Only once, down on the beach, did Mrs Lewis break the silence with a single muffled sob, which, it seemed, had it been allowed free reign, would have prised open the heavens.

Isaac was carried home to be washed and clothed, and I went to look for Izzy, to tell her the news. I found her, with some other women from the village, on the stony beach of Porth Helaeth, where two other bodies had come in. Many of the dead, however well attired when they went into the water, had been stripped to some degree by the action of the sea, particularly, in the case of the women, their loose skirts and nether garments, and it was the practice of the village women to cover them up, and make them decent, before their journey to the church.

As I made my way down the path, I heard a man calling out, in a sharp tone of prohibition, exaggerated, probably because, as in the case of most of the guardsmen and militia, he thought he was dealing with people who spoke only Welsh.

Izzy turned towards him, and seeing that he was addressing her, returned in an equally strident tone.

"Hasn`t she suffered shame enough without the likes of you gaping up her backside! Or is that what you want? Come and have a peek if you`re that curious!"

The man held up his hands and backed off.

There are certain times when a woman always has the upper hand.

I passed the man on the path as I came down and he started to make his way back up. He shook his head. "It`s almost impossible," he said. "A running battle."

"Why don`t you just let them get on with it?"

"Can you answer for it that they`re not pilfering?" he asked.

"The Rector can. Everything is handed over to him."

"So he says, and I`m sure so he thinks. But who knows? Anyway, they use it as a pretext for scratching about in the rocks, don`t they?"

"Do you have evidence for that?" I asked. "Or is it just what you`ve got from the newspapers?"

"All right, don`t get shirty, no need for that. Live and let live, that`s my motto, but I have to do my job, don`t I?"

"Yes," I agreed, for at close quarters he seemed a decent enough man.

"Well, it`s not my problem. I just do the best I can. One thing`s for certain, I won`t be getting any richer out of all this."

I continued to where Izzy was finishing her work, and told her the news. She sat down on a flat stone and looked out towards the sea, and her eyes filled slowly with tears. I put my hand on her shoulder.

"Things will never, never be the same again, will they?"

"No, I don`t think they will."

"Let`s go away, Richie," she said. "Let`s go away from here as soon as we can."

"We will," I replied, though as I thought of it, the problems gathered in my mind like an assembly of rain clouds on the horizon.

The following day, the Rector conducted a small service at the house, and then led the procession of thirty or so villagers, with Isaac`s coffin to the churchyard. The grass and rambling undergrowth and wild shrubs which normally, as at the time when my mother had been laid to rest, gave the churchyard a pleasant and cheerful aspect, had been stripped away, and the bare ground was now pitted with shadowy holes ready for use.

Isaac was buried in a quiet corner, on gently rising ground, on the far side of the church, the furthest from the sea.

For the village, it marked a turning point. The following day, new vessels appeared in the bay, anchoring just off the shore, and the salvage operation had begun. Inevitably, I suppose, the interests of the salvage engineers were not those of the villagers, and though open hostility was rare, there were antagonisms; in the main, however, the village turned back in on itself, to get on with its life,

The area patrolled by the militia marked a kind of frontier, inside which only those authorised were permitted. Once again, however, the sea proved that it is no respecter of the designs of man. After a week, the bodies began to wash up on beaches further and further afield, Benllech, Traeth Coch, Llandona, past Puffin Island, too, round to Beaumaris and even as far as Conwy, and the story went that bodies which were coming to shore now were the ones that were carrying the most gold.

Whether this was true or not, I had no way of knowing, but part of the explanation had come from Mr Jenkins, the principal diver with the salvage operation. With his full black beard and ruddy complection, Mr Jenkins, along with Captain Martin who was in charge of the salvage team and Mr Smith, the Receiver of the Wreck, had become a regular customer at the Talyfron, and his jovial character, together with the fact that he spoke Welsh had made him accepted in spite of the circumstances.

I was there, one evening the following week, about my old business of calling to pick up Dilwyn and take him home, when I heard Mr Jenkins expounding thus: "In normal circumstances, you see, a body, living or dead, tends to be buoyed up by the salt sea, and we divers, you know, we have to have lead weights put onto us to make us go down. Now, a body with lungs full of water rather than air, may begin to go down, very true, but a body with twenty sovereigns in each pocket, or a belt with gold nugget in it, now," here he made a suitably descriptive gesture of his hand, "that body will go down like that!"

He waited for the effect of this to be fully appreciated, giving himself time for another sip of his drink, and then continued. "Now," he said, "you may be wondering as to how that body, now that it is down at the bottom, and weighted down there with gold, as I say, how that body doesn't stay down there. Well, the answer is this. That body, as it lies down there, will start to do what any dead body will do, which is that it will begin to rot, and with that rotting, it will produce gases in itself that swell that body up to half its normal size again. Now, a body thus swollen, pound for pound in relation to its volume, is a lighter body than it was before, until that lightness counterbalances the weight of that heavy encumbrance, the gold, and at last, up she comes, or up he comes, if you like, for despite the different properties of the male and female body and the way they behave in salt water, the rotting process is much the same.

"Now," he continued, after another pause to sip, for it was clear that he was not yet finished, and meantime every other tongue in the house had fallen silent, "it follows, does it not, that the more gold, or other heavy substance, for it is weight and not value that is in consideration here, as I say, the more gold a body is carrying the more rotting and the more production of swelling gases it will require to reach that balance, and the longer it will take those bodies to start coming back up into the push and pull of the tides as we know them. Now, to conclude, though no man can say it for certain, but if it were to turn out that the last bodies to come up, and from what I have heard there are many yet who have not obliged in that respect, if, as I say, those bodies prove to be the mortal remains of those who sought to leave that ship with as much of their worldly fortune as they could rightly stash about them, do not tell people that it was Prothero Jenkins who told you otherwise."

His tale finished, he called for another drink, and now a hushed murmur of conversation supplied the place of his monologue. And amidst those who had been impressed by his tale, either by the substance or by the lugubrious manner of his telling it, none was more rapt than Dilwyn Jones.

Chapter 35

It is from that evening - though my perception of it may be purely incidental – that I began to notice changes in Dilwyn`s behaviour, quite apart from his periodic drunkenness, that were worrying, and, in spite of myself, I did worry about him.

"He thought he could do a deal," said Izzy. "He thought there`d be some winking of eyes with gold bullion slipped away to safe havens, and so there may be, for all we know, but if there is, he`s not part of it, is he? That`s what`s got to him."

There were tales of him wandering along the cliffs at night, after his stint at the Talyfron, sharing his bottle of brandy with the guards, trying to get in with what was happening, trying to sniff out any corruption that he could make himself part of. When this didn`t work, and by all accounts, the guards began to see him, after a while, as a figure of fun, he roamed further afield, combing the beaches in the dead of night, no doubt in search of that weightiness of encumbrance, as Mr Jenkins might have put it, that had required so much gassy purulence to bring it floating back to shore.

He was brought home one morning by the quarry master of Traeth Bychan, who had found him asleep there on the beach, soaked to the waist by the incoming tide. "I might have done better to leave him, the state he`s in," he said, though whether in contempt or compassion, I was not certain, for he was himself a sometime drinking companion at the Talyfron, and I sensed that in what he saw he read his own possible fate.

With Ivor`s help, I got Dilwyn to bed and called the doctor.

"The yellow pallor," said Doctor Jenkins, "can be a symptom of infectious jaundice, but in this case it is certainly the result of a debility to the liver caused by the excessive consumption of intoxicating liquor." Having explained this to me, he turned directly to Dilwyn. "You must cut out the brandy, man, or you`ll be dead within six months. Nothing clearer. Do you understand?"

Dilwyn nodded meekly.

"Good, then I`ll bid you good morning."

"Make sure there are no bottles in his room," I instructed Margaret. Then I took Ivor to one side, "I don`t know what is going to happen," I said, "but you had better take over the management of the farm before everything goes to pot."

Ivor nodded, as if to say it was no more than he was doing already.

"You shouldn`t worry about him," said Izzy. "You`ve already done more than he deserves."

I thought this somewhat hard hearted, but I knew Izzy had cause enough not to waste feelings on Dilwyn, and I wondered too if she saw this as a further disruption to our own vague plans.

"I wouldn`t worry about him," I explained, "if it weren`t for my mother."

She nodded in acceptance, and after that was as careful as anyone to see that his sickroom was attended to, and that he had what was needed to regain his strength.

By this time, the inquest in the village had run its course, and the Coroner, having viewed, as he must, all of the recovered bodies, and having presided over the evidence, had asked the jury to consider their verdict. Despite the confusion, for many of the Welsh speaking jurors had to have the evidence translated, and despite some vitriolic confrontations and skirmishes between lawyers and witnesses, the loss of the Royal Charter, and the loss of life resulting were deemed to be accidental. Tired of the whole business, most of the village was glad to see the proceedings moving away to Liverpool, where the Board of Trade was to hold its own enquiry.

I took my farewell of Mr Gapper outside the Talyfron two days after the inquest finished.

"Where will you go?" I asked.

"To Liverpool first, of course, then, who knows? New Zealand again, eventually, I suppose – take hold of my life again - but I have no stomach for such a voyage again now."

"The funeral?" I asked.

"Yesterday," he said. "I`ve written to her father. He may come or not, I do not know. Some families have already had bodies exhumed and taken them home. I hope not in her case. Here at least, I will remember where she lies."

We took our leave, and I watched the coach making its slow way up the hill. At the corner of the lane, I reflected, he would be able to take one last glance towards St Galgo`s church.

He had never explained to me why he had referred to Mrs Rose as his wife.

As long as Dilwyn Jones was recovering, Izzy and I did not speak about our plans to leave Moelfre. His condition improved slowly, and two weeks after the doctor`s visit, he could sit up in bed, though the yellow tinge of his skin remained, and the weakness consequent on lying in bed limited his walking, at least without assistance, to a few paces.

I gave as much help as I could to Ivor, and confided in him that I intended to leave as soon as Dilwyn could look after himself.

"You`re doing the right thing," he said. "We`ll stay here. Hold out as long as we can. Well, we don`t know anything else, really."

It was in the last week of November, as Ivor and I were bringing in the herd, that Margaret rushed out into the yard, screaming. She could not articulate the cause of her distress except by pointing, but when we went into the house, Dilwyn was lying at the foot of the stairs, his eyes writhing, and gasping for breath. We eased him onto the chair by the fireside, and after ten minutes, he slipped into a sleep. There was a strong smell of brandy on his breath.

In his room, an empty bottle lay by the bed.

"Who gave him this?"

"I swear," said Margaret, "it was locked in the cabinet."

It was clear from her terror that she knew nothing about it.

The doctor arrived half an hour later.

"Drunk," he pronounced.

"We don`t know how he got the bottle," I said.

"I`ve no doubt," said the doctor, in a matter of fact way, "he got it himself." He took in the circumstances. "He was beginning to walk, you say?"

"Yes, with assistance."

"Then, there you have it. He came down the stairs, took a bottle back with him, drank it, decided to come down for more, and fell."

He took another look at the patient. "He`ll not waken up for a good time yet. Take him up to bed. Try not to disturb him more than you have to. I`ll see him in the morning."

Ivor tipped back the chair, and I took the legs, and together we struggled up the stairs to his room, where Izzy and Margaret had re-made the bed.

"What did the doctor say?" said Izzy.

"Let him sleep until it wears off."

She looked at him critically. His face was pinched and his breathing was harsh and dry. She turned her mouth down as if doubting the doctor`s judgement.

"Perhaps we`d better sit with him."

Margaret made a fire in the room, and we drew chairs up to the end of the bed.

For two hours, his condition stayed the same, and we grew accustomed to the steady sharp intake of his breath, talking quietly to each other from time to time, and then sitting in silence. Then, quite suddenly, he started to gag in the throat, and shake so that it seemed he must wake.

"I think we should bring the doctor back," said Izzy, "I don`t think he`s just drunk, I think he`s hurt."

I called Ivor and gave him instructions.

"So, you think he`s worse," said the doctor, taking off his coat. We described the symptoms and he nodded. He lifted one of Dilwyn`s eyelids, looked into his eye, and then let it fall shut. "I`ll examine him, if you wish, but I have to warn you, in his condition, there`s very little I can do further than that."

At his bidding, we left the room, to let him carry on with his examination. Twenty minutes later, he came down the stairs, and Margaret brought him water to wash his hands. It was some time before he spoke.

"I suspect," he began, "that he has some broken ribs. To judge from the bruising on his side, that is almost certainly the case. Painful, but not in itself, in normal circumstances, dangerous. However, it may be possible that the breaking of the rib has also caused a puncture to the lung, in which case, the outcome is less certain. If there is also internal bleeding, then…well, that may be the reason for the severity of breathing you have noted."

"Is there anything we can do?" said Izzy.

He shrugged his shoulder. "Keep him still. Don`t let the room be too warm. Apart from that, nothing, until he awakens, if he awakens. That, I`m afraid to say, is not in my hands, or yours."

He put his coat on, shook my hand, and took his leave. When I came back into the room, I told Margaret to go to bed, and asked Ivor to take Izzy home.

"I`ll stay here with you," said Izzy.

"There`s no need," I said. "I`ll sit with him, I`ll probably sleep myself."

She said nothing else, but stayed, nevertheless.

The doctor had placed two pillows behind Dilwyn`s head, so that he was in a position between sitting and lying, though with his head slightly to one side, His breathing was short, but less harsh than before. Every so often, his eyes opened for a moment, but they were unfocused, and he seemed unaware of his surroundings.

"Do you think he knows we`re here?" asked Izzy.

"I don`t know."

Izzy drowsed, and her head slipped onto my shoulder. In the corner of the room, a clock, one that my mother had brought from Porthaethwy, ticked away the minutes to midnight, and then beyond.

"Do you think we should lift him a little?"

Hearing Izzy`s voice I realised that I had drowsed too. The clock had moved on to two o`clock. Dilwyn`s head had slipped further to the side, so that his body now seemed to list heavily.

"I don`t know. The doctor said not to move him."

"I think we should," said Izzy, going to the side of the bed, and rearranging the pillows so that he was again sitting upright.

"Dilwyn?" she said, close to his ear. "Would you like to sip some water?"

She offered the glass to his lips but there was no response.

"At least he looks more comfortable," she said, coming back to sit beside me.

We continued our vigil, drowsing intermittently, until five o`clock in the morning. Then, I was aware of Izzy shaking me and standing up. Dilwyn`s breath had become like a gargle, as if fluid were bubbling in his throat, and suddenly his eyes opened and bulged as if in terror.

"Do something, Richie!" called Izzy. "Help him."

I sat on the side of the bed next to him, and held his gaze; of all the sights I had seen in the last month, none was more terrible to me than that.

It lasted only a moment. I felt the tension of his shoulders lapse, and his eyes closed to show just of strip of white, and then, quite suddenly, it was all over.

Izzy, having stepped involuntarily backwards, had her hands to her mouth, and her eyes were filling with tears.

"It`s all right, Izzy, it`s over now. Go downstairs and call Ivor. Tell him that Mr Jones has died."

Later in the morning, though at what time exactly I do not recall, the doctor came again.

"It`s as I thought," he said, standing over Dilwyn`s body. "Nothing anyone could have done. Perhaps a blessing, all things considered, perhaps a blessing. Now," he went on, "it`s time for you to look after yourself."

I wondered for a moment what he meant and then realised, for the first time, that the front of my shirt was covered in blood.

Chapter 36

Later that morning, I walked out to the Swnt, and as far as the cliffs looking down over Porth Helaeth. The last autumn colours had drained, it seemed, back into the earth, and a pale winter sun was shining through thin clouds onto the bay, tranquil apart from the distant thrum of the engine of the lighter over the Royal Charter site, and a smudge of black smoke which drifted towards the horizon.

A militia man, fifty yards off, eyed me suspiciously and then came towards me.

"You a local man, are you?" he asked.

"Yes."

"Then you`ll know it`s no good trying to get any closer than this."

"Yes."

"Best get off, then, if I were you. I should search you really, that`s what our orders are, if anyone gets too near."

"My step-father died this morning. I was just trying to find a little peace and fresh air."

"I`m sorry to hear that. In that case…"

"I won`t be staying long."

"I`ll be glad to get back home, personally," he said, after a moment, as if, in the circumstances he felt he owed me some personal converse.

"Is it bad?"

"Well, not too bad, I suppose. Only in the night, down there, we hear noises, you know, just the sea, like, but the mind plays tricks, with all that that went on. Sounds like voices, crying out. Enough to make you wish you was elsewhere."

"How is the salvage operation going, then?"

"Well, they don`t really tell us anything, do they? But the masters are smiling more than they were. Mind you, they`ll never get all of it, will they?"

"No, I don`t suppose they will."

A voice shouted across to him from the path opposite.

"That`s my sergeant," he said. "I`d better get back. I`ll tell him I searched you," he added, with a wink. "Nothing to declare."

I watched him go, and then, for the last time, looked out across the bay, past the site of the wreck to Ynys Dulas, and Point Lynas beyond.

"Thank you," I said to Izzy.

"What are you thanking me for?"

"For staying last night. It made a big difference to have someone there with me."

She shrugged her shoulders. "It was only natural for me to be there with you."

"Yes. I`m still grateful, though. You more than anyone might have reason to distance yourself from him."

"Why do you say that, Richie?"

"My mother told me the reason you and your mother left the house."

She nodded and walked towards the window, where she stood for some time, thinking.

"I think," she said, at last, "you have been under a misapprehension, Richie. Exactly what your mother told you, I do not know, but the reason we were made to leave the house was that your mother discovered that Dilwyn Jones was my father."

She turned from the window to see the astonishment on my face.

"It might have remained a secret, perhaps even from myself, had not Dilwyn blurted it out himself in one of his drunken outbursts."

"I can`t believe my mother would be so uncharitable."

"Don`t cast too much blame on her. What woman wishes to live in the same house as her husband`s former mistress and his illegitimate child?"

"Why didn`t you tell me?"

"Because you would have tried to reconcile me to Dilwyn and that could never have been. Besides, I promised my mother.

It is only his death that releases me from that promise."

"But you weren`t born here, were you?"

"No. Dilwyn was a drover in those days. It was his father who was the tenant of this farm then. My mother met him in Amlwch. When she became pregnant with me, he denied that he was the father and claimed she lay with other men. Then his father grew ill and Dilwyn said that he would take her on as a servant, but only if it was understood that the child – I was two years old then – was of someone else."

"And you grew up not knowing?"

"My mother told me when we moved out of the house. But I think I always knew in my heart."

"In spite of the King of Erin on Ynys Moelfre?"

"Yes, in spite of him. When you first came here, I thought in my confused way that you might be my brother. That`s why I followed you. Do you remember?"

"Yes. I`m afraid I didn`t treat you very much like a brother."

"That`s just as well, for then I may have loved you as a brother and not as I love you now."

"Some good came of it then."

She nodded.

"So," I said, "properly speaking, you are the tenant now."

"And how long do you think it will be," she asked, "before Lord Boston comes a-calling?"

Chapter 37

Izzy was perfectly right in thinking that the situation would soon be picked up by Lord Boston, or at least, if not by the great man himself, by his land agent, Mr Dodds.

That same evening, just as we were beginning to discuss the arrangements for Dilwyn`s funeral, the distinctive knock of his cane was heard on the door.

"I`m very sorry for your personal loss," he said, "but the truth is this has merely precipitated something which was imminent. Imminent, Mr Williams," he repeated as if to give some extra weight of significance to the word, and, somewhat ominously, began to open his leather brief-case. "This," he resumed, brandishing a wad of papers, "is an order obtained from the County Court authorising the bailiff to re-possess the farmhouse, buildings, and all effects thereto, including the livestock. You may, of course, choose to contest this as to the value of the sums concerned, but, in that case, should the assets be valued at less than the debt, it would be yourself who would be liable for the shortfall."

"And what if the assets are greater than the debt?"

"If you were confident that was the case, it would be a course of action you would be well advised to consider."

"But it`s not a course of action you would recommend?"

"I am paid by Lord Boston to carry out his business, not to give advice. If, however... " he paused and took off his glasses, as if the business were all but done, "if you were to ask me for independent advice for which I was not paid, that is to say, the advice of a decent man to someone whose interest he had at heart, then, no, it is not a course of action I would recommend."

"Thank you."

"The position is this. We must get a new tenant for this farm. As you are not a farmer, and as you have no capital sum to invest, that tenant must be someone else."

"What will happen to Ivor?"

"I`m sure the new tenant will value his knowledge of the farm and his long-standing service. I think we can say that his position is not in question."

"Thank you," I said again.

We stood up and he patted my shoulder. "You`re wise to face up to these things," he said, looking from me to Izzy, "Clean break, new start. Whatever you do, I`m sure you`ll make a good fist of it. I wish you the very best of fortune."

"So, that`s that, then!"

"What are we going to do?"

"Go to Liverpool. Manchester, I don`t know."

"So long as we get away from here, Richie."

"It won`t be easy."

"I don`t remember it ever being that easy."

"I have enough money for the journey. We`ll have to get somewhere to live, which should be all right so long as I get work. There won`t be many luxuries."

We sat there for some time, each subdued in our own thoughts. Was it a picture of happiness together that we entertained, or one of labour and poverty and hardship? At the threshold of our new life together, neither of us seemed willing to voice our thoughts.

"Will you walk me to the cottage?" said Izzy, at last.

We set out. It was a clear night, with a light frost, and stars and moonlight over the bay.

"Will we be all right?" she asked.

"Yes, we`ll be all right."

"If you want the chance to go off alone, Richie, say so now. If that is your true wish, I will hold you to nothing, and claim nothing."

"I don`t have any such wish," I replied.

"Come inside for a moment," she said, when we reached the door. "I want to show you something."

She lit the oil-lamp, and then detaching its chimney pipe, moved the stove aside. Then she lifted up the stone on which it had been standing, and from beneath took a package wrapped round with sacking and string.

She sat on the bed, and unfolded the sacking to reveal a loose assortment of coins, guineas with the Queen`s head, gold sovereigns with the stamp of the Australian colony, and others, both silver and gold of varying denominations.

"Izzy," I said, making my mind up straight away, "if these are from the wreck, as they must be, we must take them to the Rector the first thing in the morning."

"But why?"

"Because it is the property of someone else."

"I swear to you, Richie," she said, "everything you see here was picked up freely from the rocks, where it lay, and belonged to no-one. If you say I must give it over, and, when the time is, let my own child starve, Richie, I say no. If you will not relinquish your Sunday School virtue, then you must relinquish me."

I turned away, knowing that her will had mastered mine, for long enough to grow accustomed to such minor loss of dignity as it caused me.

"The roads are watched. Anyone leaving Moelfre now casts suspicion on themselves. Do you have any plan," I asked, "as to how we may carry this little nest egg away without fear of arrest?"

"Yes," said Izzy. "I have a plan."

The following morning, I went to see the Reverend Stephen Roose Hughes.

"We`ll take him to Amlwch to be buried."

"Amlwch, that makes sense. In the circumstances. I remember he wanted your mother buried there."

"Yes. I came to tell you also that Izzy and I are going to leave Moelfre."

"I thought you would. I hoped you might stay until I could be the one to marry you."

"There isn`t time. They`re putting in a new tenant. Besides, a child is on the way."

"Yes. I thought that might be the case. Anyway, you know you have my blessing, don`t you?"

"Yes, I know."

We went outside, and stood a while by the churchyard wall.

"You know," he said, at last, "sometimes, when things get too much for her, my wife just cries. Just like that. It all comes out. I wish I could do that, Richie, I really do."

"Take care of yourself. You do too much."

"I only do what has to be done. It`s a simple formula. God`s formula."

Another ten minutes passed as we sat in silence.

"Do you know where you`ll go?"

"To Amlwch first. After that I don`t know."

"Don`t be like Luke," he said at last.

"Luke?"

"In the poem, `Michael`. You remember?"

"Yes. The son."

"Don`t be like him."

"No, I won`t."

"Good. Then goodbye Richie."

"Goodbye."

We stood and faced each other, our hands gripped in the clasp of a final handshake. I don`t know whether there were tears in his eyes. There were in mine.

We set out for Amlwch the next morning. Izzy, on the seat of the wagon next to me, was wearing my mother`s mourning dress, her wedding ring, and the silver necklace with my father and mother`s initials inscribed on it. Behind us were two small chests containing the personal possessions we had chosen for the journey. On the wagon itself was the coffin containing Dilwyn`s body; it also contained the sack which Izzy had uncovered from beneath the cottage stove.

As for the money itself – it was little enough. It would suffice, once we were away from Anglesey, to pay for decent lodgings, so that when the time came, Izzy`s confinement would be clean and comfortable; and it would suffice, I calculated, to save us from beginnings which might trap us forever in a life of penury.

We stayed for two nights at the Queen`s Hotel in Amlwch, and saw Dilwyn`s funeral take place in St Eleth`s churchyard. Then we sold the horse and wagon to purchase our passage on the Schooner, Maria Gurney, Captain John Hughes, out of Amlwch harbour to Holyhead; and thence, by the steam packet, across the Irish Sea to the only place in the world where I knew I had a friend.

Dublin 1860
New House 1869

Part 10

Chapter 38

29th June 2009

Hi Dad, got back from my second trip to Anglesey yesterday. Stayed on a couple of days longer than planned to have a closer look round, but didn`t really find out any more facts re. family history – I don`t think I really expected to. I managed to get someone to take me out on a boat from a place called Traeth Bychan, which is near where `The Royal Charter` went down. There were a lot of quarries there at one time, I`m told, but now it`s just the most picturesque sea-side place you could imagine, with a café and ice-cream parlour behind a sandy cove with a sailing club building at the head of the beach. The boat I went out on is moored in the tiny harbour there, which is basically a disused quarry which floods with the tide, though it`s very peaceful and sheltered, and very colourful and pretty with all the boats. We went down the coast a mile or so, past Moelfre and a tiny island which is called Ynys Moelfre, and along past the cliffs where the ship was wrecked. The coastline actually looks quite mild and undramatic. And when I was there there was just a soft misty yellow light bathing everything, but on the night when the ship was wrecked it was apparently blowing a hurricane - it was bad not just in Wales but across the whole country. The ship came around the island, and had turned the point to head eastward into Liverpool Bay when the wind changed to the north-east in the middle of the night and started blowing them towards the land. They put down the anchors, but the anchor chains snapped and the boat was blown inshore in the darkness. It was grounded in sand to begin with but the tide started to come in, about dawn, and threw the boat up onto the rocks, and it broke up. A lot of the people who were killed were smashed on the rocks rather than drowned. It must have been a bit like a plane crash. Only about forty out of five hundred survived, and there was not a single woman or child amongst the survivors. For anyone there witnessing it, it must have been truly horrific. There were stories of large amounts of gold going missing from the wreck, and of bodies being looted, but from everything I`ve read now, I don`t think it`s very likely. What does seem to be the case, though, is that if it hadn`t been for the bravery of the villagers of Moelfre who went down onto the rocks in the middle of the storm, hardly anyone would have survived at all. If our ancestor was there, I hope he did his bit!

Anyway, that`s about it. I`ll give you a call and let you know the flight times. Looking forward to seeing you all next week! Saff.

From Saffy Williams
To: Sally Whitelock
30/05/09

Hi Sal! Well, I`m back home from the great Anglesey adventure, and aren`t you just dying to know how I got on? Well, to begin with, Rob picked me up from the hotel in Beaumaris in the morning and drove me across to Traeth Bychan where he keeps his boat. We went out across the bay and he showed me all the places connected with the wreck of `The Royal Charter`. He tried to teach me some sailing techniques, too, but I was pretty useless! We were out for a couple of hours, then had to get back because of the tide. Went back to the hotel – that`s where I texted you from – and then later he picked me up for dinner. We went to a restaurant called `The Boathouse` in Red Wharf Bay, very picturesque with view out over sands and headland opposite, and amazing food, too. I really enjoyed it, and he was really good company, and it was only on the way back that I let myself start thinking about what he might say when we got back, and what I might say if he did! I mean, I did quite fancy him in a way, but then, well, it`s not always as simple as that, is it! He pulled up in The Bulkeley Arms carpark, and I just blurted out, "Look, I`d ask you to come in for a drink, you know, but I have to tell you I`m in a relationship with a guy called Charlie back home, and..." I`m not sure how I was going to end that statement exactly, but he came straight in and said, "I`ve had a really nice day, and I`d love to come in for a drink, but I have to tell you that I`m  in a relationship, too, with a guy called Tom, who`s in Brussels at the moment…" I don`t know if I was more shocked or relieved! When I got back here, Lucy said, oh, yeh – casual as you like – didn`t you realise? Anyway, we did go in for a drink, and I`ve got his e-mail address, and we`re going to keep in touch. So, there you are, Sal, maybe not what you were waiting to hear, but no harm done! I`m flying back to Jo`berg next Tuesday, and will contact you then. Saff xxx.

***

"So, you don`t think the family fortune came from the Royal Charter gold, after all, then?"

"No, I mean, there`s nothing really to prove they were even there in 1859, but even if they were, despite what the stories are, I doubt if anyone got really rich like that."

"No?"

"The site was pretty well sealed off after the first day, and there was a salvage operation which went on for months, with divers and everything."

"Did they have divers in Victorian times?"

"Apparently, yes. Not SCUBA divers, but the basic diving suit thing, you know. The remains of the wreck were dragged back onto the seabed but it was lying in shallow water, so they could get at it."

"So they got all the gold out?"

"Most of it. From the strong rooms, anyway. No-one really ever knew how much individual wealth people had on board."

"Oh, well, never mind."

"So, that explodes my theory about the argument."

"You mean the one where Stephen was so horrified to discover how Richard had come by his wealth that he ran away to South Africa?"

"Yes. Sound a bit silly when you think about it, really, doesn`t it?"

"Well, you know, I was wondering, after you first mentioned it, whether the row might be anything to do with the son not liking his father making money out of armaments. Have there been any pacifists on your side of the family?"

"Not that I know of."

"Well, I don't suppose we'll ever get to the bottom of it."

"No. I think I've got as far as I'm ever going to get! Oh, by the way, I checked out the painter, Wheeler, in Wikipedia."

"'The Churchyard at Eastry' chap?"

"Yes."

"What's Wikipedia?"

"It's an on-line encyclopoedia."

"Right. So he's in it, is he?"

"Yes. I've got it here. This is what it says: *R. S. Wheeler, [b 1815 – d 1863] Minor Victorian painter, briefly associated with the Pre-Raphaelite movement; left London in 1852 and lived and worked in Dublin until his death. Noted chiefly for his studies of horses and domestic animals. On his death, the collection was bequeathed to an unknown beneficiary, and was sold to a private collector from New York City, in 1864 for an undisclosed sum, thought to be in excess of £15,000, a considerable figure at the time.*"

"That's interesting. So 'The Churchyard at Eastry' might be worth something after all."

"Well, it might be a good idea to have it valued for insurance purposes."

"Yes, that's a good idea. I think I'll do that."

***

Text Message, from Saffy Williams to Charlie Robson [Jo'berg] 6th July, 2009, 9.40am

Hi babes. In deprtrs Mnchstr. C u thurs. Wll call from JNB. Can't wait! Luv u. Saff xxx

The End

Lightning Source UK Ltd.
Milton Keynes UK
22 May 2010

154556UK00002B/16/P